5TO

Not
for
Doctors
Only

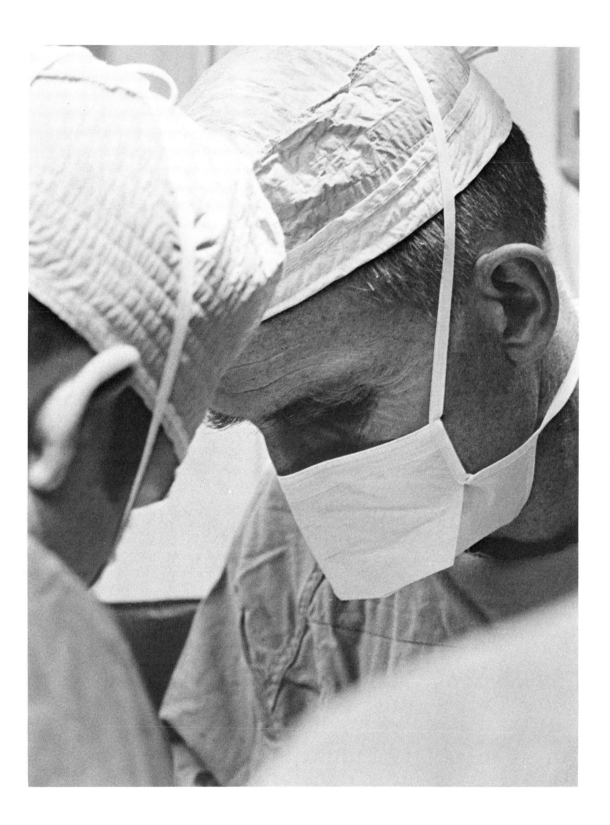

Not for Doctors Only

*Over 100 medical discoveries
even your doctor
may not know about yet*

Dr. James Wasco

Addison-Wesley Publishing Company, Inc.
*Reading, Massachusetts ▪ Menlo Park, California
London ▪ Amsterdam ▪ Don Mills, Ontario ▪ Sydney*

Library of Congress Cataloging in Publication Data

Wasco, James, 1942–
  Not for doctors only.

  Bibliography: p. 300
  Includes index.
  1. Medicine. 2. Medical innovations. I. Title.
[DNLM: 1. Medicine--Popular works. 2. Biomedical
engineering--Popular works. WB130 W312n]
R149.W37   616   80-19357
ISBN 0-201-08298-5 (Pbk)
ISBN 0-201-08297-7

Copyright © 1980 by James E. Wasco, M.D. Philippines copyright © 1980 by James E. Wasco, M.D.

Library of Congress Catalog Card No. 80-19357.

ISBN 0-201-08298-5 P

ISBN 0-201-08297-7 H

ABCDEFGHIJ-MA-89876543210

Book design by Susan Marsh.

FOR HELEN

*who, by her support and encouragement,
is a constant source of inspiration*

To our readers

We hope the information provided by NOT FOR DOCTORS ONLY will encourage you to read further, ask questions, and become a better informed patient. The medical advice contained in this book is as sound as we can make it. But like advice from your doctor or nurse, it may not always work. Many of the medical discoveries described here are still experimental and may not be appropriate for every patient with a particular condition or disease.

So here are some qualifications: If you are under the care of a physician and receive advice contrary to this book, follow the physician's advice. That way the individual characteristics of your problem can be considered. If you have an allergy or a suspected allergy to a recommended medicine, check with your doctor, at least by phone. With any medication, read label directions carefully. And if any medical problem persists beyond a reasonable period, you should usually see a doctor.

Acknowledgements

A written work is rarely the product of a single individual. Many people have contributed to this book, and I am grateful to them all.

The public relations staffs of several Boston area hospitals generously contributed their time, arranged interviews and schedules, and provided photographs. In particular, I thank Florence Schumacher, Joan Bachenheimer, and Tony Lloyd of the Beth Israel Hospital; Joe Gavaghan and Jim King of the Brigham and Women's Hospital; Ellen Barlow of the Massachusetts Eye and Ear Infirmary; David Estridge of the Children's Hospital Medical Center; Vern Woodlief of the Massachusetts Rehabilitation Hospital; Herb Fuhrmann at Lynn Hospital; Marcia Cohen from the Lahey Clinic; Peter Gerace and Kathy Murray from the Mount Auburn Hospital; Hunter McCleary of the Tufts–New England Medical Center, and Sue Gertman and Donald Giller from the Boston University Medical Center. I would also like to thank Woody Wilson of the Emory University Medical Center in Atlanta, Georgia.

Cheryl Simon spent long hours researching several sections and wading through resource information. Carol Dullea contributed her time and her typing and had the unpleasant task of deciphering my scribbling and tapes. She was always available, despite my poor attention to schedules.

My colleagues from the medical and administrative staffs of the Lynn Hospital were sources of reference, advice, and support.

Much of the credit for the completion of this book must go to Doe Coover and Anne Eldridge of Addison-Wesley. Without their constant encouragement, this project might never have left the ground.

Thank you as well to my many colleagues at WBZ–TV in Boston. Maggie Hines offered great ideas. Tim Houghton, Barry Schulman, Barry Rosenthal, Marty Dobelmeyer, Bones Fisher, and Lowry Steward gave advice and support and understood my many schedule problems. And all of them taught me a great deal about communicating health information to the public.

My greatest gratitude is to my family. My wife, Helen, helped in ways too many to be enumerated, always had a supportive and constructive word, and encouraged me every step of the way. Matthew and Emily continue to delight me, and helped in ways that they will not understand until they grow older.

Contents

Introduction

These are exciting times in medicine. In the short span of the last two decades, new discoveries and technological advancements have altered the shape of medical practice more so than during any other time in our history. Many of these discoveries astound both doctors and lay people, as seemingly impossible tasks are made suddenly possible. New drugs on the horizon promise to cure some of mankind's oldest diseases. Fiberoptic instruments, using "strands" of light, can peer into the darkest recesses of the body. Computer technology enables ultrasound, and X-ray studies to provide detailed studies of the structure and function of most of the body's organs. The operating microscope allows surgeons to perform repairs on intricate body structures that are barely visible to the eye. And bionic creations made of the latest synthetic materials can replace a leg, a hand, or an ear.

Meanwhile, investigators turn increasing attention toward the cell to solve the mysteries of disease. The electron microscope defines the miniature anatomy of the cell's interior and traces elusive chemical pathways. Genetic studies interpret the basis for life's direction and open the threshold to predictive medicine—the ability to forecast and treat illness before disease causes irrevocable damage.

Clearly, biomedical research has become a national priority, and discoveries and new developments seem to occur overnight. While the more startling and unusual developments find their way into our newspapers and magazines, hundreds more are reported—in various states of progress—each year to doctors only, at medical meetings and through professional medical journals.

The medical journal more than any other medium, perhaps, is the doctor's access to current news of experiments, research, and technological breakthroughs. Early reports of new drugs or surgical procedures often appear first in such medical journals as the *New England Journal of Medicine* or the *Journal of the American Medical Association*. Specialists have their medical journals, too, magazines such as *Annals of Plastic Surgery* or *Orthopedics Digest* that concentrate on a specific field of medicine. In fact, there are scores of medical journals published today (over ninety are listed in this book's bibliography alone), each presenting doctors with new and important information about practicing medicine.

Physicians have a responsibility to incorporate this new information into their daily practice, to keep abreast of developments that affect their patients' lives—your lives. But as patients you also have a responsibility to be as knowledgeable as possible about the conditions that affect your lives and to be as well informed as you can about the new scientific discoveries that may save your life.

This book is a people's medical journal. It attempts to bring you information about some of the more interesting—and important—innovations in medical care, as well as the controversies and debates that inevitably accompany new ideas. In these pages you'll learn how vitamin A is being used to treat acne, how monkeys have become the seeing-eye dogs of paraplegic patients, and how a new copierlike machine reads books and magazines aloud to the blind. You'll also find reports from the front—why interferon may, or may not, be the wonder drug of the future, and how computers may someday be able to restore vision to a blind person. The work of medical researchers is never ending, and as such there will always be new reports to make. While we can make no claim for this book to be an exhaustive survey, I think we have brought you the most intriguing and the most current new developments. Throughout I have also tried to include those medical developments that have some practical relevance to you as patients.

Not for Doctors Only is divided into several sections. **Discoveries** analyzes specific achievements within defined medical problems. This section describes the latest treatments and medications that promise relief for a variety of medical disorders, from persistent skin problems to difficult cardiac and intestinal conditions to cancer. **Breakthroughs** looks at innovations that have drastically affected the diagnosis and therapy of a wide range of medical conditions. Many breakthroughs originated in other disciplines and seemed revolutionary in medicine just a few years ago. Today, they are in common use. **High Tech** profiles the mechanical developments that promise more efficient and complete diagnosis and therapy. **Bionics** chronicles the many parts of the body for which there are artificial replacements. In **Perspectives** we study the ideas and attitudes that are reshaping our traditional approaches to sickness and health. And **Updates** takes an in-depth look at several major, ongoing medical problems and examines how recent medical developments altered the prognosis—and outlook—of patients with those problems.

The information in this book relies on many sources. I have had the good fortune to witness the ongoing progress of many of the projects you will meet on these pages. My medical practice, educational experience, and travel as a medical reporter for Westinghouse Broadcasting have taken me into diverse clinical and laboratory settings and introduced me to the fascinating world of medical research where whole lives are dedicated to the solution of one elusive problem.

Much of the information in this book comes, obviously, from medical journals. I have also gathered information from news releases and articles prepared by hospitals, laboratories, and the press.

I have also tried to include historical material to illustrate the changing concepts of medical treatment through time. I am, however, constantly impressed by how much our medical ancestors knew, even without the sophisticated technology and methods commonplace today. These early physicians relied only on their powers of observation, but they laid the foundations of modern medicine through their innovative study.

The case histories throughout the book are intended to show that medical conditions are not merely diseases in a textbook, but are experienced by real people, who must confront and live with these problems on a daily basis.

And finally, whenever possible I have included resource listings indicating where you may obtain additional information on the subject of that section. As I have said before, the responsibility for good health lies with both the physician and the patient. I constantly meet patients who fill prescriptions blindly or stumble into diagnostic testing areas without regard to why such treatment takes place. The well-informed patient better understands diagnosis and treatment and actively participates in his or her medical care program with a physician. The well-informed patient/consumer can also significantly reduce health-care costs, both individually and collectively. It is for this well-informed consumer that *Not for Doctors Only* has been written.

The information in this book does not, of course, suggest final answers. Each year brings new discoveries. Some are eventually proven invalid; others pass the test of time and take their place alongside findings of the past. Our understanding of disease continues to fluctuate, producing wonderment in some instances and frustration in others. All of us—doctors, researchers, and patients alike—must remember that progress is never made without a struggle, and that answers are found neither quickly nor easily. As philosopher George Santayana said, ''We must welcome the future, knowing that soon it will be the past; and we must respect the past, knowing that once it was all that was humanly possible.''

Not
for
Doctors
Only

A sound heart is the life of the flesh.

Proverbs 14:30

Heart disease is responsible for more than 700,000 deaths per year—it is the number one killer in America. Heart disease is also of particular concern because it strikes people in their middle, most productive years.

Research on heart disease has taken a twofold approach: preventing the disease in healthy people and minimizing its impact in people at risk.

Preventive measures such as attention to diet, exercise, control of blood pressure, and nonsmoking have contributed to the recent decline in the death rate from heart disease. So have medical and technological developments, which enable earlier and more accurate diagnosis and more effective therapy.

The following examples of new directions and dimensions in cardiology are not inclusive, but they do represent some of the more interesting developments that are having an impact right now.

Coronary artery bypass surgery

At a recent meeting of the American College of Cardiology, a past president of that prestigious society described coronary bypass surgery as ''the most important development of the decade in medicine.'' Another past president of the same society had a different opinion: ''Except for relatively small groups of patients, there is no evidence that the procedure prevents or postpones premature death.'' So goes the controversy over coronary bypass surgery.

In coronary artery bypass surgery a small piece of saphenous vein taken from the leg (this is the same vein that becomes enlarged and incompetent and is therefore removed in varicose vein surgery) is connected at one end to the aorta and at the other end to the coronary artery beyond the obstruction. The obstruction is therefore bypassed and blood flow restored to the heart muscle. Obstruction can occur in any or all three of the major coronary vessels. Each can be bypassed, and each requires a separate graft. In a so-called triple bypass, three separate vein grafts bypass all three coronary vessels.

Coronary bypass surgery is usually performed to relieve the symptoms of angina pectoris, a chest discomfort originating in the heart that is caused by reduced blood flow to the heart muscle. Approximately 80 percent of patients with angina pectoris are men. Patients with angina typically experience a squeezing pressure or heaviness beneath the breastbone which often shoots to the neck, left arm, or shoulder. Effort or stress generally brings on angina pectoris; rest generally relieves the pain.

Angina pectoris is closely tied to another disorder, atherosclerosis, in which deposits of fat and cholesterol narrow the arteries. As the diameter of an artery narrows, the amount of blood that it car-ries is reduced. When atherosclerosis occurs in a coronary artery, the heart muscle is deprived of blood and the oxygen and nutrients blood carries. In patients stricken with angina pectoris, the reduced blood flow may be just enough to supply the heart at rest. But any circumstances that make the heart work harder create an increased oxygen demand in the muscle; the narrowed artery cannot provide the additional blood, and the pain of angina results.

Coronary artery obstruction does not always cause pain. Weakness, heart failure, and abnormal heat rhythm are frequent complications as well. If the artery becomes completely obstructed and blood flow is entirely cut off, that area of the heart muscle dies and a heart attack results.

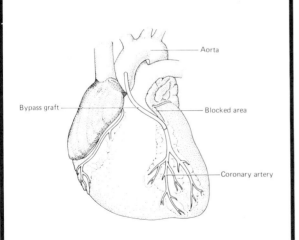

A coronary bypass graft

Aorta

Bypass graft

Blocked area

Coronary artery

CASE HISTORY

C. G. is a sixty-three-year-old manager of a fast-food chain whose history of cardiac problems dates back five years. At that time he experienced a tight, squeezing discomfort across his chest while climbing a flight of stairs. The discomfort subsided after about five minutes, and although he was concerned he did not visit his physician. Several weeks later he experienced more prolonged

The Anatomy of the Heart

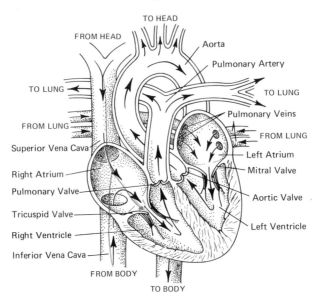

The heart, the body's most powerful muscle, consists of four chambers — — the upper right and left atria and the lower right and left ventricles.

The heart's function (detailed above, left) is to maintain an even blood flow to the body. The right atrium receives blood from the body through two large veins (the inferior vena cava and the superior vena cava). Blood is passed through the right ventricle and pumped to the lungs by the coronary artery. The lungs oxygenate the blood and return it through the pulmonary veins to the left atrium, on to the left ventricle, and into the aorta for body circulation.

The coronary arteries (detailed above, right) supply blood to the heart. Oxygenated blood from the lungs is carried from the aorta through the coronary arteries, which terminate in smaller surface arteries that ensure blood flow throughout the heart.

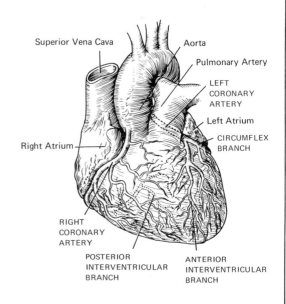

chest pain while shoveling snow outside and went to the local hospital, where he was admitted for observation. During medical evaluation he was found to have early high blood pressure and high blood cholesterol. Chest X rays were normal. His electrocardiogram was abnormal but blood determinations and subsequent ECGs over several days failed to document a heart attack. He was placed on nitroglycerin and a medication called Inderal. Over the next three days he had numerous bouts of chest pain that became more frequent. His symptoms were so pronounced that he had to take a medical leave from his job. His doctor recommended cardiac catheterization, which demonstrated that two coronary arteries were 70 to 80 percent closed because of arteriosclerosis. Coronary bypass surgery was performed, in which two vein grafts were placed in the left coronary artery. One year after surgery, C. G. is working again and is free of symptoms. He walks two to three miles each day, takes no medication, and has had no chest pain since the surgery.

Coronary artery bypass surgery clearly improves the quality of life. In a recent medical journal article, Dr. J. Willis Hearst, chairman of the Department of Medicine at Emory University in Atlanta, summarized the results of coronary artery bypass surgery around the country. He found that 60 percent of people who have the operation have no more angina pain. Another 30 percent have less pain than they had before the operation. The operation thus helps at least 90 percent of those who undergo it. Their pain is relieved, and they are able to lead more active lives.

Initially, some skeptics related this improvement in life-style to the psychological effect of the operation itself. Others felt it might be caused by accidental nerve cutting at the operation or the complete closure of the artery during the operation, leading to a heart attack during the operation itself. (Patients who have had a heart attack often become free of pain, as the offending area of heart muscle is now completely dead.)

Recent direct evidence that bypass surgery improves coronary blood flow has disproven these challenges. There is an initial narrowing of the grafts within one month, but 70 to 85 percent of them, according to most studies, are open and moving blood one year after the operation. Thereafter, 2 to 3 percent of the grafts close each year, up to five years. The return of angina pain correlates with the narrowing of the graft. Patients with open and functioning grafts are generally free of symptoms; those whose grafts have closed down begin to develop symptoms again.

Whether coronary artery bypass surgery always prolongs life more than medical therapy is a moot point—and a complicated one because medical therapy has also continued to advance and evolve. Encouraged by the spectacular relief of symptoms the operation sometimes provides, surgeons have frequently gone ahead with it, assuming the benefits will be greater than those medicine alone could provide. (One is reminded of the interdiction from *Alice in Wonderland:* ''No No, said the Queen, sentence first verdict afterwards.'')

The controversy was brought to the forefront in 1977 when a Veterans Administration hospitals study found that

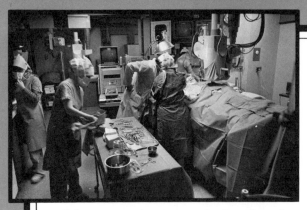

Before coronary bypass operation is performed, an X-ray study is performed to pinpoint exact location of blocked artery. (Photo by Bradford F. Herzog, courtesy Beth Israel Hospital, Boston)

matched groups of patients, whether treated medically or surgically, had similar survival rates. Commenting in the same *New England Journal of Medicine* issue in which the article appeared, Dr. Eugene Brownwald, professor of medicine at Harvard University Medical School, cautioned against excessive enthusiasm for bypass surgery while the effect of its treatment on longevity is unresolved. In the editorial he called for more comparison of medically and surgically treated patients.

Stirred by the challenge of the VA study article, medical centers have continued to analyze their results with coronary artery bypass surgery. Most now feel that its benefits relate directly to proper patient selection. All patients with angina pectoris are not alike. Some may have obstructing plaque (build-up of cholesterol) in only one of the major coronary vessels; others in all three. The location and the degree of obstruction are definite factors in patient survival and the operation's effectiveness. Atherosclerotic obstruction of 50 percent or more in the left main coronary artery before it divides into its two branches has a particularly ominous sig-

nificance. This artery supplies the main pumping chamber of the heart—the left ventricle. Over half the people who develop significant obstruction in that vessel die within a year, but coronary bypass surgery reduces this percentage dramatically. Similarly, obstruction in the right coronary artery and both branches of the left coronary artery, or any two of these, is almost as lethal, but coronary bypass surgery has increased the survival rate for patients with these problems as well. The operation seems to offer no prolongation of life to people with single-vessel disease that does not involve the left coronary artery.

In the opinion of most cardiologists, each patient must be considered as an individual in treating coronary artery disease. Most patients can be managed successfully with medications to increase coronary blood flow and attention to general factors such as proper diet and the elimination of smoking. Surgery may be the treatment of choice if the chest pain is disabling and cannot be controlled by drugs, if there is significant disease in the left main coronary artery, or if there is obstruction in more than one coronary artery. In most centers where the bypass operation is frequently performed, the mortality rate for the operation itself is less than 1 percent, and surgical patients clearly have more relief from symptoms than those who are treated with medication alone.

But coronary artery bypass surgery is an expensive procedure. To date the operation carries a price tag of $12,000 or more. This figure must be put into perspective, however. Unstable angina often results in frequent and repeated admissions to the hospital to rule out heart attacks. The cost of intensive care unit monitoring and frequent ECG and blood determinations that accompany these admissions is also high—in many cases, several thousand dollars per year. Cardiac surgeon Dr. John Collins at Boston's prestigious Peter Bent Brigham Hospital recently evaluated 100 patients who had coronary artery bypass surgery. His study showed that these patients spent so much less time in hospitals after their operation that the savings over a period of four years equaled the cost of the surgery. And, of course, the loss to society of people with disabling angina who are unable to work must be considered.

In fact, over the long term, surgical treatment may be more cost effective and therefore cheaper than medical treatment. In any event, both medical and surgical treatments of heart disease can be costly—but it is not always in the best interest of the patient to let cost be the determining factor.

All heart specialists agree that surgery for angina pectoris should never be considered until the exact location and degree of coronary artery obstruction is determined. This is done with an examination called angiocardiography. A long, flexible tube called a catheter is inserted into an artery in the arm and threaded toward the heart. Then a contrast material that shows up on X rays is injected into the coronary arteries to outline any obstruction. Whereas angiography does have certain risks, new techniques have made it relatively safe. Angiography is not considered, however, unless it will really affect the patient's care by answering any one of several questions. Does the patient really have coronary artery disease? Why is medical therapy not working? Does

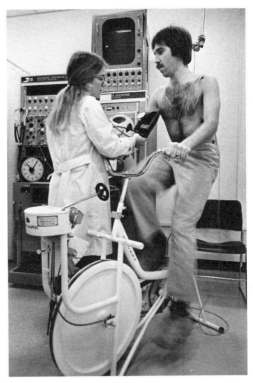

Patient undergoes ECG stress test, one of the many tests given to determine the need for coronary bypass surgery. (Photo by Don Robinson, courtesy Beth Israel Hospital, Boston)

the patient have a problem which surgery can repair?

Some heart specialists order angiograms on every patient with angina pectoris. Most are less aggressive and order the procedure only when the condition does not respond to medical treatment, so-called unstable angina, or when they suspect obstruction in the left main coronary artery. As X-ray techniques continue to become safer and the implication of coronary artery obstruction becomes more defined, coronary angiography will be used in more and more situations.

Not all patients with angina pectoris

are candidates for coronary artery bypass surgery. Dr. W. Dudley Johnson, cardiovascular surgeon at the Medical College of Wisconsin, puts it this way: "Patients do not die of angina pectoris; they die of obstruction in their arteries." Simply put, angina is a symptom, a squeezing pain in the chest. The symptom alone should not be treated, but rather the disease process behind the symptom, in this case coronary artery obstruction. As we shall see in the next section, a new treatment has been developed to do just that. Angina pectoris is sometimes incorrectly diagnosed, up to 10 percent of the time in some studies, because other medical conditions may mimic its symptoms. Some angina is caused by minor coronary artery obstruction of less than 50 percent. In other cases vessel obstruction is present in a small, less important vessel. Surgery has no benefit over medical therapy in such cases.

PTA—the balloon treatment

At the core of heart and blood vessel diseases is atherosclerosis, and insidious condition featuring progressive narrowing of blood vessels and resultant poor circulation to limbs and vital organs. In the wake of current controversies over medical versus surgical treatment for many conditions, alternative methods of treatment are generating new interest. One promising new technique, percutaneous transluminal angioplasty (PTA), involves using a balloon at the end of a long tube or catheter to open up arteries and improve circulation to the heart, kidneys, and legs, relieving such problems as angina, hypertension, and gangrene.

As we have seen, arteries can become obstructed by a buildup of fats and cholesterol along their inner walls. During PTA treatment, the expanding balloon actually compresses or flattens the plaque against the wall, effectively enlarging the artery opening and allowing blood to flow through more freely. However, long-term obstructions, where calcium has formed in the plaque, may be more difficult—and perhaps even impossible—to relieve with this technique.

The story of balloon treatment of artery obstruction begins in 1963, with Dr. Charles Dotter, a radiologist from the University of Oregon. After fourteen years of research with balloon catheters in lab animals, he presented his experiments to an international radiology meeting in Czechoslovakia, where he suggested the potential of the balloon catheter for relieving atherosclerosis in humans. He realized his own hopes and suggestions one year later, when he successfully used the technique on ten people whose legs were destined for amputation because of poor blood flow. By relieving atherosclerosis in the femoral artery in the groin, he restored circulation. There were no complications.

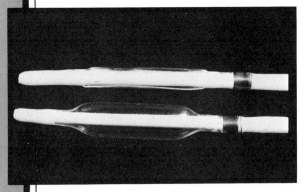

The PTA balloon expands (bottom) to compress plaque against an artery wall. (Courtesy Victor Millan, M.D.)

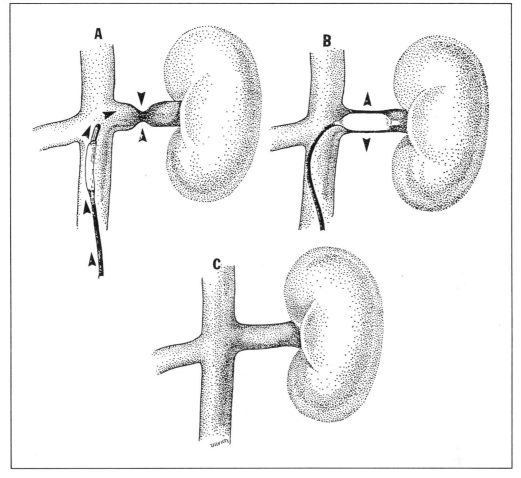

Balloon treatment for artery obstruction.
(A) balloon is guided to point of obstruction;
inflated (B); artery is cleared (C). (Courtesy
Victor Millan, M.D.)

CASE HISTORY

A. W. is a sixty-year-old executive with
a two-year history of chest pain, diag-
nosed as angina pectoris. Despite nitro-
glycerin and a variety of other medica-
tions, his condition worsened quickly.
Chest pain occurred with even minimal
exertion, in cold weather, even while
climbing a flight of stairs. During a
treadmill stress test he developed chest
pain after only four minutes and had a
heart rate of 95 beats per minute. His
physician ordered an X ray of his coro-
nary arteries which shows 90 percent
obstruction of the left anterior descend-
ing coronary artery, the artery that sup-
plies blood to the major muscle of the
heart, the left ventricle.

Several options for treatment were
discussed. He decided to forgo coronary
artery bypass surgery and instead chose
balloon catheter treatment. In the car-
diac study laboratory, a one-eighth-inch

catheter was inserted into an artery in his leg and guided up toward the heart while the physician watched with fluoroscopy (by which an X-ray image is transmitted to a television monitor). The catheter tip was positioned at the narrowed coronary artery, wedged, and the balloon inflated. The medical team watched on monitors in the laboratory as the circulation immediately improved in the heart artery. X rays taken shortly afterward showed that the obstruction was gone.

After the procedure, A. W. had no chest pain and returned to work. The treadmill stress test was repeated and was normal. His heart rate reached 150 beats per minute, and even after 10 minutes on the machine he was free of pain. One year later, he works at active physical labor and still is free of symptoms.

Successful balloon treatment of coronary artery narrowing was first performed in 1977, by Dr. Andreas Gruntzig at the University Hospital in Zurich, Switzerland, and was greeted with amazement by his colleagues the world over. Recently his pioneering group reported on fifty patients who selected this form of therapy as an alternative to coronary artery bypass surgery. Thirty-two patients were treated, and twenty of them, or about 64 percent, had excellent results, with improvement in their symptoms and treadmill stress testing. They were able to return to their normal work free of pain. In most of the untreated eighteen patients the catheter could not reach the proper location because of anatomical peculiarities of the patients' coronary arteries. In others, the catheter was positioned properly but the procedure just didn't work.

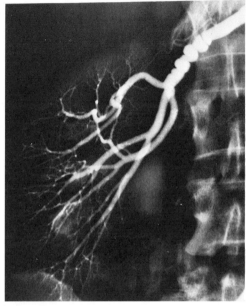

X-ray photo of obstructed artery before balloon treatment.

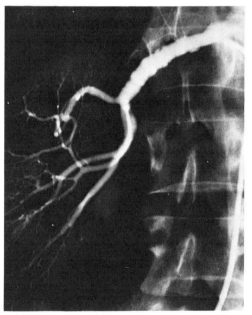

X-ray photo taken after balloon treatment, showing cleared artery.

Many other United States medical centers who are also using the technique reported their results at a recent national conference on PTA. The success rate in the 300 or so cases has consistently been about 60 percent, and most patients have done well in follow-up for a year or more.

But heart surgeons are careful to point out that not every patient with coronary artery disease is an appropriate candidate for this procedure. After careful selection, perhaps two or three out of every ten might be considered. Patients must have angina pectoris that cannot be managed medically. The artery obstruction must be discrete, well localized, and fairly close to the beginning of the coronary artery so that the balloon catheter can easily reach the blockage. The patient must also understand that coronary artery bypass surgery is a possibility if the procedure fails. In the reported studies, 7 percent of the patients required the open-heart operation immediately because of failure in the catheterization laboratory.

Balloon catheter treatment is only experimental today, but it certainly gives new meaning to coronary angiography, the X-ray study developed twenty years ago which outlines the coronary arteries and reveals obstructions. The potential of PTA is exciting because, as one surgeon put it, "many patients can be treated for coronary artery obstruction right here in the catheterization lab at the time the diagnosis is made on X ray." Another surgeon added, ". . . and at 10 percent of the cost of coronary bypass surgery."

The balloon catheter treatment has been modified since Dr. Dotter's work in the mid-sixties, and it is now also used for a variety of artery obstructions, including those in the pelvis. Perhaps the most exciting use is in patients with hypertension. Of the 20 million people who have hypertension, about 5 percent have the renovascular variety, in which the increased pressure is caused by an obstruction in the artery that supplies the kidney. Surgical correction is the standard treatment to restore kidney circulation, but not every patient with the problem is a candidate for surgery. Many have severe kidney failure and are quite ill, and there is the distinct possibility of losing the kidney¯ should the operation fail.

PTA offers few such risks. According to a recent review of PTA in the *Journal of the American Medical Association*, 90 percent of patients with renovascular hypertension can potentially benefit by PTA. Half will be "cured"; that is, they will no longer need medication to control their blood pressure. The other half will require less medication than before.

Dr. Donald Schwarten of St. Vincent's Hospital, Indianapolis; Dr. Charles Tegtmeyer of the University of Virginia Medical Center, Charlottesville; and Drs. Victor Millan and Nicolaos Madias of the Tufts–New England Medical Center, Boston, have the most experience with the technique. Among them, they have treated 200 patients successfully.

In the Tufts study, one patient's blood pressure went from 180/115 to 120/80 immediately as the circulation was restored to the kidney. Some patients have required two or three treatments to achieve success.

The complication rate for PTA has been very small when treating hypertension. It is done under local anesthesia,

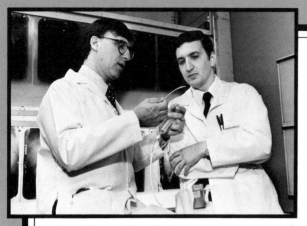

Drs. Victor Millan (left) and Dr. Nicolaos Madias, pioneers in PTA research for hypertension, examine the balloon and catheter. (Courtesy New England Medical Center, Boston)

thus avoiding the expense and danger of an operation.

Though not in standard use yet, PTA is a procedure with a potentially great future. Dr. Madias of Tufts explains: "From a medical perspective it is close to a perfect treatment. It gets to the root of the problem and corrects it anatomically, without the expense or risks of surgery." Surgeons apparently agree. At a recent meeting of the American College of Surgeons, PTA was listed as one of the great advances of the decade in surgery.

The Holter monitor

Half of the 700,000 people who die each year in the United States from heart attack die before they reach the hospital. As we have seen, angina pectoris or atherosclerosis can cause heart attack if the flow of blood to the heart is severely restricted. But sudden death from heart attack is most often the result of an abnormal heart rhythm that begins spontaneously and prevents the heart from pumping blood. Finding the individuals who are prone to this lethal heart rhythm is a major challenge in cardiology.

That challenge is being met today for many people with a continuous electrocardiogram recording technique called the Holter monitor.

Ever since the British physician Dr. Augustus Waller invented the electrocardiogram in 1887, heart specialists have been fascinated by the interpretation of the heart's electrical activity. Today the ECG is one of the major diagnostic devices in cardiology, permitting the diagnosis and monitoring of many rhythm disturbances, heart attacks, muscle enlargements, and chemical or electrolyte problems. But despite its widespread acceptance, the ECG is limited as a diagnostic tool. Stories abound of people who die suddenly from heart failure, despite having recently had a "normal" ECG. The reason the ECG fails to record all abnormal and potentially lethal heart rhythms is that it does not record *every* heartbeat. Although the heart beats more than 100,000 times each day, the standard ECG records only 50 to 100 of these beats at one time. If an abnormal rhythm is intermittent, brief, or unpredictable, there is great chance that the ECG will not detect it.

CASE HISTORY

A. M. is a sixty-year-old florist who had been bothered by palpitations for years. Often during the day, her heart would race. "It feels as if it is jumping out of my chest," she explained to her doctor. The episodes were irregular and did not occur every day, but they were beginning to occur more often.

The feeling sometimes passed innocently within minutes. Occasionally it would last for hours. During these longer spells, A. M. grew very weak and nearly passed out.

No cause was found for the palpitations. Several complete physical examinations and electrocardiograms over several years were all normal. Her physician advised her to come to the office or a hospital emergency room during one of the "spells" to see if her heart was indeed "racing." Each time she tried to do that, the feeling subsided before she arrived or before the electrocardiogram was taken.

Finally she was referred to a cardiologist who suggested twenty-four-hour heart monitoring with the Holter monitor. During the day that she wore the recording device while going about her activities at the store, she experienced two of her "spells." Analysis of the Holter recording showed brief runs of paroxysmal atrial tachycardia, during which her heart was beating 180 times per minute.

The cardiologist prescribed digitalis, an oral medication to slow her heart. Now, two years later, she is free of her palpitations.

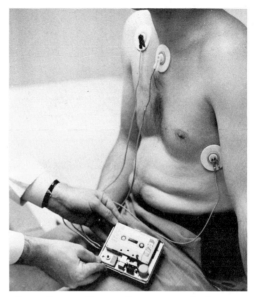

Electrodes on adhesive discs are attached to skin. Wires from electrodes connect to Holter monitor cassette-recording unit. (Photo by Joseph Murphy)

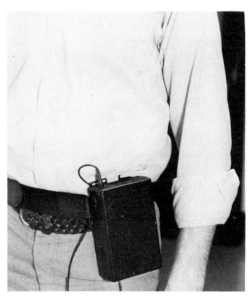

With Holter monitor in place, patient can resume normal activities while the device monitors twenty-four hours of activity. (Photo by Joseph Murphy)

The Holter monitor is a continuous twenty-four-hour electrocardiogram. It records every beat of the heart *without exception* during the day and night while the patient is working, relaxing, eating, and even sleeping. Developed by Dr. Norman J. Holter twenty years ago, the first ambulatory ECG monitor was a heavy, cumbersome transmitter worn across the shoulders like a knapsack, sporting a large antenna which directed the signals to a separate, equally large receiver. Today's version is a small,

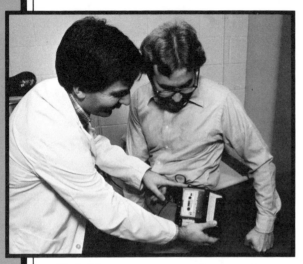

Technician removes cassette from recorder after full day of monitoring. (Courtesy Mt. Auburn Hospital, Cambridge, Massachusetts)

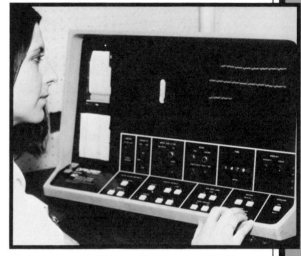

Technician reads high-speed replay of patient's twenty-four-hour heartbeat, recorded by Holter monitor, and looks for any irregularities. (Courtesy Mt. Auburn Hospital, Cambridge, Massachusetts)

compact, portable recorder, weighing less than a pound, that is able to record a full twenty-four-hour ECG tracing on a slow-moving, self-contained cassette tape. Special adhesive electrodes are attached painlessly to the patient's chest and connected to the recorder with thin wires. The unit is comfortable to wear on an adjustable belt around the waist or shoulders, and it does not interfere with daily activities.

The recorder also has a time channel so that any specific heartbeat or groups of beats can be related precisely to the time they occurred. The patient is given a logbook and encouraged to record the events of the day and any symptoms that might be important, such as weakness, dizziness, chest pain, or palpitations. Later, when the recording tape is processed by a high-speed computer and reader, any irregularities of rhythm can be plotted in relation to time of day, medications, or activity.

Many patients may have elusive and unpredictable symptoms caused by abnormal cardiac rhythms; Holter recording during such episodes is valuable to guide therapy. If a rapid, potentially lethal rhythm is documented, medications can be prescribed to slow the heartbeat or make the heart less irritable. If a slow rhythm is documented, a pacemaker may be recommended. Rapid and slow rhythms may both produce the same symptoms in the patient; since the treatment for each differs, the importance of distinguishing between the two is obvious.

Cardiologists also use Holter monitoring to evaluate the effectiveness of prescribed cardiac medications, which can be quite toxic if used incorrectly. This applies particularly to patients who are convalescing from heart attack or who have coronary artery disease; these patients have a relatively high incidence of sudden lethal heart rhythms.

When it was first reported, the Holter monitor was greeted with some skepticism. So was the electrocardiogram itself. The noted cardiologist Dr. Paul Dudley White, one of the pioneers in the use of the electrocardiogram, was told by his colleagues only fifty years ago, "Forget this heart business. No one can specialize in such a narrow line of work. You'll go broke. And for heaven's sake, stop tinkering with those electric recording devices; they'll get you nowhere." The electrocardiogram is, of course, a very accurate and useful diagnostic tool, and the Holter monitor is expanding its role for the future.

Preventing sudden cardiac death

The Holter monitor is useful for diagnosing heart malfunctions and treating them accordingly. But what about the recent victim of a heart attack? What is being done to ensure that the patient doesn't have a second or a third attack? Or die from the first one?

Much of the recent effort to reduce cardiac mortality has been directed at the first months following a heart attack, when the risk of dying is highest. While the death rates from a heart attack decrease with time after the attack, they remain extremely high for the first six months, long after the protective hospital monitoring period is over and the patient has returned home. Most of the patients who die during this time are stricken suddenly with an abnormal heart rhythm.

It now appears that sulfinpyrazone, a medication used in gout treatment, may play a promising new role in the prevention of sudden death from heart attack by suppressing fatal arrhythmias, or irregular heartbeats.

Sulfinpyrazone (trade name Anturane) has been used to treat chronic gout for many years. The drug is a uricosuric agent—that is, it helps the kidney eliminate or filter uric acid from the blood. In the 1960s journal reports suggested that sulfinpyrazone might also be used to treat vascular disease. Various investigators found that sulfinpyrazone reduced blood clotting in patients with artificial heart valves and peripheral circulatory disease, and diminished the mortality rate of elderly patients recuperating from stroke or heart attack.

These early findings prompted the formation of a formal group to study sulfinpyrazone's exact effects among patients who had a documented heart attack. Traditionally, this group of patients had high mortality rates. In 1975 an Anturane (sulfinpyrazone) Reinfarction Trial Research Group (ARTRG) was formed under the direction of Temple University cardiologist Dr. Sol Sherry, consisting of investigators from twenty-six hospitals around the United States. Although subsidized by the pharmaceutical manufacturer of the drug, CIBA/Geigy, the study was independently designed and conducted and has since been hailed as a model research project.

Sixteen hundred patients who had suffered heart attacks volunteered to participate in the study. Half of them were given Anturane tablets four times daily, beginning one month after their heart attack; the remaining patients were given a placebo. The patients were selected randomly, and neither the patients nor the investigators knew which patients were taking the placebo and which were taking Anturane. The pills were coded, and the codes were known only to the coordinating center.

After two years the code was broken and the ARTRG published the long-awaited results in the *New England Journal of Medicine.* During the two-year study, there were fifty-nine sudden deaths out of one hundred cardiac deaths in the study group. The Anturane-treated patients had 50 percent fewer deaths than the placebo group and 75 percent fewer sudden deaths. (A sudden death is the unexpected development of an abnormal heart rhythm that is incompatible with life.) Statistically, the benefit of Anturane seemed to occur entirely during the second to sixth months after the infarction (heart attack); there-after, there seemed to be little benefit.

In discussing their findings, the investigators noted that the statistics on the placebo-treated group were similar to standard mortality rates for heart attack patients. In the January 31, 1980, *New England Journal* report, the study group noted: "The period of the highest risk was early after the acute event, and the risk substantially decreased with time." Anturane reduced the risk: the sudden death rate for the placebo group was 10 percent, but only 5 percent for the Anturane group. No side effects from Anturane were reported.

The ARTRG suggested that Anturane appeared to make the heart muscle more resistant to abnormal rhythms. The drug may also have a role in the inhibition of platelets, blood components important in the blood-clotting mechanism.

If Anturane was shown to be so successful in preventing sudden cardiac death why is it not more widely used?

The main reason is that despite the encouraging results of the ARTRG study, sulfinpyrazone must undergo further testing before the drug meets Food and Drug Administration standards. In May 1980 the FDA refused to approve sulfin-pyrazone for use in preventing abnormal heart rhythms in patients who have had a heart attack. Dr. Richard Crout, director of the FDA's Bureau of Drugs, said, "The Anturane reinfarction trial provides suggestive evidence that sulfin-pyrazone may be effective in reducing the rate of deaths in patients who have heart attacks, but this study does not provide us with the quality of scientific evidence the law requires to approve the drug for this use."

The FDA apparently disputed the classification of patients in the placebo group in the "sudden death" category. Dr. Marion Finkel, the FDA's associate director for new drug evaluation who directed the review, felt that some of the so-called sudden deaths in the placebo group were actually patients who had suffered another heart attack and therefore should not have been included in the comparison. "Removing this group of patients from the sudden death category substantially changes the conclusions of the report," Dr. Finkel explains. Responding in the May 21, 1980, *Medical Tribune,* Dr. Sherry defended the study group report and noted that two independent review bodies substantiated its findings.

The FDA's dramatic challenge to the ARTRG's equally dramatic report typifies the controversy that accompanies any new medical advance—a dispute that protects the consumer from premature use of an unproven drug.

Other studies on sulfinpyrazone are

scheduled, and the drug will undoubtedly take an appropriate place in the treatment of heart disease. And if the long-term results follow the pattern established by the ARTRG study group, several hundred patients per week across the country may have a reprieve from the devastating aftereffects of a heart attack.

Mitral valve prolapse

With the growing scope of medical knowledge comes the unfortunate tendency to be complacent about "how much we know." As a prominent physician once said, "Remember that one-half of everything the medical profession considers correct today will eventually be proven wrong. Our problem is, we don't know which half."

So it is with a condition called mitral valve prolapse. Unrecognized in 1960, today it is considered the most common form of cardiac valvular disease in the United States, affecting some 5 to 10 percent of the population. Its most common symptoms can be vague: palpitations, fatigue, shortness of breath, chest pain, and fainting spells, so nonspecific that patients with the condition were recently thought to have psychological problems instead.

Refinements in diagnostic techniques in the last fifteen years have led to the recognition and understanding of mitral valve prolapse. Many individuals with mitral valve prolapse experience no symptoms and suffer no ill-effects from the condition. However, the long-term prognosis is still uncertain. An increasing number of reports associates the disorder with sudden death among seemingly healthy young people, as well as stroke, heart attack, heart infection, and congestive heart failure. In any event, early diagnosis of mitral valve prolapse is certainly important.

CASE HISTORY

M. D. is a thirty-five-year-old lawyer who was ambitious, successful, and recognized in her field. She sought medical attention because her heart was "beating so fast."

M. D. had had occasional "skipped heartbeats" for as long as she could remember. "It's your nerves," her doctors told her. The "skipped beats" never interfered with her work or social life, so she gave them little attention. Once, during a college physical examination, doctors detected a heart murmur, but chest X ray and ECG were normal.

When her father died suddenly, the skipped heartbeats became more prominent. Gradually M. D. became tired and run-down. Her physician couldn't help her, and she was referred to a psychiatrist who thought that she was suffering a prolonged grief reaction, in part due to unresolved conflicts she had had with her father.

With psychotherapy she improved and was able to work a full day at the office. But the skipped beats continued. "You're doing too much too soon," the psychiatrist said. She went to bed earlier and cut down her hours at work. She became even more tired.

Six months ago M. D. had the sudden onset of a rapid, forceful heartbeat with anxiety and shortness of breath. She again visited her physician, who found her to have normal blood pressure and a pulse of 80. He also heard a faint and intermittent "clicking sound," but no murmur. The electrocardiogram was normal. She was referred to a cardiologist, who performed an echo cardiogram, a relatively new technique using ultrasound to observe the heart's activity (see pages 122–123), which demonstrated mitral valve prolapse. She was started on propranolol (trade name Inderal).

Today M. D. has trouble remembering what the "skipped beats" were like. "I haven't felt once since the medicine was started," she says. She is working a full schedule in court and the office and has resumed teaching at the university. She no longer sees the psychiatrist and exercises regularly. "My diagnosis became my cure," she said. "I feel great knowing that, during all these years, the problem was not in my head after all."

Mitral valve prolapse occurs commonly in women and can apparently be inherited, although the disease's exact cause is unknown. When the disease strikes, the mitral valve, which separates the left atrium (which receives blood from the lungs) from the left ventricle that pumps blood to the rest of the body, seems to be too large for the ventricle. During systole (the period when the heart contracts), the valve billows backward into the atrium, like the spinnaker on a sailboat. Pressure from the heart's contraction can eventually weaken the valve so that it becomes incompetent in the later stages of the condition, and some blood can flow backward into the atrium rather than forward through the aorta.

Later in life, a patient with a prolapsed mitral valve can develop heart failure and endocarditis, an infection of the heart that typically occurs on deformed heart valves. A further complicating problem can be stroke, which occurs when bacterial growths on heart valves that accompany endocarditis flake off the valve, pass through the circulation, and eventually obstruct blood vessels in the brain. The sudden death that has been associated with the condition may be a result of the unexpected occurrence of a fatal abnormal heart rhythm.

For many years, physicians were aware of and reported on patients who had peculiar clicking sounds during systole. The familiar "lub-duh-dub" sound was given many names but was generally thought to originate outside the heart. The corresponding symptoms of palpitations, weakness, and fainting were also recognized and were called a variety of names; asthenia, effort syndrome, and soldier's heart were among them.

In 1961 South African physicians Drs. J. V. Reid and J. B. Barlow solved the mystery when they conclusively showed that the curious sounds originated in a "deformity of the mitral valve."

In fairness to the generations of physicians who misdiagnosed mitral valve prolapse through the years, only the recent diagnostic techniques of echo cardiography and angiography have permitted the condition to be witnessed. The classic clicking sounds vary considerably in intensity, are sometimes (but not always) accompanied by a murmur, and are often completely inaudible as the patient assumes different positions.

In a recent issue of the *Journal of American Medical Association*, University of California cardiologist Dr. J.

Michael Criley commented: "Since most people with mitral valve prolapse have no symptoms, they probably require no therapy, except for antibiotics before surgery . . . to lessen the possibility of heart valve infections." He noted that when symptoms do occur, most physicians use the medication propranolol (Inderal), which increases heart size and reduces the strength of its contraction, thus compensating for the larger mitral valve. Surgery to correct or replace the valve is also possible in severe cases.

Since diagnosis of the condition is relatively new, further studies are needed before the true implications of mitral valve prolapse are known. Only then will physicians know with assurance what to do when they diagnose it.

Resources

■ Referrals for cardaic diagnosis and treatment are best obtained from your doctor, hospital, or state medical society.

Information on heart disease and the latest research is always available from the local and state offices of the American Heart Association, listed in your telephone directory. The national coordinating office is:

American Heart Association
National Office
7320 Greenville Avenue
Dallas, Texas 75231
214-750-5300

■ National Heart Research projects are coordinated by:

National Heart, Lung, and Blood Vessel Institute
Public Inquiries Office
Room 4A21, Building 31
National Institutes of Health
Bethesda, Maryland 20205
301-496-4236

National Academy of Sciences/National Research Council
Washington, D.C. 20418
202-393-8100

■ Another source of information on heart disease is:

Consumer Information Center
Pueblo, Colorado 81009
303-544-5227, ext. 370

■ Sulfinpyrazone (Trade name Anturane) is manufactured by:
CIBA Pharmaceutical Company
Summit, New Jersey 07901
201-277-5000

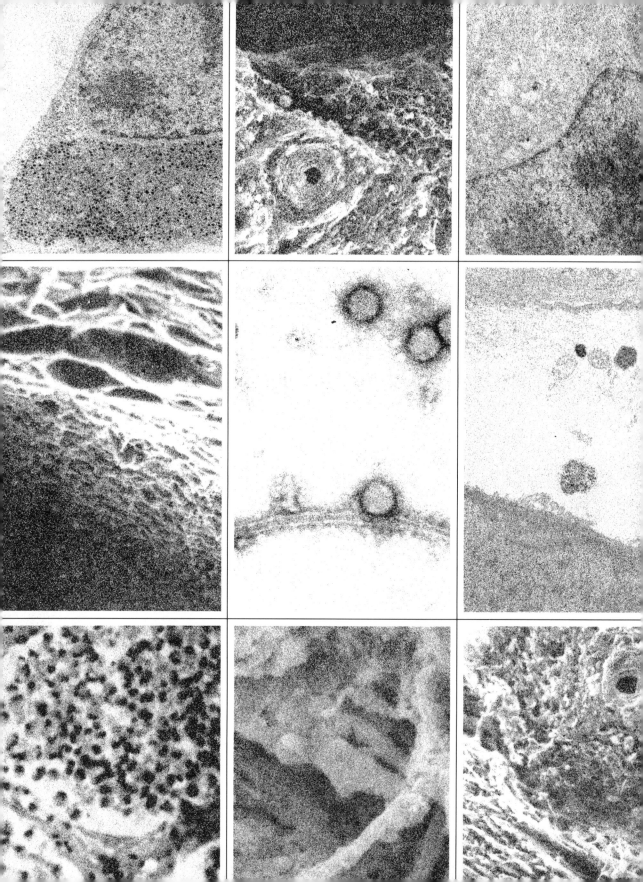

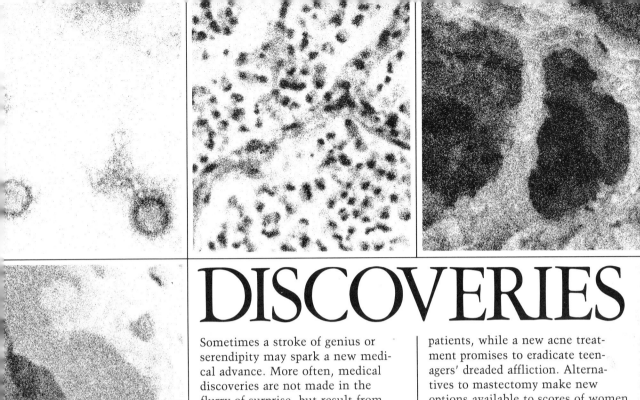

DISCOVERIES

Sometimes a stroke of genius or serendipity may spark a new medical advance. More often, medical discoveries are not made in the flurry of surprise, but result from years of painstaking observation and experimentation involving a myriad of researchers, physicians, and technicians. Around the world these medical personnel struggle to develop new drugs, new treatments, new cures. They fight to prove the accuracy of such advances and to test the dangers of drugs and practices once considered safe.

A single such discovery may touch the lives of thousands. A vaccine for pneumonia offers hope to elderly patients, while a new acne treatment promises to eradicate teenagers' dreaded affliction. Alternatives to mastectomy make new options available to scores of women with breast cancer today. And everyone will be grateful for a drug that may finally get rid of those annoying cold sores.

In any discovery, advances are made in minds that are open to change, and by scientists who refuse to be satisfied with current knowledge. In the words of Martin Fischer, ''Every discovery in science is a tacit criticism of things as they are. That is why the wise man is invariably called a fool.''

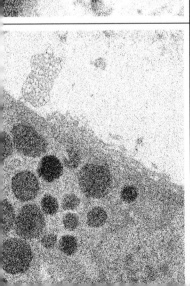

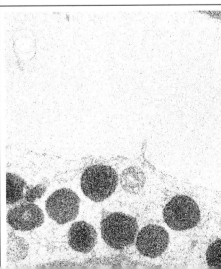

Vaccinating against pneumonia

If we believe a thing to be bad, and if we have a right to prevent it, it is our duty to try to prevent it and to damn the consequence.

Alfred Lord Milner, 1909

According to a recent United States surgeon general's report, pneumonia is the fifth leading cause of death in the United States. Three million people have pneumonia each year; more than 10 percent are hospitalized; and they lose over 15 million days from work. The government estimates the total cost of pneumonia at $2 billion per year.

Pneumonia is an infection of the lung caused by a variety of bacteria, mycoplasma (atypical organisms that are neither bacteria nor viruses), and viruses. A severe and common form of the disease is pneumococcal pneumonia. The pneumococcus, which causes it, is a virulent bacteria that grows in pairs or in very short chains and exists in eighty-three known varieties. It alone accounts for more than 50,000 deaths per year and is particularly dangerous to older adults and individuals with chronic disease such as emphysema. At the turn of the century, Sir William Osler called pneumonia "the old man's friend." The disease commonly brought a speedy end to the misery of people with serious and debilitating diseases, mostly older adults.

For many years the treatment of pneumonia was based on antibiotics (predominately penicillin), but despite their promise antibiotics have not always cured the infection. Now, however, a vaccine for pneumonia raises the hope that mankind may be spared this dread disease.

About pneumonia

Pneumonia strikes individuals over forty years of age three to four times more often than those under thirty and is more common in men than in women. Two-thirds of people with pneumonia have underlying

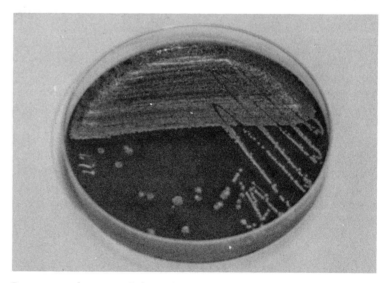

Pneumococcal pneumonia bacteria culture. Each white speck is a bacteria growth. (Photo by Joseph Murphy)

conditions that impair their resistance; half of all pneumonia patients, for example, have emphysema, and many abuse alcohol.

The respiratory defense system presents a set of obstacles that stop most bacteria from entering the trachea, or windpipe; when these defense mechanisms break down, pneumonia can be the result. Normally, the epiglottis, a sort of trap door that closes over the trachea opening, keeps out postnasal secretions. Tiny hairs on the airway walls called cilia beat in a wavelike motion to move mucus, bacteria, and other foreign particles back toward the mouth, where the cough mechanism removes them explosively.

Often a virus cold or flu lowers a person's resistance by altering the properties of normal secretions and the bacteria that normally live in the airways. Harmful bacteria, in these circumstances, have a more hospitable environment in which to grow. Cold weather or chilling of the body can lower the temperature of the trachea environment and decrease mucous and ciliary activity. Fatigue and illness

also lower resistance. Diabetes, emphysema, anemia, and other chronic infections make pneumonia more likely, as do chemical pollutants, cigarette smoke, and alcohol.

Once bacterial infection occurs, the victim experiences the familiar symptoms of pneumonia: high fever, coughing up thick mucus, and occasional pain with coughing. The physician diagnoses pneumonia by reviewing the patient's history, hearing the typical sounds of congestion and infection in the lung (called rales), and seeing an elevated white blood cell count and a shadow on the X ray. The doctor may also take a sample of the sputum for laboratory analysis of bacteria.

Dr. Kevin Wilson, a pulmonary specialist at Baylor College of Medicine in Texas, explains the degrees of severity of pneumonia: "Most patients have 'walking pneumonia'— they can easily be treated with antibiotics at home. Those with underlying chronic infections, or who are actually and seriously ill, may need to be hospitalized. Diagnosis and treatment can be much more complicated in these patients."

Finding a vaccine

The interest in a vaccine for pneumonia stemmed from Edward Jenner's discovery in treating smallpox that immunization can successfully ward off infection. Efforts to develop a vaccine against pneumonia began at the turn of the century in South Africa. Soon afterward, proof was found that the injection of a carbohydrate from a pneumococcal bacteria could induce antibodies against pneumonia. But when penicillin became available, interest in developing the vaccine waned. The antibiotic was cheaper, nontoxic, and promised to eradicate the infection.

That promise was never realized, however. Many of the eighty-three pneumococcus varieties are resistant to penicillin, and today there are still almost half as many annual pneumonia deaths as there were in 1900. In older adults, the mortality rate for pneumonia is well over 25 percent. Drug treatment does not remove the factors that determine mortality in infectious disease. Sixty percent of all the deaths from pneumococcal

Chest X ray of patient with right upper lobe pneumonia, shown by white patch across right lung (left side of chest in photo). (Courtesy Eli Lilly and Co.)

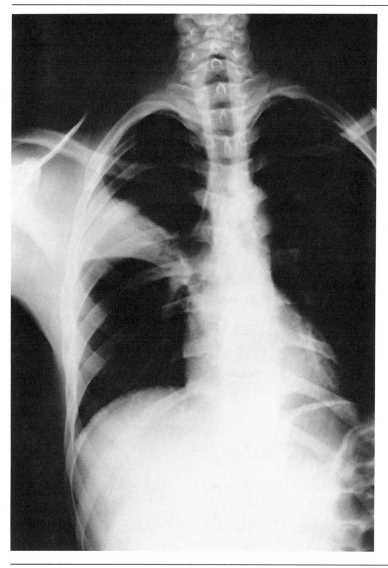

pneumonia occur in the first five days of the illness despite penicillin treatment. Autopsies of pneumonia victims who were treated with penicillin show no evidence of any infection remaining; the penicillin did its job. Severe and irreversible damage to the body occurred early in the infection, before the antibiotic was begun.

With all this in mind, Dr. Robert Austrian of the University of Pennsylvania rekindled an interest in a pneumonia vaccine in the early 1970s.

How the pneumonia vaccine works

In 1977, the Merck, Sharp and Dohme pharmaceutical company released a pneumonia vaccine called Pneumovax. More recently Lederle Laboratories entered the picture with Pnu-imune. Both vaccines contain carbohydrates from the capsules (the outer membranes) of the fourteen types of pneumococcus that cause over 80 percent of all pneumococcal infections. Once in the body, the carbohydrates act as antigens: they induce the body to develop antibodies that prevent subsequent contact with

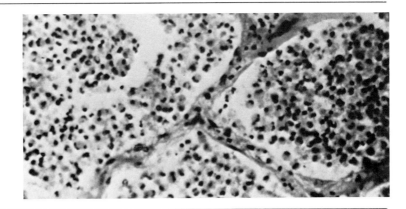

Bronchial tubes filled with pneumonia bacteria. (Courtesy Eli Lilly and Co.)

any of those fourteen types of pneumococcus from developing into serious infection. They have been shown to be highly effective.

Shortly after its introduction, the vaccine was first administered in the United States as part of a formal voluntary program at the Don Orione Home in East Boston, Massachusetts. The Don Orione Home is a 200-bed skilled nursing facility run by an international Catholic order, and like other institutions for the elderly, its inhabitants have suffered the ravages of pneumonia.

More than 3 million doses of the vaccine have now been given across the country with positive results. The vaccine offers high-grade protection from pneumococcal disease and produces few adverse reactions, such as low-grade fever and irritation. That the first testing of the vaccine took place in Massachusetts is significant; influenza followed by pneumonia as a cause of death is 30 to 40 percent higher in that state than in the United States as a whole. In fact, in 1973 Massachusetts ranked first in the country in deaths

from this infection. Since the introduction of the pneumonia vaccine, however, that death rate has fallen drastically.

CASE HISTORY

C. G. has lived at home alone for the past five of her seventy-two years. While basically healthy, she does have chronic congestive heart failure, which is well controlled with medications and a low-salt diet. She eats poorly, however, often not taking the time to prepare food for herself.

Three years in a row she was treated for pneumonia, with symptoms of high fever, chills, and rapid breathing; once she had to be hospitalized. Two years ago, C. G. received the pneumonia vaccine. She has been well since.

Will pneumonia now be eradicated?

In 1978 the World Health Organization announced that smallpox, a previously dreaded disease, had finally been eradicated as a result of a worldwide immunization program. Can we expect the same of

pneumococcal pneumonia? Unfortunately, the answer to that is probably not, because there are so many pneumococcus varieties. The fourteen strains in today's version of the vaccine may not always be the major cause of serious infection; other types may become dominant. Constant monitoring and possible vaccine alterations will almost certainly be necessary. And, of course, the vaccine is not effective against those forms of pneumonia caused by other bacteria, viruses, and mycoplasma.

Yet the vaccine offers enormous potential. Until recently, immunization programs have been directed mostly at children and the usual childhood diseases, such as measles and whooping cough. Adults usually received immunizations only of tetanus toxoid after injury or to protect them from disease endemic to an area of travel. Elderly patients have been virtually ignored, yet they are very susceptible to serious infection. The vaccine's manufacturers cite persons fifty years of age and older as one group who should get the pneumococcal vaccine. According to the package inserts, the vaccine is also recommended for people whose spleens function poorly or have been removed (they have less capacity to respond to infection because their antibody production is reduced) and those with chronic lung or liver disease. People who work in occupations associated with an excessive risk of pneumonia, such as mining, would also be candidates, as would some children with severe anemia, lung infection, or other chronic debilitating diseases.

Even though the package inserts specifically list diabetics as likely candidates for receiving the vaccine, many diabetes specialists disagree. In their experience, well-controlled diabetes presents no greater risk of infection, and diabetes per se is not an absolute indication for the vaccine. Poor control or complicated diabetes may, however, present problems. Each case should therefore be treated individually after consultation with the appropriate physician.

When Edward Jenner developed vaccination in the late 1700s, many colleagues who could not agree with the concept of prevention ridiculed him. British physician John Haygarth agreed with Jenner, but advised that smallpox should continue to be studied. He stated that vaccination "was the most fortunate and beneficial improvement that medical science ever accomplished. It cannot, however, preclude the necessity of investigating the variolous poison [the poison of smallpox] and of considering by what regulations its propagation may be prevented."

Haygarth's warning is a good lesson for today. Dr. Harry A. Feldman, an infectious disease specialist at the State University of New York, recently commented on the pneumonia vaccine: "An important advance has been given to us, but its effectiveness will reflect the intelligence with which it is utilized."

Resources

- Pneumonia vaccines are administered by your doctor, local hospital or state sponsored immunization programs.

Information about such programs is generally available from your state Department of Public Health and city or county Department of Public Health.

- The following pharmaceutical companies manufacture pneumonia vaccines:

Merck, Sharp and Dohme
West Point, Pennsylvania
19486
215-699-5311
(Pneumovax)

Lederle Laboratories
Wayne, New Jersey 07470
201-831-2000
(Pnu-imune)

- Immunization information is also available from:

Center for Disease Control
Bureau of State Services
Technical Information Services
Atlanta, Georgia 30333
404-452-4021

National Institute of Child Health and Infant Development
National Institutes of Health
Office of Research Reporting
Room 2A34
Building 31
Bethesda, Maryland 20205
301-496-5133

Fighting cancer with heat

If I had the means to cause fever, I could cure all illness.

Parmenides, fifth century B.C.

The beneficial effect of heat on chronic illness, and on cancer in particular, has been known for generations. Throughout ancient and modern medical literature, scattered reports tell of tumor regression following a febrile illness and attempts to reduce tumors by heating the body or causing a febrile illness, usually erysipelas (an infection of the skin caused by the bacteria *streptococcus*). Even though some evidence of success can be found, heat treatment eventually was replaced by more effective methods, including surgery, radiation, anticancer drugs, and immunology, which are now considered to be the four standard treatments for cancer.

Despite limited success in treating cancer with heat—or hyperthermia—researchers have continued to study the effect of temperature on cancer cells. In the past five years there has been a resurgence of interest in heat treatment for cancer, and many cancer centers are now conducting studies of the effects of heat and other standard therapies.

Heat treatment for cancer is still experimental and is usually reserved for cases that respond poorly to other forms of treatment. But the initial encouraging results suggest that in the years to come heat treatment may very well become the fifth standard treatment for cancer.

Cancer's Achilles heel

Do cancer cells contain some metabolic "Achilles heel" that makes them more sensitive than normal cells to the effects of heat? Although the actual mechanisms are unclear, evidence suggests that the answer is yes. An elevated temperature may inhibit cell division, a well-known feature of rapidly growing cancer cells. It may damage the cell membrane, the hard sheath that surrounds the cell, making it easier for the body's own "killer lymphocytes" or certain drugs to attack and remove the cancer cells. Or heat may just kill the cancer cells directly in some yet unknown way by arresting the chemical reaction within the cells.

CASE HISTORY

A. E. is a fifty-three-year-old executive in an insurance company. One year ago a routine chest X ray during a physical examination for life insurance revealed a tumor in his right lung.

A. E. was surprised because he had no symptoms. He did, however, smoke two packs of cigarettes per day and had worked with asbestos insulation materials for several years before his promotion to a management position within his company.

A. E. was immediately referred to an oncologist, a cancer specialist, who biopsied the tumor. It was found to be a mesothelioma, a highly malignant form of cancer. Although mesothelioma is quite rare, it does appear often in people with a prior history of asbestos exposure who smoke cigarettes as well. Because of the poor response of mesothelioma to standard cancer therapies, A. E. was referred to the Tufts–New England Medical Center in Boston, where specialists suggested using heat treatment along with radiation. The specialists explained that the treatment was only experimental and the results could not be predicted. A. E. volunteered for the treatment and therapy was begun.

Three times per week, for several weeks, A. E. lay under a transparent plastic canopy with his head exposed. A diathermy unit slowly raised his body temperature to 105 degrees Fahrenheit. After forty minutes at this temperature he was removed from the chamber and taken to the radiology department, where he received a standard dose of external radiation. He was then returned to the heat chamber for another fifteen minutes. Two other days per week he had radiation therapy alone.

Six months after the treatment, A. E.'s mesothelioma has regressed markedly.

Since A. E., three other patients have undergone tumor treatment in the New England Medical Center's environmental chamber for hyperthermia, and all have shown encouraging results.

Edward S. Sternick, a physicist and the director of medical physics at the Boston hospital, designed and built the chamber. He notes, "After years of research on the radiobiology of cancer in our institution and the effects of heat on the cancer cell, we attempted to find a way to heat the patient's body in a limited way so as to minimize the serious effects of extreme hyperthermia—namely, liver, brain, and cardiovascular system damage—that had been noted in previous attempts to treat cancer with heat."

Sternick's unit uses diathermy, a special frequency of radio waves that preferentially heat body tissues having a high percentage of water and low electrical resistance, such as blood. The radio waves, which come from the mattress on which the patient lies in the chamber, increase the body temperature by rapidly vibrating the molecules within those tissues. A microcomputer, also designed for the chamber, monitors the patient's respiration, pulse, blood pressure, and rectal and skin temperatures, and balances the power input in the chamber to limit the patient's temperature rise to 105 degrees Fahrenheit (40.5 degrees Celsius).

The saying "Primum non nocere" (First of all do the patient no harm) has guided physicians since 15 B.C., when it was first written as part of an oath for practitioners of the healing arts. It applies also to the Tufts heat therapy project, as Dr. Bahman Emami, a professor of therapeutic radiology and a partner in the heat therapy study, explains: "We are now in the first stage of a multipart investigation. Once we have studied twenty patient volunteers to assess what, if any, tissue damage occurs, only then will we move on to the next phase, that of comparing hyperthermia with conventional cancer therapies to evaluate the results in a scientific way."

Water beds and wax baths

Most of the early work with heat treatment for cancer involved the induction of bacterial infections to produce fever. In 1883 German microbiologist Friedrich Fehleisen injected the streptococcus bacteria into the skin of five patients with lymph node tumors and noted tumor re-

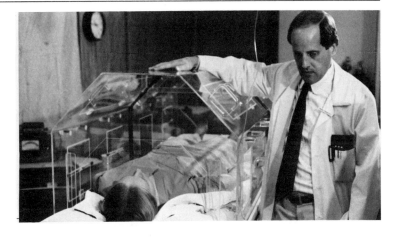

Dr. Edward A. Sternick checks temperature while administering heat treatment to patient in heat chamber.

gression. Ten years later, New York Surgeon William B. Coley injected the fever-producing toxin of the streptococcus into eighty-three cancer patients, twenty-one of whom eventually showed cancer regression. Similar reports followed through the years, but became less evident in the literature as other forms of cancer therapy became more popular.

Several modern investigators have suggested a reconsideration of induced infection to provide heat therapy. "The careful work of the last century cannot be casually dismissed as 'archival' and 'irrelevant,'" writes Dr. D. F. H. Wallach, chairman of therapeutic radiology at the Tufts University School of Medicine. "Rather, at a time when stable antibiotic-sensitive streptococcal strains are available infections with such organisms should be assessed for their effects on tumors by stringent medical conditions."

However heat therapy works, it does kill cancer cells. Dr. Beppino Giavanello of the Stehlin Cancer Center in Houston published a study in 1973 showing that tempera-

tures of 107 to 109 degrees selectively kill cancer cells while leaving normal ones intact. In other studies ingenious ways are being used to reproduce that fever level.

At the National Cancer Institute in Washington, D. C., under the direction of oncologist Dr. Joan Bull, cancer patients selected for heat treatment are wrapped in plastic blankets through which water circulates at 113 degrees. Plastic bags over the hands and feet and a plastic suit over the patient's body act as a vapor barrier to prevent heat loss by perspiration. A variety of cancers have been treated in this way, all of them refractory or

not appropriately treated by conventional methods. The results are encouraging.

Dr. Robert Pettigrew of Edinburgh's Western General Hospital in Scotland is one of the pioneers in hyperthermia. Since 1969 he has used paraffin baths heated to 113 degrees and has reported dramatic remissions, particularly of liver tumors, some of which have lasted three years or more.

Dr. Leon Parks at the University of Mississippi Medical Center has taken a page from kidney dialysis and open-heart surgery manuals in his technique for creating hyperthermia. Blood diverted outside the body in a type of plastic

Many doctors feel that cancer cells are more sensitive to radiation when body temperatures are raised. Here a patient undergoes radiation therapy immediately following heat treatment.

shunt passes through heating coils and returns at a temperature of 113 degrees. Dr. Parks's series of more than 120 patients with "widely spread" cancers of the lung, colon, and breast have had "remarkable survivals, considering the type and magnitude of the particular malignancies." Similar heating methods are also being used at the Stehlin Center in Houston.

Many other medical centers noted for their work in cancer treatment, including Memorial Sloan-Kettering Cancer Center in New York City and the University of California at Los Angeles, have used radio waves that cause total body heating without damaging normal tissues. Patients with metastatic melanoma (a skin cancer) "whose survival is usually measured in weeks," according to UCLA oncologist Dr. Kristian Storm, "have lived for a year or more after heat therapy. This has previously been unheard of with malignant melanoma."

Microwave and ultrasound wave treatments are ways of increasing body heat that are being used in other institutions.

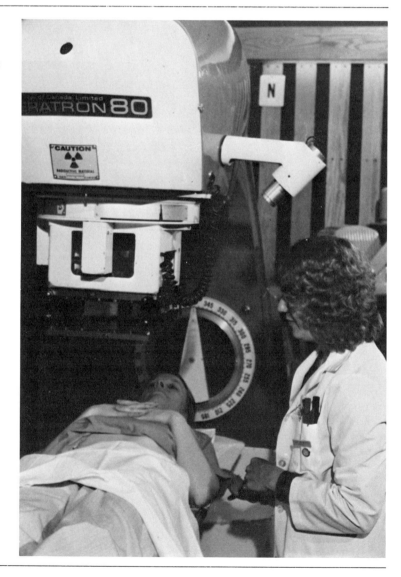

Explaining sudden infant death syndrome

The drawbacks

There are demonstrated drawbacks to hyperthermia. One difficulty is that temperatures greater than 106 degrees Fahrenheit (41 degrees Celsius) may damage heart, brain, liver, and kidney tissues. The pulse rate may rise to 200 beats per minute or more, which puts a severe strain on the heart. Such temperatures also cause great pain or even seizures and therefore require that the patient be anesthetized, which may further complicate therapy. These effects are compounded in cancer patients whose physical condition has deteriorated from the ravaging effects of the disease.

Hyperthermia is not yet a standard treatment for cancer. Even though heat alone has been shown to cause damage to cancer cells and regression of tumors, it is used today mainly as an adjunct to other treatments. "We must answer a number of questions before definite statements about its clinical effectiveness can be made," says Dr. Sternick.

No cancer patient has yet been cured with heat, but the treatment has extended survival for many.

Till now the babes oft died with ills unknown, for none was there with skill to aid.

Anonymous, 1470

S hock. Disbelief. Anger. The severe reactions of families to the tragedy of an infant who dies suddenly, mysteriously, often in the middle of what seems a peaceful night of sleep, are often accompanied by uncontrollable grief that may last for years.

Sudden infant death syndrome (SIDS) is a mysterious phenomenon defined as "the sudden, unexpected death of an apparently healthy infant for whom an autopsy fails to establish a reason." SIDS is the largest cause of death among infants between the ages of one and twelve months, killing 7,000 infants per year. The disease, often called crib death because its victims usually die while sleeping, has for years posed a completely baffling problem to the medical world. The past several years have brought forth many promising clues, largely because of an intense effort by investigators from various medical disciplines sponsored by the National Institute of Child Health and Human Development; but even today the mysteries are not completely solved.

CASE HISTORY

M. W. was a six-month-old female child who had always been in good health. Her mother had taken her for regular visits to a pediatrician, who provided only routine medical care. Only two weeks after one of these visits, at which M. W. had been found to be in good health, M. W.'s mother was out working in the yard. She brought the baby with her to enjoy the beautiful May day, and when the child became tired she brought the crib into the backyard and placed it underneath a tree. M. W. fell asleep quickly while the mother went about her gardening chores. Twenty minutes later M. W.'s mother returned to check the baby. She had ceased breathing and had turned blue. In panic, the mother rushed the baby into the house and called the rescue squad. They arrived within three minutes and instituted cardiopulmonary resuscitation, but without success. M. W. was transferred to the emergency room, where continued cardiopulmonary resuscitation was not effective, and she was pronounced dead. At autopsy the diagnosis was sudden infant death.

Apnea and SIDS

For years SIDS was assumed to be caused by a failure in one of the body's life support systems—but which one? Investigators were handicapped because most of today's diagnostic tools require living subjects, and SIDS was never identified until after death.

In 1972 Dr. Alfred Steinschneider at the Upstate Medical Center in Syracuse, New York, reported prolonged periods of cessation of breathing (apnea), which had been described in adults years before, in several infants who later became victims of SIDS. Since poor control of respiration during sleep leads to underventilation of the lungs, this was certainly a possible mechanism for SIDS.

Investigators Daniel Shen and Dorothy Kelly of the Chil-

dren's Hospital Medical Center in Boston have also observed prolonged periods of apnea in SIDS babies. Research has gone in that direction ever since.

Dr. Richard Naeye is chairman of the Department of Pathology at Pennsylvania State University College of Medicine. Assuming that chronic underventilation of the lungs would lead to other pathological changes, Dr. Naeye and his colleagues began detailed microscopic studies of the organs of SIDS victims at autopsy. He found the following results, reported recently in *Scientific American*, all of which could be expected in low-oxygen states:

■ Sixty percent of SIDS victims have increased muscle in the pulmonary arteries, the vessels that deliver blood to the lungs. This could be caused by diminished oxygen in the air spaces, or alveoli, in the lungs.

■ When the pulmonary arteries become thicker, they resist the flow of blood. This pressure, in time, forces a pressure rise in the right ventricle, and heart muscle thickens accordingly. Autop-

sies of SIDS victims show increased muscle in the right ventricle of the heart.

■ Under the microscope, the fat surrounding the vital internal organs of SIDS victims has a characteristic brown appearance at birth because of the abundant presence of particles called mitochondria in the cells. Normally they are lost in the first year of life, but in SIDS victims mitochondria and brown fat remain.

■ Diminished oxygen requires a higher level of metabolism to compensate and a correspondingly higher level of adrenaline. SIDS victims have an abnormal increase in the size of the gland tissues that make adrenaline, which is responsible for much of our metabolism.

■ Production of red blood cells by the liver and increased production of red blood cells in the bone marrow are common in SIDS victims and can be expected from chronically low oxygen levels.

■ Victims of SIDS may have normal birth weights but lag in growth after birth, similar to experimental animals that are maintained in low-oxygen environments.

- SIDS victims show increased levels of cortisone, typically seen in low-oxygen states.

In addition, Dr. Naeye's study reported that parents of SIDS victims often recount that their SIDS child had an abnormal cry and less intense reactions to environmental stimuli than their other children. Subtle brain damage caused by low oxygen levels could account for this.

All of this evidence strongly suggests that the normal physiological mechanisms to control breathing are altered in sudden infant death victims.

In all children (in all humans, in fact) there is a period of sleep known as REM (rapid eye movement) when the eyes move rapidly under the eyelids. During this phase of sleep an interesting phenomenon also occurs in the chest. The intercostal muscles, which move the chest wall, stop functioning, and breathing is slowed or even stopped. Because of the cessation of breathing, the normal carbon dioxide–oxygen exchange is severely restricted, and a low oxygen level in the blood results. A carotid body, a chemical sensor in the neck, picks up the low oxygen–high carbon dioxide levels and automatically restarts breathing. That breathing is restricted during REM sleep is proven by the fact that infants typically have partial lung collapse during this period.

The Children's Hospital Medical Center group found that SIDS infants respond poorly to inhaling carbon dioxide. In the normal child or adult, carbon dioxide inhalation results in increased frequency and depth of breathing to compensate for lack of oxygen. Dr. Naeye's group found that over half of sudden infant death syndrome victims had poorly developed carotid bodies. If this organ functions poorly, an infant may not be able to sense the altered oxygen–carbon dioxide exchange and therefore not be able to restart its breathing during a prolonged apneic period.

The causes of these breathing abnormalities do not appear to be genetic. If they were, the identical twin of an SIDS victim would have a greater tendency to the condition than a fraternal twin. They do not. Yet, interestingly, all twins have a higher overall rate of SIDS between them than non-twin siblings, suggesting that factors during pregnancy may contribute to SIDS.

Four factors affecting pregnant women are currently felt to be related to sudden infant death: (1) bacterial infection of the amniotic fluid, which can directly cause brain damage; (2) anemia in the mother, often associated with excessive fetal and neonatal deaths; (3) cigarette smoking during pregnancy, which can lead to restricted placental blood flow and retarded fetal growth; and (4) the ingestion of barbiturates, known to retard brain growth (a single dose of a narcotic can reduce ventilation in an infant for more than twenty-four hours).

In addition, researchers have isolated two factors common to SIDS victims themselves: (1) blood type B, for unknown reasons; and (2) crowded housing—children living in a crowded environment usually have upper respiratory infections, which have been known to increase the frequency and duration of apneic spells in children prone to apnea.

What lies ahead?

All this compelling evidence is common to two-thirds of SIDS victims; one-third show no such evidence of respiratory malfunction. Cardiac arrhythmias, accidental strangulation, and acute infections have all been held responsible, but evidence has been inconclusive.

Still, Dr. Naeye is optimistic. "The long-term prospect for preventing sudden infant death is promising," he claims. "Investigations are now in progress to determine whether abnormalities can be detected in newborn babies that will identify infants who are at high risk for sudden infant death syndrome." If such high-risk infants can be detected, infant breathing monitors, which are attached to a baby's chest and sound an alarm if the baby's breathing becomes abnormal, may prevent some deaths by warning of the slowing or stopping of breathing. Current "apnea monitors" are cumbersome for a baby's use, but technology such as the miniature monitor

(see "High Tech," page 155) will undoubtedly change that.

Drugs might also be given to stimulate respiratory centers and prevent apneic periods in susceptible infants. Pharmaceutical research has produced no such drug yet, but strides are being made yearly in new pharmaceutical products.

Whatever treatment or preventive measure is employed need be used only for several months. Apneic spells usually disappear after twelve months, and those infants who have been saved by apneic monitors show no sign of brain impairment.

After years of frustration, spinning medical wheels, and following blind research alleys, researchers appear to be unraveling the mysteries of SIDS—at last.

Resources

There are widely distributed regional offices of the Sudden Infant Death Foundation, usually listed in the telephone directory under Sudden Infant Death Regional Center. There are also national information sources.

- National Sudden Infant Death Foundation
310 South Michigan Avenue
Chicago, Illinois 60604
312-663-0650

- Office of Maternal and Child Health
Bureau of Community Health Services
Department of Health and Human Services
Room 736 Parklawn Building
5600 Fishers Lane
Rockville, Maryland 20850
301-443-6600

- International Guild for Infant Survival
7501 Liberty Road
Baltimore, Maryland 21207
301-944-2502

Mending the heartbreak of psoriasis

Her skin was white as leprosy
The nightmare life-in-death
was she.

Samuel Taylor Coleridge
*The Rime of the Ancient
Mariner*, 1798

Two to 3 percent of the world's population, several million people in the United States alone, suffer from the flaking, disfiguring skin lesions of psoriasis. Individuals with the disease often refuse to go swimming or to wear shortened summer attire. Many scholars believe that the leprosy of the Old Testament is actually psoriasis; the description of the leper's affliction closely matches the symptoms experienced by the sufferers of psoriasis today.

About psoriasis

The cause of psoriasis is still unknown. We do know, however, that the thickened, red, scaly, and flaky areas occur because of skin cells that multiply and grow faster than normal ones. Normal skin cells complete a growth cycle every nineteen days, during which they grow, mature, and flake off. In psoriasis the cycle is completed in only one and a half days, causing the extensive white patches and flaking so typical of the condition.

Psoriasis cannot be cured, but it can be suppressed with exciting treatments now available. Perhaps the most promising is PUVA—Psoralen ultraviolet A, the controlled use of ultraviolet irradiation with a sensitizing chemical called a psoralen.

CASE HISTORY

E. M. is a twenty-three-year-old graduate student in history who has had psoriasis for six years. It began as flaky patches of skin on her elbows, but within several months it involved her knees, lower back, and scalp. During her stressful early college years, she gained thirty pounds and her condition worsened. Psoriasis was now a part of her life, and she learned that any stressful event, infection, or minor accident would lead to more flaking, roughness, and itching. It was difficult to keep from rubbing and scratching away the flakes; yet new ones appeared even before the old ones were gone. On summer vacations, however, she seemed to improve. E. M. had been to sev-

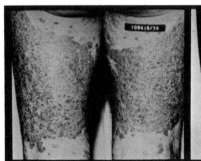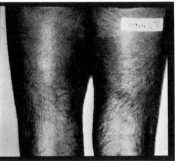

(Left) Patient with severe psoriasis and (right) same patient after PUVA therapy has cleared the skin. (Courtesy Beth Israel Hospital, Boston)

eral dermatologists through the years. Her medicine chest was filled with cortisone creams, tars, and a variety of pills, all of which occasionally helped, but none of which worked with any consistency.

Four months ago, her dermatologist recommended PUVA. Twice a week she took a pill at home, then came to the hospital to sit in an ultraviolet room for fifteen minutes. For the first time in six years she is free of all psoriasis and now has only monthly maintenance therapy.

PUVA

Sun exposure has long been recognized as helpful in treating psoriasis. Adults and children alike notice frequently that their psoriasis lesions disappear or at least improve during summer vacations or with sunbathing. Some experts feel that the year-round exposure of the face to the sun is the major reason why that part of the body is least affected with psoriasis.

Even though sunlight has potential benefits, many people cannot or will not expose their skin in public for fear of embarrassment. Furthermore, most people are busy at work or at home and cannot afford the time for regular sunbathing. Others have prominent lesions on breast or genital areas that make sun exposure inappropriate.

Dermatologists for years have used ultraviolet boxes in their offices where patients with psoriasis could regularly come to expose their skin to its healing rays. In recent years sixteen medical centers have been studying the effect of controlled long-wave ultraviolet light treatments on psoriasis patients whose skin has been previously sensitized with a psoralen, a drug known to reduce skin cell overgrowth.

Psoralens are a group of chemicals that by themselves are inactive. In the presence of ultraviolet light, however, they attack the DNA (chromosome and gene material) in the skin cells and disrupt normal DNA activity and regeneration, a necessary element in skin cell growth.

Initially psoralens were used topically on the skin, but the treatment frequently caused blistering and patches of increased pigment. Orally administered psoralens sensitize the skin even to sunlight. But sunlight is not always available, and its daily and seasonal variations make it an unreliable light source. Long-wave ultraviolet radiation is more intense than standard commercial sources and more practical than sunlight.

In PUVA treatment, the patient takes an oral dose (determined by body weight) of the chemical psoralen. Two hours later, when the psoralen has been absorbed into the bloodstream and delivered to the skin, the patient is exposed to long-wave ultraviolet irradiation in a specially constructed light room or box. The procedure is repeated two to three times weekly until the psoriasis clears, which usually takes sixteen to twenty treatments. The patient then assumes a maintenance schedule.

In 1974 the first evidence of complete clearing of psoriasis with this treatment was reported in a twenty-one-patient study originated at the Harvard Medical School and the Massachusetts General and Beth Israel hospitals in Boston.

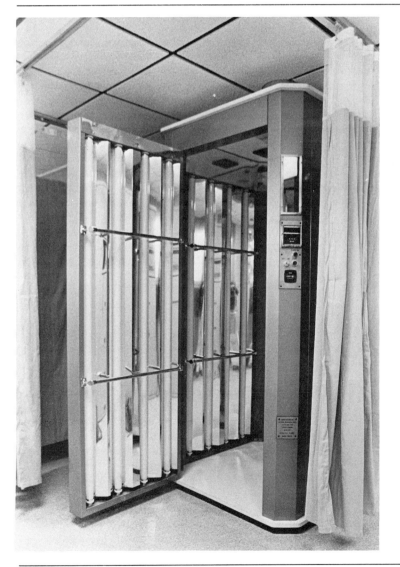

Some patients received treatment of the entire body; in others, half of the body was treated with PUVA, the other half with conventional ultraviolet therapy alone for comparison. Since that study many thousands of people have been treated.

The sixteen medical centers that are now cooperating in an evaluation of PUVA are generating data that are greatly encouraging about the eventual place for this therapy in the treatment of refractory psoriasis.

What are the problems?

Psoralens have been around for more than twenty years; they are commonly used to treat vitiligo, a skin condition characterized by white, depigmented areas. During all this time, no harmful side effects of psoralens have been noted; it was and is a safe drug. Ultraviolet light exposure, however, has been implicated as a cause of skin cancer. According to Beth Israel dermatologist Dr. Robert Stern, who

Ultraviolet light box, where PUVA therapy is conducted. (Courtesy Beth Israel Hospital, Boston)

is active in the PUVA study, "The sun's ultraviolet rays are felt to be the major factor in basal cell and squamous cell cancer, the two most common types. All patients in the PUVA study, therefore, have been carefully followed to see if skin cancer would appear." Dr. Stern and other physicians have been careful to notify patients of this risk when they begin therapy.

The results from the sixteen cooperative centers demonstrate that 2 percent of the patients on PUVA therapy did develop skin cancer, about two and one-half times the rate of the rest of the population. Close statistical analysis shows that the increase in skin cancer is most prominent in those patients who had previous skin cancers, had received extensive ultraviolet treatments in the past, or whose skin was very fair and tended to burn more easily.

Psoriasis itself does not predispose a person to skin cancer. Patients with psoriasis are exposed to many types of treatments, however, some of which may increase their tendency to develop skin cancer. PUVA itself is felt to be slightly carcinogenic, perhaps because of its interference with normal DNA function.

What are the alternatives?

There is no perfect treatment for psoriasis. Most of the time psoriasis can be controlled on an outpatient basis, but the treatments are expensive, time-consuming, and often inconvenient. Tar preparations are irritating to the skin and messy to use. Topical cortisone used over a long period of time may injure the skin. Methotrexate, an oral medication that also inhibits DNA synthesis, is widely used and effective, but it is toxic to the liver.

PUVA appears to be the most effective treatment for psoriasis developed so far, but it is still in the investigational stage and not approved for general use. Dr. Stern and others emphasize, "PUVA should only be used after carefully weighing its risks, particularly in patients with light skin, or previous history of irradiation or skin tumor."

Further work will unearth more information on PUVA, but dermatologists are generally excited about its potential.

Resources

The U.S. medical centers cooperating in PUVA research are:
- Baylor College of Medicine, Houston
- Beth Israel Hospital, Boston
- Columbia University College of Physicians and Surgeons, New York City
- Dartmouth Medical College, Hanover, NH
- Duke University Medical School, Durham, NC
- Massachusetts General Hospital, Boston
- Mayo Graduate School, Rochester, MN
- Mount Sinai Medical Center, New York City
- Stanford University, Palo Alto, CA
- Temple University, Philadelphia
- University of California, San Francisco
- University of Miami, FL
- University of Michigan Medical School, Ann Arbor
- University of Pennsylvania, Philadelphia
- Washington Hospital Center, Washington, D.C.
- Yale University Medical School, New Haven, CT

The
continuing
war on
bacteria

Microbes will have the last word.

Ascribed to Louis Pasteur

Pasteur's microbes were bacteria, and the diseases they cause—infections—have always been major challenges in medicine. In 1940 infection caused 25 percent of all deaths; in 1977 that number was only 3 percent. Penicillin and the variety of antimicrobial agents it spawned have overcome many of the worst

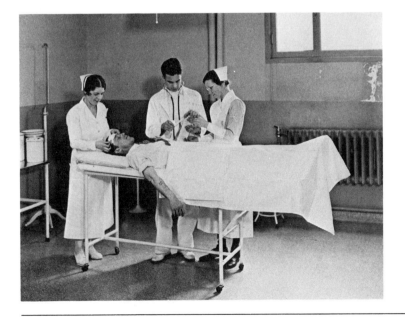

infections. But forty years after the "miracle" of penicillin Pasteur's words haunt us again. Bacteria, in many cases, have developed resistance to the antibiotics that had promised to eradicate them. Even as new, more potent antibiotics are developed to replace the traditional ones, bacteria are learning to tolerate them as well. "Physicians are being repeatedly warned that they may soon be faced with pathogens that are resistant to all available antimicrobials," stated

Dr. Richard Dixon of the United States Center for Disease Control in a recent article on antibiotic resistance. While admitting that completely resistant bacteria are rare, infectious disease specialists nonetheless agree that the problem of resistance is growing.

Mutant bacteria—resistant to antibiotics?

New generations of bacteria reflect the experience of their ancestors, just as we reflect our own. Like humans, bacteria have DNA and genes, the strands of protein that are the code of life. Although every individual's DNA structure is remarkably constant, many environmental factors can evoke a change or mutation in the structure that can be passed on to the next generation.

So it is with bacteria. As generations of bacteria are exposcd to a particular antibiotic, they can mutate, or change, and develop resistance

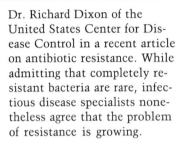

When patients were treated in the 1920s, antibiotics were not yet available, and many individuals died of complicating infections. (Courtesy Lynn Hospital, Massachusetts)

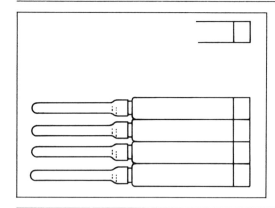

(Top) 300,000 units of penicillin cured a case of gonorrhea in 1950. (Bottom) Today, because of growing bacterial resistance, 4.8 million units of penicillin are needed for gonorrhea therapy, and bacteria may still resist treatment.

to that antibiotic. The more an antibiotic is used, the faster resistance develops. For this reason infectious disease specialists have long warned against the use of antibiotics "just to be safe" or "just in case" bacterial infection is present. Instead, they recommend that doctors obtain proof of specific infection (by testing a culture of the germ) before starting antibiotic therapy.

Bacteria can also become resistant to antibiotics because of plasmids, small bits of DNA that are not part of the bacteria's normal genetic makeup. "Plasmids are parasites that live off bacteria and can use the bacteria's reproductive machinery to create bacteria with new characteristics," explains Dr. John Baxter, geneticist at the University of California in San Francisco. Plasmids containing the gene for resistance to several antibiotics can move freely from one bacterium to another, thereby transferring antibiotic resistance. They were first identified in an epidemic of resistant bacterial dysentery in Japan in 1959 and have since been found elsewhere. Just as bacteria can enter different human beings

and yet produce a similar infection, so the same plasmid can enter or infect different bacteria. In fact, a given gene, such as the one for bacterial resistance, can also leap from plasmid to plasmid.

If a group of bacteria, some with antibiotic-resistant plasmids and some without, is exposed to that antibiotic, only the plasmid-containing bacteria survive. They subsequently reproduce, and a whole new generation of resistant bacteria results.

The problem of resistance

In the 1950s the first signs of antibiotic-resistant bacteria appeared in hospitalized patients. An increasing number of staph infections (caused by the bacterium *staphylococcus aureus*) did not respond to penicillin, the antibiotic of choice for staph at that time. Somehow the bacteria had learned to deactivate the penicillin; later it was learned that the bacteria produced beta-lactamase, an enzyme that rendered penicillin harmless to them. New forms of semisynthetic penicillin and antibiotics called cephalosporins (Keflin and Velosef, commonly used to-

day, are examples) solved the problem temporarily. But in the past ten years resistant staph have been on the rise again. According to the Center for Disease Control in Atlanta, 50 percent of hospital staph infections are now resistant to penicillin.

Other resistant bacteria are appearing with alarming frequency. Gonorrhea is one case in point. Because of the growing resistance of *Neisseria gonorrhoeae*, the bacterium that causes it, to penicillin, the amount of the drug required to treat this venereal disease has risen from 300,000 units, which was sufficient to cure a case in 1950, to 4.8 million units, which cures most, but not all, cases of gonorrhea today. Furthermore, today's doses are given with probenecid, a chemical that raises the blood level of penicillin two to four times. Blood and tissue levels of penicillin are, therefore, thirty or more times what were needed thirty years ago.

As if this wasn't enough of a problem, the Center for Disease Control reports the appearance of strains of gonorrhea that are totally resistant

In middle ear infections, common to children, fluid accumulates behind eardrum and obstructs passage to back of throat (Courtesy Eli Lilly and Co.)

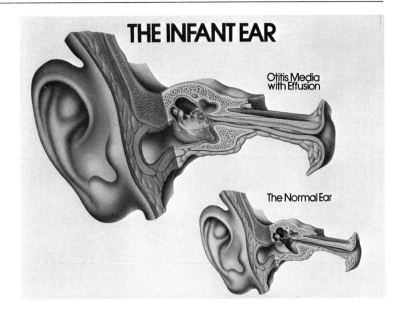

THE INFANT EAR

Otitis Media with Effusion

The Normal Ear

to penicillin. These strains, which also produce the beta-lactamase enzyme, were first discovered in Philippine Islands prostitutes in 1976 and have apparently found their way to the United States and Europe. The public health problem is potentially serious and officials remain vigilant for new cases.

Resistant bacteria are also a frustrating problem in children's ear infections. Pediatricians now find that their traditional treatments are no longer adequate. By the time they are three years old, 70 percent of all children will have had otitis media, a middle ear infection. By age five, that figure is close to 100 percent. Next to the common cold, ear infection is the most common childhood illness and one that may have a long-range effect on the child's ability to hear.

Middle ear infections are more common in children than in adults because of the anatomy of a child's ear. The eustachian tube, which connects the back of the nose and throat to the middle ear, is more horizontal in children. As a result, postnasal secretions easily find their way to

the ear, aided by the increased pressure when children blow their nose or cry. In the relatively closed confines of the middle ear space, infection begins easily.

"Because fluid may persist in the middle ear seven or eight months after the pain and fever have gone, a child with an ear infection may develop serious hearing impairment," notes Dr. Charles Bluestine, ear, nose and throat professor at the University of Pittsburgh. Hearing loss is serious in all ages, but never so much as for young children, who are learning language skills in those years.

For years the standard treatment of ear infections in children has been ampicillin, a semisynthetic form of penicillin. In 1974 Dr. Sidney Ross, a pediatrician at the Children's National Medical Center in Washington, D. C., reported that he had found a few cases of resistance to

ampicillin in *Haemophilus influenzae* (H. flu), the second most common bacterial cause of ear infection in children. Alarmingly, Dr. Ross's 1979 studies reported that 35 percent of all H. flu ear infections in the Washington, D. C., area were resistant to ampicillin. (Fully 8 percent of *all* ear infections resisted the standard treatment.) Although not as high, similar resistance figures for H. flu appear across the country: 16 percent resistance in Boston, 22 percent in Oklahoma City, 13 percent in Dallas. And the figures rise each year.

Until recently, H. flu was considered a problem only in ear infections of children under five years of age. Now, however, studies report it in individuals of twenty years and occasionally older. Pediatricians and primary care physicians are responding to the growing problem of H. flu resistance by closer observation, more frequent follow-up visits, and more vigorous attempts to identify the specific bacterial pathogen in cases of ear infection.

Treatment protocols for ear infections are also changing in response to bacterial resistance. More frequently physicians order combinations of antibiotics or newer antibiotics such as cefaclor (trade name Ceclor) that can kill a wider range of bacteria. They are also on the alert for signs of hearing impairment, and they insert tubes to drain middle ear fluid to prevent a hearing loss. "Circumcision is probably the only surgical procedure more common than ear tube insertion," states Dr. Bluestone, commenting on the growing use of this technique.

The problem today

Have the warnings against overdependence on antibiotics been heeded? Critics would answer no, citing the amount of penicillin given for sore throats that are actually virus-caused and the prophylactic use of antibiotics before surgery. Others would say these and other similar circum-

stances are appropriate. "If a physician is worried about infection," one primary care provider explains, "that is the time to give antibiotics." There is little to prove or refute either side. The only hard information is the number of antibiotic prescriptions written: 250 million per year in the United States.

If frequent exposure to antibiotics leads to resistant bacteria, the animal food industry may be contributing to the problem. Antibiotics are used in animal food with what many experts fear is alarming regularity. According to the United States Food and Drug Administration, 40 percent of the 20 million pounds of antibiotics produced in the United States each year are put in animal food, allegedly to prevent infection and promote growth in animals that are to be used for human consumption. A task force called by the FDA to study the problem recommended that since humans are exposed to these antibiotics when they eat the animal meat, penicillin, tetracycline, sulfonamides, and other antibiotics should not be used in animal food. Their recommen-

dations have still not been acted upon.

It is fair to say there is controversy over this issue. Consultants to the food industry claim that food antibiotics contribute little to bacterial resistance compared with prescription antibiotics. In Europe, however, where tetracycline is no longer used in animal feed, bacterial resistance to that antibiotic is less.

What is the solution?

In response to bacterial resistance to traditional antibiotics, new antibiotics are developed each year. Realistically, though, the problem of fighting bacterial resistance cannot forever depend on new antibiotics.

A better approach would be to attack the methods by which plasmids transfer resistance to bacteria—in other words, to block the chemical action that inactivates the antibiotic. Researchers at Pfizer pharmaceutical laboratories in Connecticut have recently done just that: they have isolated a chemical that stops the enzyme beta-lactamase. The several bacteria that produce this enzyme (it is,

New treatments for herpes

remember, the one that inactivates penicillin) have been tested with the agent, and they seem to lose their ability to become resistant. "This agent just might give a new lease on life to the older penicillins," speculates a Pfizer researcher. But he adds, "Until, that is, the bacteria become resistant to it as well."

As therapy becomes more sophisticated and scientific probing reaches deeper levels, ever more is revealed about the nature of bacteria and their incredible resolve to survive. As Francis Bacon said in his *Essays* in 1625, "Nature is often hidden, sometimes overcome, seldom extinguished." Progress is clearly being made; but it is slow.

Resources

■ Center for Disease Control Public Inquiries Office Building 4 B2 Atlanta, Georgia 30333 404-329-3534

■ Information may also be obtained from your state health department.

"Herpes is from the Greek word for serpent, and herpes viruses really are creeps."

André J. Nahmias
Medical World News, May 12, 1980

Mention the words *cold sore* and virtually everyone will immediately recall a familiar blistering, painful area on the lip. Cold sores are an infection caused by the herpes virus that half the population, young and old, have experienced sometime during their lives. Some people get a cold sore only occasionally; others have the infection several times each year. Cold sores are the most common herpes infection, but the virus is also associated with more serious problems, among them chicken pox, infectious mononucleosis, shingles, and an increasingly common venereal disease, herpes progenitalis.

There is no cure for herpes virus infections, as those unfortunate people who are afflicted with them can attest. Most people have tried remedies recommended by their doctor and well-meaning friends alike, all with the same

result: the infection runs its course unaffected by any treatment.

But a promising new weapon for herpes infections, acyclovir, is on the horizon. Developed by a pharmaceutical laboratory in the United States, acyclovir is a topically applied ointment currently being tested in two major medical centers, and the preliminary results are encouraging. Dermatologists are also having good success with an amino acid, lysine, commonly available without a prescription.

About herpes

The herpes virus enters the body through a small break in the skin. The first infection usually occurs in childhood and lasts one to two weeks before it heals spontaneously. Even though the cold sore has healed, however, the virus itself remains in the body, withdrawing to a nearby nerve where the body's defenses keep it at bay. During times of stress, when those defenses are weakened, the infection reappears, usually in the same general area each time.

"A variety of stresses can trigger recurrent infection,"

says Dr. Kenneth Arndt, chief of dermatology at the Beth Israel Hospital in Boston. "Sun exposure is the most common trigger, but infections such as cold and flu can also do it." Periods of emotional upset also commonly lead to herpes infection, as harried students and adults know well. Dr. Arndt adds that "a few unfortunate women even get herpes infection with each menstrual period."

The exact reason that stress triggers recurrent herpes problems is unknown, but lowered body resistance probably plays a role. Patients whose resis-

tance is purposefully suppressed by medication, as it is for those undergoing organ transplantation to prevent rejection of the donor organ, have a serious problem with herpes infection.

While the common cold sore is an aggravation, other herpes infections can be disabling and sometimes fatal. There are five types of herpes infections.

■ *Herpes simplex I* causes the common cold sore and infections of the cornea; it can also cause a frequently fatal brain infection called encephalitis.

■ *Herpes simplex II* causes the painful blistering venereal infection herpes progenitalis, which is seen in both men and women one and a half days after sexual contact and lasts three weeks or more. The primary infection is painful enough to prohibit sexual intercourse. Repeat infections are usually mild, however, but they are just as contagious and constitute a serious public health hazard. It may be the most common venereal disease.

■ *Herpes zoster* causes chicken pox in children, then lies dormant. Decades later it can reappear as shingles, painful sores on the face or trunk.

■ *Epstein-Barr virus* causes mononucleosis, an infection most commonly seen in young people characterized by fever, sore throat, and weakness. This type of herpes virus is also linked with a type of facial cancer, Burkitt's lymphoma, seen almost exclusively in Africa and New Guinea, and nasopharyngeal

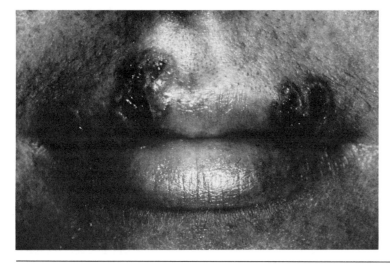

Herpes simplex I causes the familiar cold sore that recurs at the same spot following physical or emotional stress. (Courtesy Howard Goldberg, M.D.)

cancer, which arises in the membranes of the nose.

■ *Cytomegalovirus* causes sore throat, headache, and fever in adults. Newborns affected with it may have serious deformities and brain damage.

Acyclovir

Antiviral therapy has always been a "catch-22." Through the years many treatments have been effective against viruses, but all have been dangerous or toxic to normal cells. This has been true, for example, of dye and light treatments, which were common in virus therapy in the recent past. Early work with acyclovir, however, has demonstrated beneficial effect on viruses without toxicity to normal cells.

According to antiviral researchers at the Burroughs-Wellcome Company, the United States pharmaceutical manufacturer that developed the drug, acyclovir enters cells that have been infected by viruses, destroys the viruses by interfering with their growth, and has little or no effect on the cell itself.

Dr. Clyde Crumpacker, an investigator at the Beth Israel Hospital, one of the medical centers now studying the drug, comments, "Acyclovir is the first effective and safe treatment we have seen for herpes infections." In Crumpacker's study, volunteer patients with cold sores applied an ointment containing acyclovir directly to the sore four times daily for five days. They returned several times for follow-up. An equal number of patients in the study were given a placebo, an ointment without acyclovir. The National Institutes of Health in Bethesda, Maryland, is coordinating the study, and although the final test reports are still unknown, preliminary reports are encouraging. Cold sores heal quickly with acyclovir therapy, and few recurrent infections have been noted. The use of acyclovir is also being studied at the University of Utah Medical Center. If the final results there are as good, the drug could be released for general use within a year.

Current research with acyclovir involves herpes simplex I, the cold sore variety. The hope is that similar results will be shown with all the other varieties as well. If that happens, states Dr. Arndt, "acyclovir could turn out to be a very important find indeed."

Lysine

Another possible treatment for cold sores is lysine, a naturally occurring amino acid that may be purchased in tablet form in health food stores. Tablets of lysine taken three to four times daily (300 to 1,200 mg), have been effective in suppressing herpes, according to studies by Drs. Richard Griffith and Arthur Norins in Indianapolis. They found that lip and genital herpes sores disappeared overnight in over 90 percent of their patients, who ranged in age from four to sixty. Dr. Christopher Kagas of the University of Southern California has had similar results in a smaller study. Lysine has not been harmful to the patients.

Lysine originates in the cell. For twenty years or more, laboratory studies have indicated that when a virus invades a cell it somehow "encourages" the cell to make proteins that help the virus grow. The cell begins to make arginine, an amino acid helpful to viral growth, and reduces its production of lysine, which inhibits that growth. Using this information, some investigators have looked into foods that contain these amino acids. Some think that chocolate, nuts, and seeds, all of which are high in arginine and low in lysine, may be more favorable to herpes virus growth and recommend that people with frequent herpes infections eliminate those foods from their diet. Similarly, dairy products with high lysine levels may be less favorable to virus growth. (This may explain why children who drink lots of milk get fewer herpes infections.)

Advocates of lysine do point out, though, that lysine is not a cure for cold sores, as acyclovir may well prove to be. Lysine is only a suppressive, and the sores may reappear once the intake of lysine has stopped.

Treating cold sores

Since acyclovir is still in the testing stages, cold sore sufferers must rely on other methods of treatment for now. In addition to lysine, here's what dermatologists suggest as treatment for the common cold sore:

- At the first sign of swelling, tingling, or numbness, apply ice frequently and directly to the area. This seems to lessen the severity of the sore. Hourly cortisone cream applications may also be effective at this stage, but should be stopped if blisters appear.

- When blisters form, use rubbing alcohol, calamine, salt water, or any acne lotion to help dry them more quickly.

- Use zinc oxide or antibacterial ointments such as Bacitracin two to three times per day to prevent complications such as bacterial infections. They can be used once crusts have formed, but they don't affect the viral cold sore treatment.

- Use a sunscreen with PABA (para-amino-benzoic acid) on the lip before sun exposure to reduce the risk of herpes.

Herpes infections are still a problem, but with lysine, and the promise of acyclovir, help may be on the way at last. And at many medical centers in the U.S., work progresses on developing a herpes virus vaccine which may prevent herpes infection altogether.

Resources

Your family doctor can refer you to a dermatologist for refractory cases of herpes infections; hospitals and state medical societies are also good referal sources.

- Acyclovir (Trade name Zovirax) is manufactured by:

Burroughs-Wellcome
3030 Cornwallis Road
Research Triangle Park, N.C. 27709

- Other sources of information on herpes include:

Center for Disease Control
Public Inquiries Office
Building 4, Room B2
Altanta, Georgia 30333
404-329-3534

- National Institute of Allergy and Infectious Diseases
Office of Research Reporting and Public Response
Room 7A32, Building 31
National Institutes of Health
Bethesda, Maryland 20205
301-496-5717

The tragedy of DES

Some drugs have been appropriately called wonder drugs. . . . One wonders what they will do next.

Dr. Samuel E. Stumpf
Annals of Internal Medicine,
1966

W hen a pregnant woman in the 1940s was known to have had a miscarriage or other problem with an earlier pregnancy, her doctor was likely to prescribe DES (diethylstilbestrol) during a new pregnancy. This synthetic estrogen was given "just to be on the safe side" to enrich uterine tissues, make for a healthier pregnancy, and increase the chances of a normal delivery. It was all supposition. There was no proof of the value of DES, yet its use continued and even increased into the 1950s, when a randomized study finally showed that it had no effect in preserving a pregnancy. Even so, physicians continued to prescribe DES. It is estimated that 2 million women received DES during the 1940s and 1950s.

Between 1966 and 1969, Dr. Arthur Herbst, an obstetrician then working at the Massachu-setts General Hospital in Boston, found seven cases of clear cell adenocarcinoma (a vaginal cancer) in young women between the ages of fourteen and twenty-two. Dr. Herbst explains his concern: "So rare was this cancer that these seven cases exceeded the total number that had been reported previously in this age group in the entire world literature." Further study of the cases demonstrated that they all had one thing in common—their mothers had all taken DES during pregnancy.

This initial work, published in 1970 in the *New England Journal of Medicine* by Dr. Herbst, turned out to be the proverbial "tip of the iceberg." Extensive reviews of patients known to have been exposed to DES since then have demonstrated a wide range of problems, from infertility to breast and reproductive cancers and anatomical malforma-tions. And although most attention has been given to alerting daughters of DES mothers, it now appears that male children also are encoun-tering genital problems as a re-sult of DES exposure in utero. A national registry for research on hormonal transplacental carcinogens has been formed and continues to collect data on all problems with DES.

Ironically, DES has been successfully used to treat pros-tate cancer in men and meta-static breast cancer in women. But in healthy individuals, DES may pose long-term health hazards. Yet millions of people today are unknowingly exposed to the drug, which is still approved as a grain additive to fatten sheep and cattle. And unbelievably, DES is com-monly used as a "morning-after pill" to prevent pregnancy.

The effects of DES—and what to do

In 1951 and 1952, a random-ized study was carried out at the University of Chicago to evaluate the effects of diethyl-stilbestrol treatment to pre-vent pregnancy problems. Sixteen hundred women parti-cipated in the study, beginning in the first half of their preg-nancies; one half received diethylstilbestrol, the other half a placebo. This study re-vealed that DES was not effec-tive for the reasons that it was being prescribed.

When the problems with

DES began to emerge twenty years later, the patients in the 1950s study were all contacted to evaluate their health and their children's health. This study is the only one that has evaluated scientifically the long-term results of DES exposure. Now working at the University of Chicago, Dr. Herbst reports the following problems with diethylstilbestrol, none of which appear to be related to the amount of DES that the patient actually took—it seems that even small amounts of DES can have harmful effects.

■ *Mothers:* A slightly increased risk of breast cancer and cancer of the reproductive tract was noted in mothers who had taken diethylstilbestrol. Breast cancer in particular developed sooner and with greater malignancy in these patients.

What to do: Dr. Herbst and others recommend rigorous attention to breast self-examination and adherence to the guidelines of the National Cancer Institute (see "Cancer: The Personal War," pages 294–297).

■ *Daughters:* The Registry for Research on Hormonal Trans-

placental Carcinogens has reported more than 350 cases of vaginal clear cell cancer. Over two-thirds of these cases, who range from seven to twenty-nine years of age, are known to have been exposed to DES in utero. Ninety percent of the patients with this cancer are over fourteen, and a peak incidence seems to occur at around age nineteen.

"We have calculated the risk and feel that a DES-exposed daughter has a 1 in 600 chance of developing vaginal cancer," explains Dr. Herbst. The treatment for this type of cancer is radical if not mutilating surgery: removal of the uterus, fallopian tubes, vagina, and often ovaries as well. Although over 80 percent of the patients have survived five years after this surgery, the psychological effects have been all-consuming.

Though malignant tumors are relatively uncommon in DES-exposed females, non-malignant changes are very common. Many DES-exposed daughters have vaginal lining overgrowth, called adenosis, which may be a premalignant change. They also have an abnormally shaped uterus with

high frequency, and some uteruses are poorly developed. Ten percent of DES-exposed daughters have irregular menstruation at three times the normal rate. Many have fertility problems. Those who are able to conceive show much higher stillbirth and miscarriage rates.

What to do: DES-exposed women should have a thorough examination by age fourteen and Pap tests frequently, at least yearly, thereafter. Those who are pregnant should be monitored frequently during pregnancy.

■ *Sons:* In 1975 researcher John McLachlan reported in the *Journal of Science* that male rats injected with DES experienced reproductive tract problems; 60 percent became sterile. He warned that this problem may occur in humans. Additional data indicate the truth of his prediction.

Addressing an adolescent medicine conference, Dr. Henry Abrahms, a urologist at the Long Island Jewish–Hillside Medical Center, warned that the media have neglected to point out the danger of DES exposure to males. He further noted that 1 million males born between 1940 and 1971 received DES exposure in utero and are at risk. Several studies he cited show that 30 percent of DES-exposed boys and men have scrotal cysts, 10 percent have poorly developed testes, and 20 percent are infertile.

Cancer has not been seen, "but male cancers of the reproductive tract typically do not appear until the sixth to eighth decade of life. Further development in these patients is certainly a possibility," comments Dr. Abrahms.

What to do: Because of the possibility of serious problems developing in later years, men who have been exposed to DES must be warned and seek frequent medical evaluation from a physician.

Learning from the DES experience

All patients with known or suspected DES exposure, men and women alike, must be warned about potential problems. DES action groups in most larger cities and hospital ob/gyn and pediatric departments are good sources of information.

DES is one of the great tragedies of the past three decades in medicine. Millions of women took a drug to prevent a problem (which the drug did not really prevent) and thereby unknowingly exposed themselves and their unborn children to a potentially more serious problem. And all the while they were reassured by the medical profession that what they were doing was safe.

Sir William Osler once said, "A desire to take medicine is, perhaps, the great feature which distinguishes man from other animals."

Resources

■ Coordination of medical cases involving DES exposure is being handled by:

International Registry of Transplacental Hormonal Carcinogens
University of Chicago
Pritzker School of Medicine
950 East 59th Street
Chicago, Illinois 60637
312-941-1000

■ The best place for information about DES is from a DES action group. There are several throughout the country and their activities are coordinated by the New York area group that can refer you to similar groups in other locations:

DES Action Group
Long Island Jewish/Hillside Medical Center
New Hyde Park, New York 11040
212-470-2000

TPN:
Total
nutritional
therapy

The ravages of any illness
no matter how localized,
take their toll on the entire
body, destroying its reserves
and interfering with normal
function. Just as nutrition is a
key factor in maintaining
health, so it is essential in re-
covering from illness. Harvard
Medical School nutritionist
George Blackburn says, "No
medical condition is treated
well when the patient is
poorly nourished." Typically
and most efficiently, nutrition
is accomplished with a balanced oral intake.

But what about the person
with anorexia nervosa who
will not eat; the person with a
severe attack of ulcerative colitis who should not eat; or the
person in coma who cannot
eat? How can people with
severe or chronic illnesses be
properly nourished when the
stomach is not accessible?

Simple intravenous fluids with
sugar and electrolytes are not
the answer. They can provide
only 400 to 500 calories a day
and fail to supply fat, protein,
minerals, and trace elements
such as zinc and copper. When
the body is deprived of nutrition it deteriorates rapidly.

Fortunately, providing complete nutrition through the circulatory system is a reality today. This technique of total
parenteral nutrition (TPN) is
known as hyperalimentation.
(Parenteral refers to any fluid
that enters the body without
going through the gastrointestinal tract.)

William Harvey first discovered the circulation of the
blood in 1616, and with it the
concept that blood is the vehicle for transporting nutrients
to all the cells of the body.
Getting those nutrients into
the circulation in appropriate
amounts has been the major
challenge through the years.
Architect and astronomer Sir
Christopher Wren first introduced intravenous feeding in
1656, when he infused wine
and ale into the veins of dogs
using a goose quill attached to
a pig bladder as his intravenous administration set. Two

hundred years later physiologist Claude Bernard infused
sugar into animals' veins for
the first time; many similar
experiments followed.

Sugar and electrolyte solutions continued to be the
mainstay of intravenous fluid
therapy until the mid-1960s.
Their therapeutic value was
limited, because they supplied
little energy and had little
effect on healing. In fact, they
merely replaced fluids.

Attempts to provide more
complete nutrition by vein
were frustrating. Amino acids
could be added to the sugar
solution, but contributed little
to tissue growth because they
had insufficient energy to complete the reaction to make protein. Concentrated fats and
sugars could provide that
energy, but because they irri-
tate veins they had to be discontinued.

In the 1960s University of
Pennsylvania researcher Dr.
Stanley Dudrick demonstrated
a technique for infusing intravenous fluids into a large central vein, the subclavian vein
in the neck. With its large—
and therefore fast—blood flow,
this vein was not subject to
the irritation of caustic fluids,

and solutions with more nutrients could now be administered. Since then, Dudrick's technique of parenteral nutrition has been refined, and balanced intravenous nutrition that nourishes and heals is now possible.

CASE HISTORY

F. C. is a thirty-year-old housewife with a five-year history of regional enteritis (Crohn's disease). She had many periods of cramping abdominal pain and diarrhea, often requiring hospitalization. After one particularly troublesome and refractory attack, surgery was recommended. Parts of the small and large intestines were removed surgically and a colostomy was performed, draining the intestinal contents to the outside. Three weeks after the operation F. C. gradually worsened. Fever and pain returned, and the surgical wound began to drain. An X ray showed a large abscess with a fistula, or drainage tract, opening between the bowel and the skin. The intestinal contents began to leak out even around the colostomy. She lost more than twenty-five pounds. All foods and liquids were then withheld and hyperalimentation (TPN) was begun. Within two weeks the drainage stopped and the wound healed. Within two months the abscess healed and F. C. began to gain weight, even though she had had nothing to eat by mouth. After discharge from the hospital she returned home at her normal weight and one year later continues to do well.

How does TPN work?

The important relationship between nutrition and disease has been well known for some time. When a person is unable to eat for an extended period of time, the gastrointestinal tract loses its ability to function properly. Food moves through more slowly, while absorption of fats, carbohydrates, and proteins is reduced. Nausea, bloating, and diarrhea develop from this malabsorption, and the patient loses the desire for food. The continual need for energy leads the body to reach into the proteins of muscles and organ tissues, the so-called lean body mass, which is quickly reduced. For lack of nutrition, the seriously ill person literally wastes away.

Total parenteral nutrition interrupts this cycle by providing energy in the form of calories and all the important body nutrients. The nutrients are fed directly into the circulation, and therefore to the body tissues, through a major vein, concentrated in a volume of fluid that is equal to the normal daily water requirement. The nutrient fluid, a carefully mixed combination of amino acids for protein, dextrose, vitamins, minerals, and trace elements, is given through a catheter placed in the subclavian vein, a large vein just under the collarbone which drains blood from the head and upper body directly into the heart. The contents of the nutrient solution can be varied according to the clinical team's assessment of each patient's needs.

Assessing a patient's needs

The average healthy adult needs about 1,500 to 1,800 calories a day to carry on the body's work. Physical exertion and emotional stress increase the calorie needs. Fever, gastrointestinal and other inflammatory infections, major surgery, and other similar physical stresses can also dramatically increase the calorie needs. Severely ill people often require 4,000 to 5,000 calories of nutrition per day. In TPN solutions, dextrose, like all carbohydrates, provides energy at the rate of 4 calories per gram. Carbohydrate calories prevent the further breakdown of body proteins for energy, and fat infusions can also be given. Fats are the most efficient sources of energy at 9 calories per gram, but they aren't quite as effective as carbohydrates in reducing protein breakdown. For a time ethyl alcohol was considered as an energy source because of its 7-calorie-per-gram production, but the inebriation and liver toxicity of alcohol made it inappropriate for use in hyperalimentation. Most of the calorie energy in TPN comes from fats and carbohydrates.

The average daily water requirement for adults is about 35 cc per kilogram (about ½ ounce per pound of body weight), or about 2,400 cc (2½ quarts) for a 150-pound person. Children's requirements are different, and high fever and sweating can increase the figure considerably.

Essential amino acids are the protein sources in the TPN solution. The combination of protein and calories counteracts the lean-mass breakdown and ensures that body tissues can continue to grow and function normally. Most nutritionists use a ratio of 200 calories for each gram of protein provided.

A person without food as a source of energy is also deprived of vitamins, minerals, and trace elements. Typically, preparations of vitamins C, A, E, and some of the B vitamins are added to the TPN solution, as well as sodium, potassium, calcium, magnesium, zinc, and other trace elements. If trace elements are neglected, the patient on long-term intravenous nutrition often develops blood or skin problems.

Who benefits from total parenteral nutrition?

As the nutritional needs of chronically or seriously ill patients become more defined, TPN becomes more helpful. Several indications are currently accepted, all medical conditions in which patients can typically lose 10 percent or more of their normal body weight in a short period. They are:

- Inflammatory bowel disease, such as ulcerative colitis or regional enteritis. When acute attacks occur, TPN enables the bowel to be put to complete rest for long periods of time, enabling it to heal.

- Intestinal obstruction.

- Major surgery. TPN is effective pre-operatively to "tune up" patients whose disease has left them in a deteriorated state. After the operation, it shortens the recovery period.

- Cancer, radiation therapy, or chemotherapy, which typically cause nausea and loss of appetite in addition to loss of strength from the cancer alone.

- Coma, major burns, severe infections, and anorexia nervosa, nonsurgical conditions that require supportive nutrition.

- Congenital or malabsorption problems in infants and premature babies.

What are TPN's limitations?

A person can be kept on TPN for years. Patients whose esophagus can no longer route food to the stomach because of major surgery have undergone five- to ten-year treatments with total parenteral nutrition. Modifications of the technique permit outpatient or home use; patients pick up their intravenous solutions at the hospital each day, then go home where a portable pump slowly infuses the TPN solution.

Surgeons and nutritionists, however, attempt to start the patient on oral feedings or at least on tube feedings into the stomach as soon as it is feasible. The longer TPN continues, the longer it takes for the bowel to readapt to food once it is started again. Progress is very slow in those cases because intestinal cells atrophy with disuse. Nausea, diarrhea, and vomiting are common for a week or so once food is restarted. Infection can be a problem with TPN, particularly if meticulous attention is not paid to sterile techniques. Remember that the food is infused through a catheter that is placed directly through the skin and into a vein. The long-term presence of this catheter in the vein can of course lead to infection at that site that can eventually enter the bloodstream. Severe metabolic problems can also result if the patient on TPN is not monitored for levels of blood sugar, electrolytes such as sodium and potassium, and fluids as well as trace elements.

Critical care specialists feel that TPN is potent therapy and that refinements in technique will surely increase its usefulness. Continued nutritional research will increase understanding of its role. The great improvement in critically ill patients and their shortened disability time point out just how important nutrition is to health. TPN is an important way of continuing and providing that nutrition.

The "if" of interferon

Healing is a matter of time, but it is sometimes also a matter of opportunity.

Hippocrates
Precepts I, fifth century B.C.

The past two decades have witnessed the emergence of several powerful weapons in the war against cancer. Varying combinations of chemotherapy, radiation, surgery, and hormones have cured many patients with cancer and put countless others into temporary abatement or remission. Cancer patients today live longer, and the quality of their lives is improved.

But the cancer war still has many frustrations. Surgery is often mutilating and requires long convalescence. The side effects of radiation and chemotherapy—vomiting, hair loss, profound weakness, skin rashes, and others—are debilitating. Virtually all anticancer regimens also destroy a certain amount of normal tissue and are inconsistent in their effects on the cancer. Despite great progress in the past ten years, two-thirds of all cancer patients still die from their disease.

An antiviral substance called interferon may change all that. Interferon is not a drug, but rather a glycoprotein found naturally in the body that is produced by certain body cells in response to virus attack.

When first discovered at the National Institute for Medical Research in London by researchers Alick Isaacs and Jean Lindenmann in 1957, interferon was found to prohibit the multiplication of viruses and therefore reduce their ability to cause infection. The excitement that followed this discovery stemmed from the hope that interferon might be the long-sought answer to all viral illnesses, from the common cold to hepatitis.

In subsequent experiments, interferon was also found to inhibit the growth of several types of cancer. Though much skepticism remains, some researchers say that interferon may indeed be the next breakthrough in the treatment of cancer.

The ultimate value of interferon depends upon a number of ifs. *If* long-range studies on substantial numbers of patients corroborate the results

of preliminary, more limited work. . . . *If* interferon proves to be safe in doses that are still effective in therapy. . . . *If* it can be produced in large enough quantities and at a reasonable cost so as to be available when needed. It is entirely appropriate, then, even if coincidental, that scientists abbreviate interferon IF.

How interferon works

Interferon is a protein that the body produces naturally in response to strong stimulation or attack, most commonly by a virus. Three kinds of cells produce interferon: white blood cells, cells from the body's defense system called T-lymphocytes, and connective tissue cells called fibroblasts.

When a virus attacks and enters a cell, it changes the chemistry of that cell to produce millions of duplicates of itself. As enormous numbers of viruses are produced within the cell, the cell swells and explodes, splashing its contents of viruses all over adjacent cells, and the cycle repeats itself again and again.

The initial virus infection stimulates various cells to produce interferon. The interferon then passes out through the membrane surrounding the cell and enters adjacent cells, somehow notifying them of the impending virus attack. Interferon has been described as a sort of chemical Paul Revere because of this role of delivering messages between cells. These adjacent cells then respond by producing antiviral proteins, which prevent the virus from entering and duplicating itself within the cell, and the infection cycle is broken.

Interferon also slows division of normal and abnormal cells and stimulates the body's defense system to pick up and destroy foreign material, another way of strengthening it to repel attacks from invading agents and substances.

The origins of interferon

Isaacs and Lindenmann discovered interferon when they set out to investigate a phenomenon known as viral interference.

Doctors had known for many years that a patient with one viral illness almost never fell victim to a second viral infection at the same time, as though one virus somehow prevented or interfered with infection by another virus.

Isaacs and Lindenmann exposed cells from the membrane that lines the inside of a chicken egg to the virus that causes influenza. The cells became infected, as expected. When a second virus was added, however, the membrane cells resisted the infection. The researchers then removed the viruses and the membrane cells from the liquid medium in which the experiment was performed and added a new, healthy group of cells and another virus. These cells also resisted the virus attack. It was obvious that the original cells produced something in response to their infection that made subsequent cells immune to virus attack. That "something" was separate from the cells, because it remained in the solution when the original cells and viruses were removed. Isaacs and Lindenmann named their discovery interferon, because of its ability to interfere with virus infections.

Interferon and cancer

The relationship of viruses to cancer has been studied for years. Certain viruses can clearly cause leukemia and other cancers in laboratory animals. No human cancer virus has yet been identified, but there are some prominent suspects. The Epstein–Barr virus, a herpes virus that causes mononucleosis, has also been found in a facial tumor known as Burkitt's lymphoma. Another herpes virus, type II, which causes genital infection, seems to render those women with the infection more prone to develop cancer of the cervix.

Among the first to report success with interferon and cancer was Ion Gresser, an American-born scientist working at the Institute for Cancer Research in Villejuif, France. In the late 1960s he infected a group of laboratory mice with a virus known to cause leukemia in mice. He injected half the mice with interferon as well. Within one month, the mice that had received interferon and the cancer virus were free of all traces of leukemia. The mice that had received the cancer virus alone developed leukemia. News of Gresser's work reached oncolo-

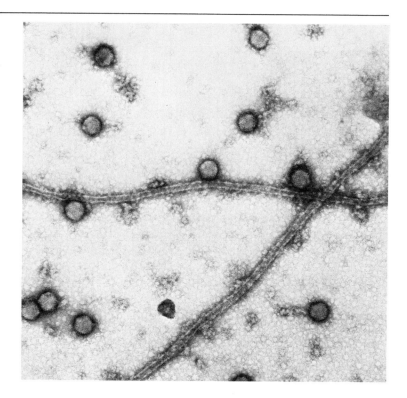

Extreme magnification (100,000x) of mouse tumor virus in a cell. Long strands are part of the cell's supporting structure. (Courtesy Worcester Foundation, Massachusetts)

gists (cancer specialists) across the world, and many of them began to try interferon in human patients with cancer.

The most if not the most impressive data on interferon and its cancer effects come from the Karolinska Hospital in Stockholm, where Hans Strander and his group have been using the agent since 1972 on selected patients with osteogenic sarcoma, a particularly virulent form of bone cancer that ordinarily has a 70 percent mortality rate over two years with traditional anticancer therapy. Despite surgery to remove the cancerous area and subsequent treatment with anticancer agents, osteogenic sarcoma metastasizes, or spreads to other parts of the body, early. Evidence of spread to the lungs often shows up in a year or less. At the Karolinska Hospital, interferon is given intramuscularly daily for a month after surgery, then intravenously three times weekly thereafter. With this protocol, 70 percent of patients with osteogenic sarcoma were alive and free of metastastis two years later, a remarkable figure.

Strander has expanded his research to include patients with lymphomas (cancers of

the tissues that produce white blood cells) such as Hodgkin's disease and has noted improvement in them as well. Smaller studies at Stanford and at the M. D. Anderson Hospital in Houston, Texas, have provided similarly encouraging results. Nineteen of thirty-eight patients with cancer of the breast and lymph tissues at the Houston hospital have improved, according to Dr. Jordan Guttermann, an oncologist at M. D. Anderson. From Roswell Park Memorial Institute in Buffalo, New York, a prestigious cancer research treatment center, comes evidence that interferon can cause regression in breast cancer and malignant melanoma. These studies demonstrate a wide range of sensitivity to interferon injection. Some tumors became up to 50

percent smaller within one month; there was no effect on others; some tumors vanished completely. Some patients noted a reduced tumor size within two to three days. Although many critics say these studies are too small to be valid, the results are certainly encouraging.

There have also been many negative and disappointing results in interferon research. Dr. Elliott Osserman of the Columbia University College of Physicians and Surgeons in New York City reported that only four of fourteen patients with a type of cancer called multiple myeloma responded to interferon. "With traditional chemotherapy, we would expect eleven of fourteen to respond," he said. At Memorial Sloan-Kettering,

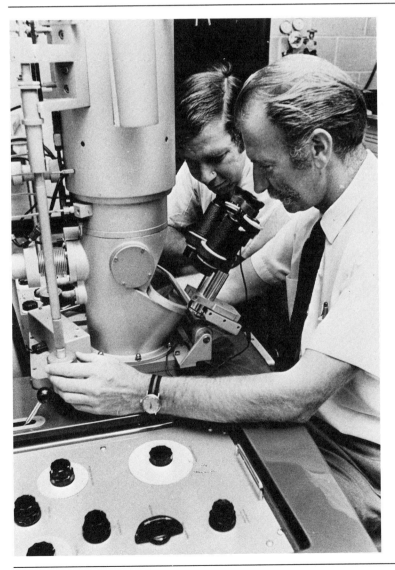

another prominent cancer center in New York, twenty patients with lung cancer have shown no effect of interferon after six months.

The American Cancer Society and National Cancer Institute have decided that because of the potential anticancer properties of the substance, a larger clinical trial is in order. "It's time to bite the bullet on interferon and cancer," says Frank Rauscher, research chief of the American Cancer Society. The two institutions have agreed to buy several million dollars' worth of interferon and distribute it to ten cancer research centers so that they can continue their investigation of its effectiveness.

One of the most exciting features of interferon and cancer treatment is that interferon occurs naturally and can therefore be expected to cause few, if any, side effects. Experience thus far has shown this to be true. Interferon occasionally causes fever, chills, loss of

The electron microscope is being used to study how viruses cause disease, particularly cancer. (Courtesy Boston University Medical Center)

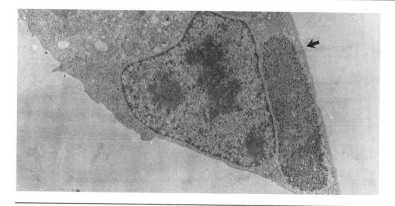

A virus, which possesses the ability to change cells' chemical machinery to duplicate the virus. The hundreds of virus particles on the righthand side of this cell (arrow), magnified 50,000x, are known to cause cancer in mice. (Courtesy Worcester Foundation, Massachusetts).

appetite, and bone marrow and skin changes, but some investigators feel these are actually caused by impurities in the current interferon preparations.

Interferon and viruses

Interferon has benefited cancer patients even when their tumors have not regressed. Many cancer patients have poor ability to ward off viral infections because their defense systems are depressed. Shingles, an infection of the nerve endings by the herpes zoster virus, is commonly seen in adult cancer patients. Chicken pox, caused by the same virus, is common in children with cancer. In a study at Stanford University, Dr. Thomas Merigan, a virologist and interferon researcher, found these conditions less frequently and in a less severe form in his cancer patients who were given interferon. At the same institution evidence is also accumulating that interferon may help to control infectious viral hepatitis.

Patients who undergo organ transplantation may also benefit from interferon's antiviral properties. Medications given to prevent organ rejection reduce the body's ability to fight virus infection. Infection with the cytomegalovirus is common during the three months after transplantation, when suppression of the patient's defense system is at its highest. At the Massachusetts General Hospital in Boston, interferon injection before and after kidney transplantation decreased the incidence of cytomegalovirus infections.

Not all viral studies with interferon have been positive. Some laboratory animals on which it was used have developed liver toxicity, impaired growth, and kidney disease, raising questions about interferon's potential hazards in infants or young children.

Interferon production

If the potential for interferon is so great, why isn't it in greater use? Although the results of interferon studies seem strongly positive, they have included only a small number of patients. Larger clinical trials are necessary before its true potential is realized. Expanded interest has also been handicapped by the limited availability of the substance.

Cells produce interferon in infinitesimal amounts, and the substance is species specific; that is, interferon works only in the animals that produce it. We cannot, therefore, produce large amounts of interferon in laboratory animals and expect it to work in humans. Only human interferon works in humans.

Most of the world's supply of interferon today comes from Finland, where Kari Cantrell of the Central Public Health Laboratory of Helsinki devised a way of producing the substance from the white blood cells left over from the Finnish National Blood Bank. In the Cantrell method, unneeded white blood cells are separated from the rest of the blood and exposed to a virus to produce the interferon.

As evidence of the minuscule amounts involved, the Helsinki laboratories are able to produce only about 100 mg of interferon (less than 4 ounces) from 65,000 pints of blood. This is enough to treat only 500 patients, and the expense is prohibitive. At current prices, about $2,000 to $3,000

Interferon is obtained by exposing white blood cells to a virus. Here a technician removes white blood cells from blood samples that have been centrifuged at high speeds to separate components. (Photo by Michael J. Lutch, courtesy Beth Israel Hospital, Boston)

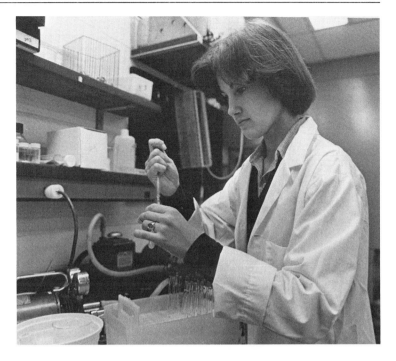

worth of interferon would be needed to treat the common cold in one patient.

Now that cancer agencies have made substantial money available for interferon research, commercial companies are getting into the act. Upjohn, Abbott Laboratories, Merck, Sharp and Dohme, Warner-Lambert, and G. D. Searle are a few companies that have committed large facilities and equipment to interferon production.

We must learn how to produce more interferon at a lower cost if it is to become a practical form of therapy. Cantrell's methods have been the most popular thus far, but by everyone's admission, in addition to being expensive, they are crude and inefficient. The interferon produced from white blood cells in this way is 99 percent impure. Less than .1 percent of the substance is actually active interferon.

Ultimately the production of large quantities of a purer substance will depend on chemical synthesis of the 150 amino acids that are arranged in a row to make up the protein interferon. Investigators at

the California Institute of Technology and other institutions are currently experimenting with sophisticated sequencing equipment which may soon enable mass production of interferon outside the body at 1/20 the present cost.

Genetic engineering may also play a role in producing interferon. In this rapidly expanding field, researchers have had a difficult problem. Interferon researcher Charles Weissmann of the Institute of Molecular Biology of the University of Zurich and the Swiss firm Biogen recently reported isolating the interferon gene from among the 1,000,000 or more pieces of DNA in human white blood cells. In the Weissmann experiments, the DNA that codes for interferon was isolated, planted into a small biological package called a plasmid, and put into an *Escherichia coli* bacterium. The bacterium then used its own reproductive material to make more of the substance. Finding the interferon gene was an awesome task that one researcher likened to "finding a paragraph in an encyclopedia without knowing what the paragraph says."

Now that genetic engineering has isolated the gene, it will be possible to produce interferon with a living bacterial assembly line. Dr. Walter Gilbert of Harvard University, a pioneer in interferon research, comments, "Even though there is evidence that this interferon is not exactly the same as the kind produced by human white blood cells, it did protect cells against the viral activity in the laboratory. This is the crucial test of its biological activity."

When Weissmann and Biogen announced the discov-

Obesity surgery

ery in the spring of 1980, the stock of Schering-Plough, a part owner of Biogen, went up eight points on the stock market, demonstrating the interest in interferon among the financial community. As one researcher commented in a spring 1980 issue of *Time* magazine, "There's gold in interferon. Those who learn to produce and sell it the cheapest will reap enormous benefits from their research investment."

Interferon has been a tantalizing agent since its discovery more than twenty years ago. The implications of a natural and therefore presumably nontoxic protein that has both antiviral and anticancer properties are enormous. The initial reports of interferon's true role in the treatment of illness are exciting—will it be a major therapy instead of merely an adjunct to traditional and problematic therapies? But only further and more extensive studies will demonstrate whether interferon can live up to its potential and provide the opportunity for healing.

Imprisoned in every fat man a thin man is wildly signaling to be let out.

Cyril Connolly

America is the land of excess. Unfortunately, for up to 50 percent of Americans that is also true of their weight. Tufts University president and nutrition expert Dr. Jean Mayer has reported that one person in five is at least 30 percent above the desirable weight for his or her height, age, and sex. Although metabolic and internal body factors are sometimes responsible, the most common reasons for obesity, according to Dr. Mayer, are underexercise and overeating. What internal factors create the desire to eat? The answer is simply not clear.

Mild to moderate obesity has been successfully controlled in a variety of ways, including behavioral, dietary, and drug aided. But for the morbidly obese—100 pounds or more overweight—most medical attempts have been unsuccessful. Morbid obesity interferes with social and work activity and hygiene, and is a threat to health and life. With

the high failure rates for medical treatment, increasing numbers of such patients seek surgery as a solution to their obesity. Sixteen thousand patients in 1976, and undoubtedly more each year since, had a surgical procedure for weight control. A review of the different types of operations show many successes, but also many risks.

CASE HISTORY

F. P. is a thirty-four-year-old store owner who has been overweight all his life. At age twelve he weighed 200 pounds and by high school graduation topped 300 on his 6-foot, 2-inch frame. Into his twenties, working became more and more difficult as he was required to be on his feet, and he developed shortness of breath quite easily. He had been to diet clinics, nutritionists, and his family physician; with each treatment he lost 30 to 40 pounds, only to regain the weight quickly. Five years ago he registered at a protein-sparing fast clinic and lost 90 pounds, bringing his weight down to 220. Within three years the weight returned, and by age thirty F. P. again weighed 350 pounds. His blood pressure was 200/110, and severe low back pain was interfering with his work.

Last year he visited a clinic that suggested intestinal bypass surgery. He underwent a personality evaluation and was thought to have the emotional stability necessary to deal with the operation. Intestinal bypass was performed, and after nine months he has lost 70 pounds and is feeling stronger. He recently returned to work and completes his day easily with less fatigue.

The numbers of centers and surgeons offering surgical relief from morbid obesity rises each year, and several kinds of operations are performed. Most are variations of procedures that were originally intended for another purpose, where weight loss was a side effect of surgery. But in the case of morbid obesity, the side effect becomes the very reason for the operation. Fifteen percent or more of people who undergo surgery for obesity have significant problems thereafter. Because of these and the risks involved, obesity surgery is now restricted in most centers to people who (1) are twice their ideal weight or 100 pounds or more overweight; (2) have tried medical treatment that has failed; (3) are less than fifty years old (to minimize complications); and (4) have a cooperative, determined attitude and are willing to return for frequent follow-up visits for well over a year.

There are three basic types of operations: jaw wiring, intestinal bypass, and gastric bypass and stapling. Each has its advantages and disadvantages.

Jaw wiring

This procedure, commonly performed on people with broken jaws, involves wiring the upper and lower jaws together. It makes chewing impossible and restricts solid food intake, thus greatly limiting calorie intake. Once the jaw is wired, the patient is placed on an 800-calorie liquid diet of juices and milk with vitamins and mineral supplements, taken through a straw.

Severe obesity is a lifetime problem, and many people resume their old eating habits when the wires are released.

And because it impairs oral hygiene and leads to more dental cavities, jaw wiring can only be temporary. The determination of morbidly obese people to eat is reflected in the many reports of people with wired jaws who successfully force solid food through the wire mask and therefore defeat the purpose of the operation.

Intestinal bypass

This operation was originally developed for patients with severe inflammatory bowel disease, such as regional enteritis (Crohn's disease). Many feet of small intestine are bypassed to reduce significantly the space for absorption of food nutrients; controlled malnutrition is the result. Dr. J. Howard Payne, surgical professor at the University of Southern California Medical Center, who developed its use for obese patients, and many other surgeons still perform and champion this procedure. Others, though, are abandoning it because of the high complication rate.

Weakness, fatigue, and severe diarrhea are the rule in patients with intestinal bypass for obesity, since food and nutrients are not fully absorbed. They often have four to eight watery stools per day and develop a severe skin irritation at the rectal opening. Many patients have resulting bone disease and arthritis because of poor calcium absorption. Even more important, others develop kidney failure or liver cirrhosis.

According to Dr. Payne, patients who have had intestinal bypass are satisfied and would ''do it again.'' They feel and look better, show improved blood pressure and heart function, and return to their previous occupations. They can also eat all they want. Weight loss can approach 100 pounds in two years with intestinal bypass, but the severe alteration in health and life-style makes this a risky alternative in the opinion of many obesity specialists. Yet it remains the most commonly performed operation for obesity.

Gastric bypass and stapling

The gastric bypass procedure is similar to an operation performed for duodenal ulcer disease. A 2-ounce pouch is created in the stomach with sutures and then connected to a loop of small intestine, bypassing most of the stomach and duodenum. In another procedure, a 2-ounce pouch is created with staples across the stomach and a small opening is left for drainage by the normal duodenal route. The object in both operations, which are quite new, is to restrict food intake by altering the stomach so that it is able to handle only 2 ounces or less with each feeding. Unlike the intestinal bypass, what the person *does* eat is digested normally.

With gastric bypass and stapling operations 80 percent of the patients lose weight. The average weight loss approximates 100 pounds in the first year. Over longer periods, some have lost 300 pounds or more.

Gastric bypass and stapling are still untested in the long-term arena, and long-term findings often modify what appears to be an excellent initial result. Those centers currently performing gastric procedures for obesity report occasional obstruction of the small opening from the stomach, requiring a repeat operation.

Whether the staples hold over many years is also a matter of debate that only time can answer.

The determined obese patient can defeat the gastric bypass and stapling operations by simply outeating the small pouch. By eating 2-ounce amounts frequently or even constantly, the patient can achieve a high twenty-four-hour calorie intake. Proper psychological screening can reduce this problem, however.

Alternatives

Medical treatment of morbid obesity has produced dismal results. Drugs that reduce the appetite are effective for only a month before the body becomes insensitive to them and the appetite returns. Therapeutic starvation and behavior modification techniques have also been extensively used, but they require what amounts to lifelong discipline, and few people can make that commitment. Most studies confirm that one-third to two-thirds of people who are 100 pounds or more overweight can stay on restrictive diets long enough to show significant weight loss. But of those

Dissolving gallstones

who do lose weight by dieting, only 10 to 20 percent maintain that loss. In time they are back where they started.

It's important that these patients not be left there. The complications of morbid obesity include hypertension and heart disease, cirrhosis, blood clots, back pain, and cancer of the uterus and breast. Only one of seven persons with morbid obesity reaches normal life expectancy.

Surgical therapy is obviously not the ultimate weapon against obesity, since it treats only the symptom and not the cause. As one surgical specialist states, ''A disease which is not mechanical in origin should not be treated mechanically.'' But because medical treatment has thus far failed, surgery remains a valid alternative until we understand obesity more fully.

A financial footnote

While surgery for obesity is effective it is also expensive. Costs for intestinal bypass and gastric procedures including the hospitalization and long-term follow-up approximate $6,000.

Fair, fat, female, forty.

Anonymous origin
Adapted from Sir Walter Scott,
St. Roman's Well

Medical and nursing students through the years have been taught the four *F*'s that typify the individual most likely to develop gallbladder disease, a major health problem that affects about 10 percent of all Americans. Current knowledge is, of course, more sophisticated than that, and the latest research has deepened the understanding of how, why, and in whom gallstones form.

One outgrowth of this work has been the recent discovery of chenodeoxycholic acid (CDCA), a substance that appears to dissolve gallstones with about 75 percent efficacy. CDCA is still an experimental drug, although many gastroenterologists feel that the Food and Drug Administration will almost certainly approve it when the results of a national cooperative gallstone study are released late in 1980.

The study is funded by the National Institutes of Health and is being coordinated by the Cedars-Sinai Medical Center in Los Angeles. Ten other major United States medical centers are participating.

About gallbladder disease

Gallstones resemble small pebbles and are usually composed of cholesterol or a pigment substance called bilirubin, both found in the bile. They form when the cholesterol or pigment substance becomes so concentrated in the bile that it precipitates, or separates out of solution into solid particles.

The accurate incidence of gallbladder disease is unknown because many people have

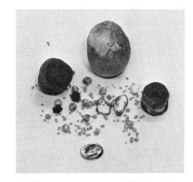

Gallstones can vary widely in size, as shown by this photo. CDCA is most effective on smaller stones.
(Photo by Joseph Murphy, courtesy Alan Diamond, M.D.)

An abdominal X ray showing multiple small gallstones that completely fill the gallbladder and outline its shape. (Photo by Joseph Murphy)

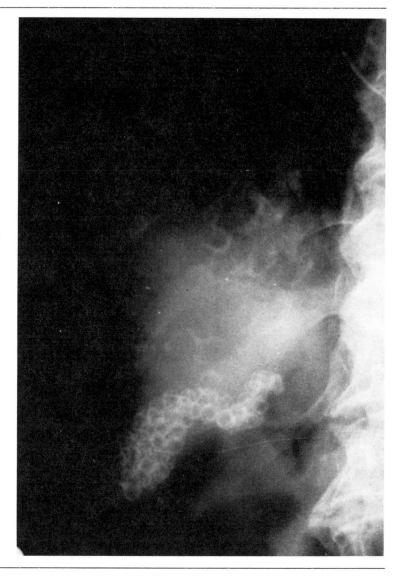

gallstones without any symptoms. Gallstones have been found incidentally at autopsy in patients known to have no gastrointestinal complaints.

The accepted treatment for gallstones today is surgery. Gallbladder surgery is the most common abdominal operation, performed half a million times per year. It has a 1½ percent mortality rate overall, but that approaches 5 percent in patients over sixty.

CASE HISTORY

E. M. is a thirty-six-year-old housewife who had a long history of vague gastrointestinal complaints, including bloating, fullness, and cramping pain in the upper abdomen after a meal. After many unsuccessful attempts to control the problem with diet and drugs, her physician suggested a more complete workup. Gallbladder X rays demonstrated many small gallstones.

Because she was resistant to surgery and her physician was participating in the CDCA gallstone study, E. M. was started on CDCA at 2,500 mg per day. Within six months her symptoms subsided, but gallstones still appeared on an X ray. Eighteen months after the start of therapy, the gallstones had dissolved and the medication was discontinued. Two years later, a few small stones were again seen, although she still had no symptoms. She took CDCA again, and the gallstones disappeared within six months.

E. M. has been free of symptoms for five years.

The CDCA alternative

Almost half of all people with gallstones may soon have this same alternative to surgery. CDCA is a bile salt that reduces the saturation of cholesterol in the bile, a factor in the formation of up to 80 percent of all gallstones. Clinical trials of CDCA in patients with cholesterol stones at the Mayo Clinic and elsewhere show that 75 percent dissolve completely in two or three years. Very small stones may dissolve in six months or less; larger stones take longer. Very large single stones sometimes never completely dissolve. The progress of the therapy is followed by oral cholecystogram X rays repeated at six- to nine-

month intervals; the patient takes several small tablets of a substance secreted in the bile that is visible on X rays, and the next morning X rays are taken.

CDCA is given as an oral medication in tablet form, with the dosage based on the patient's weight. The medication interferes with an enzyme responsible for cholesterol production in the liver and therefore lowers the cholesterol content of the bile. When bile cholesterol saturation is reduced, cholesterol stones do not form, and previously formed stones begin to dissolve. In order for CDCA to dissolve gallstones, the gallbladder must be functioning well and the stones must be made of cholesterol.

CDCA is most effective when used for:

■ *Cholesterol stones:* Eighty percent of all people with gallstones have this type of stone. Women on oral contraceptives or estrogen who develop gallstones most likely have this type.

■ *Silent gallstones:* Those discovered incidentally on medical evaluation and pro-

ducing few or no symptoms.

■ *Many small gallstones:* The larger the stone, the less effective the therapy.

CDCA has a frequent side effect: abdominal cramps and watery diarrhea, which develop because of high bile salt concentration in the large intestine. The amount of diarrhea is related to the CDCA dosage, so very obese people who need large amounts of the medication may be unable to take it because of loose stools. This is unfortunate, because their size also makes these patients poor surgical risks. In clinical trials so far, diarrhea was severe enough in 10 to 20 percent of patients that the optimum dose of CDCA had to be reduced.

CDCA can be expected to work in only about half of patients with gallstones. For others, surgery remains the treatment of choice. According to Dr. Jonathan Thistle, a gastroenterologist at the Mayo Clinic, in an article recently published in the *Journal of the American Medical Association*, the types of patients listed on page 66 should not be treated with CDCA therapy.

Cholesterol

Chenodeoxycholic acid

Note the similarity in the chemical formula of cholesterol and chenodloxycholic acid, one reason CDCA is effective in dissolving cholesterol gallstones.

■ Those with pigment gallbladder stones, containing calcium and the breakdown products of hemoglobin, the oxygen-carrying protein in red blood cells. Twenty percent of people with gallstones have this type.

■ Patients with a history of acute cholecystitis and gallbladder inflammation.

■ Those whose gallbladder does not function well, usually because of advanced disease.

■ People with medical problems that could be aggravated by the side effect of diarrhea. This is unfortunate for people with Crohn's disease (a regional enteritis marked by recurring episodes of diarrhea), as they frequently have a higher incidence of gallstones than the general population.

■ People with liver disease.

Once the gallstones dissolve and the CDCA is stopped —usually anywhere from six months to three years—the gallstones may recur because the basic problem that caused the stones is still present. Most patients are advised to eat a low-cholesterol, high-fiber diet which may reduce the re-formation of gallstones. In the studies done so far at Guy's Hospital Medical Center in London, stones re-formed in 25 percent of patients on CDCA in about three years once the medication was stopped. In about 50 percent, stones recurred in five years. Long-term CDCA therapy may therefore be recommended as a prophylaxis, but confirming results are not available yet.

In the research trials so far, the CDCA cost to the patient is about $1 per day, or more than $300 per year. (The cost to the pill manufacturer is currently fifty cents per day.) If the FDA approves the drug, as expected, increased production may reduce the daily cost. If not, the need certainly exists for a lower-priced analog of the medication.

A recent article in the medical journal *Hospital Practice* commented that the jury on CDCA is still out, a feeling most gastroenterologists today share. Obviously, many patients will continue to be best treated by surgery for gallstones, but many, given the choice, will want to try medical therapy before consenting to the scalpel. The expected availability of CDCA as an alternative to surgery will surely change the way medicine is practiced on patients with gallstones, and the 1,000-patient national cooperative gallstone study report is eagerly anticipated.

A new understanding of dyslexia

If I should not be learning now, when should I be?

Lacydes
Diogenes Laertius, 241 B.C.

Mother says there is something wrong with me, because you could say anything to me and I'd get it right away, but if I read it myself I couldn't get it."

The sixteen-year-old high school student who uttered those words read at a first-grade level and was a participant in the first major study of dyslexia, undertaken in 1925 by Dr. Samuel Orton at an Iowa mental health clinic.

Dr. Orton's case reports are generally credited with stimulating the world's interest in dyslexia. Today we recognize the condition as a major cause of academic failure that involves specific retardation in reading, writing, and spelling. Through the years the causes of this unusual disorder have eluded neurologists, who have variously called it an environmental, social, or emotional disorder.

But in 1979, Harvard Medical School researchers demonstrated for the first time that dyslexia might be related to specific anatomical differences in the brain. This important discovery may lead to a new understanding of this troubling and heretofore baffling condition.

About dyslexia

The major manifestation of dyslexia is a child's inability to read. All dyslexics are not all the same, however. Some may have difficulty with language, others with memory, and still others with spatial relationships. The popular concept of dyslexia is a condition in which individuals see letters backward. The eyes are not the problem in dyslexia, though; rather, it is the brain that has trouble interpreting what the eyes see.

"Dyslexics cannot deal with the arbitrary labels that make up language," states Dr. Martha Denckla, a neurologist at the Children's Hospital Medical Center in Boston. "They have difficulty in learning that when there's a bump on the right it's a *b*, and when it's on the left it's a *d*." When one of her young patients was being asked to distinguish

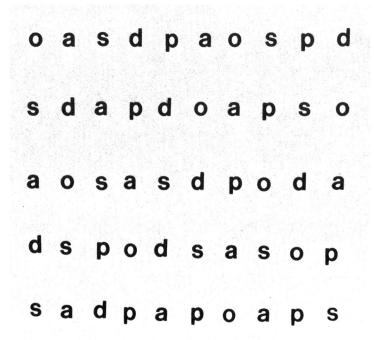

o a s d p a o s p d

s d a p d o a p s o

a o s a s d p o d a

d s p o d s a s o p

s a d p a p o a p s

among several similar letters, the eight-year-old said: "I have no trouble telling these things apart. It's when I meet one of them alone that I can't remember his name." Dyslexics may also reverse the order of letters in syllables, of syllables in words, and of words in sentences to the point of mirror reading. The sentence *The man saw a red dog*, for example, might appear as *A red god was the man* to a dyslexic. The learning problems of dyslexia can extend to math as well. A dyslexic will often transpose numerals.

Dyslexic individuals generally have no other reading or hearing problems, are usually of average intelligence, and may be socially well adjusted despite their handicap. But dyslexics labor with written language tasks and usually remain poor readers throughout their lives. Children with dyslexia inevitably suffer humiliation as they lag behind in school.

CASE HISTORY (BY A MOTHER)

Our son was quite normal early in life—talking at nine months, running at twelve months, quick to understand new situations. In retrospect, he had a short attention span, quite at variance with his apparent abilities.

In the first grade the teacher reported that he was energetic and well liked but "was not working up to potential." He printed his name in mirror images and confused many letters—b with d, p with q, for example. He was frustrated by attempts to learn. "Not to worry," the teacher said. "Such problems are common in the first grade."

In the second grade, reading and spelling were still a problem, and we consulted reading specialists. "He'll grow out of it," they said. He was unhappy in school and had trouble concentrating.

In the third grade he became disruptive, walked around in class, and didn't complete assignments. "He lacks discipline," the teacher reported. He ate and slept poorly, openly expressed hatred for school, and cried frequently at home. "I'm dumb," he said when special reading classes didn't help.

Unable to find help at school, we turned to our pediatrician. She referred us to a neurology clinic, where tests revealed dyslexia. Several classroom approaches were suggested with success. He got A's, for example, when allowed to give his test answers aloud rather than writing them down. His teachers were amazed, and he was relieved to find out that he wasn't "dumb."

We have changed schools to one with a specific learning

disabilities program. He gets
A's and B's and seems happy.

The Galaburda/Kemper research

Understanding the anatomical basis of a problem is the first step toward correcting it. But in the past, the cause of dyslexia was not known.

In 1979 Beth Israel Hospital neurologists Drs. Albert Galaburda and Thomas Kemper made some startling observations on the brain of a twenty-year-old accident victim who was known to have dyslexia. This was an unusual opportunity because dyslexia is not a fatal condition, and tissue samples are therefore rarely available for study. The individual was known to have dyslexia at age six, when he entered elementary school. His father and three brothers were slow readers, and all were left-handed. He had difficulty distinguishing right from left and was judged to be clumsy since early childhood. Although his birth and early childhood were normal, his speech was delayed and he had difficulty with reading and spelling. At

---

Error patterns in dyslexia

Reversals
Of letters: d-b, g-p, u-h, t-f
Of letter sequences: was-saw, felt-left, plea-peal, dog-god, toad-boat

Confusions
Between letters that look the same: m-n, k-h
Between similar small words: it-at, if-of, we-me

Omissions
Of letters and syllables: Brad (brand), beliv (believe), stad (strand), bicle (bicycle)

Substitutions
Of words with similar meanings: wealthy-rich, auto-car, forest-woods, a-the

---

age eighteen he had fourth-grade skills.

Even though the young man's brain appeared normal under routine pathological study, careful microscopic techniques revealed an abnormality not seen before. In the left cerebral hemisphere, where language functions are thought to be located, the normally well-organized layers of cells were disorganized, convoluted, and misplaced. Furthermore, the language area was smaller than would normally be expected. The land-

mark findings were discovered through a technique known as cytoarchitectonics, the study of the location or architecture of cells. It is a very specialized technique known to few researchers. Says Dr. Galaburda, "Unless you study the brain in this excruciating detail, you might miss something very important." The Harvard neurologist does not know and won't speculate whether all dyslexics have this brain structure abnormality. "General conclusions will have to await the study of

Language area of the brain. Abnormal area shown by arrows has many convolutions; should resemble normal area at right. This may be a factor in dyslexia. (Courtesy Beth Israel Hospital, Boston)

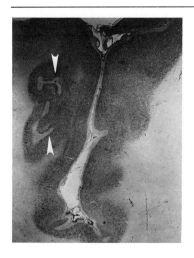

more brains of dyslexics," he says. Galaburda's work, published in the *Annals of Neurology*, was an important finding.

Experts estimate that there are 2 to 15 million dyslexics in the United States today. The exact figure is difficult to pin down, since as recently as the 1960s few physicians recognized that a language disability could have its roots in a medical problem. Instead, they frequently blamed emotional conflicts, and as a result their patients got little help. Unfortunately, many schools today still do not recognize dyslexic children.

Coping with dyslexia

While there is no cure in sight for dyslexia, individuals disabled by the disorder may learn to overcome their handicap in a variety of ways. Their true problem must be recognized, lest they be mislabeled failures, unteachables, or emotionally disturbed. Such individuals often react in self-defense with compensatory and unattractive behavior patterns.

According to Paula Dozier Rome and Jean Smith Osman, co-directors of the Reading Center in Rochester, Minnesota, as noted in the medical journal *Pediatric Annals*, "If a child is seriously retarded in reading and has normal intelligence, chances are about nine in ten that there is a specific language disability."

Mrs. Rome and Mrs. Osman have been helping dyslexics for twenty-five years; their students range in age from five to sixty-five. Their diagnosis of dyslexia is a fairly simple procedure, concentrating on five elements: school history, family history, estimate of intelligence, oral reading, and spelling. "The dyslexic will continue to suffer from the affliction from the first attempts to learn the ABCs until the last days of life," they note. According to the women, the treatment for dyslexia is basically education. A good program should involve a multisensory approach using visual, auditory, and tactile presentations. In a visual presentation, words are supplied for the student to memorize and use subsequently in reading. The phonic units of the language (*ea* and *ou*, for example) and the rules and generalizations of speech and writing must be stressed. And the program must be structured to progress from the simple to the complex.

Not too long ago there were clinics that treated dyslexia by exercising eye muscles, prescribing large doses of vitamins, or excluding food additives and sugar from the diet. Today all responsible dyslexia treatment centers, like Rome and Osman's, follow the pioneering multidisciplinary approach that Dr. Orton originally developed.

With proper guidance, many people with dyslexia have made their way into learned professions and positions.

New treatments for peptic ulcer

Former Vice-President Nelson Rockefeller, General George Patton, Thomas Edison, and Danish fablist Hans Christian Andersen are just four well-known people who have succeeded despite their learning disabilities.

Resources

■ Your pediatrician is the best source for a referral to a center that evaluates learning disabilities. Such centers are usually located in major medical centers that have pediatric and neurology departments. Progressive school departments may also have such information.

■ The National Orton Society is an excellent dyslexia resource and has many regional and local state chapters. For information about the one nearest you, contact:

National Orton Society
8415 Bellona Lane
Suite 115
Towson, Maryland 21204
301-296-0232

I must be successful; I have an ulcer to prove it.

Anonymous executive

Often called the "badge of success," peptic ulcer disease affects over 20 million Americans. While some physicians say ulcer incidence is decreasing, peptic ulcer disease accounts for 2 percent of all hospital admissions and remains a major health problem. And contrary to popular belief, ulcers are not unique to stress-torn, hard-driving male executives. With increasing frequency, ulcers are seen in housewives, working women, and children.

Known to be related to excess stomach acid, ulcers for years were treated with bland diets, antacids, and drugs such as belladonna. Newer understanding of ulcer disease has led to a decreasing role for these mainstays of therapy, and the old traditions are now being replaced by cimetidine, a drug that specifically blocks acid secretion.

About peptic ulcer

An ulcer is an erosion or sore that arises, in 80 percent of cases, in the lining of the duodenum, the first part of the small intestine, and with less frequency in the stomach. It occurs mainly between ages twenty and fifty and with three to ten times greater frequency in men, although before puberty and after menopause the frequencies of occurrence in men and in women are equal.

Acid has been recognized for years as a major factor in ulcer disease, and although the precise relationship of acid to ulcer is not completely understood, several facts are now known.

The stomach contains large parietal cells that secrete hydrochloric acid to aid in the digestion of foods. Chief cells alongside these secrete pepsinogen, a precursor of pepsin. It is believed that pepsin and acid together somehow lead to destruction of the delicate intestinal lining. People with duodenal ulcer disease have an increased number of parietal cells and can therefore produce more acid. They also seem to respond more vigorously to foods that normally promote acid secretion and put out ever increasing amounts. Acid secretion is regulated by gastrin, a hormone produced in the upper part of the stomach, and by the vagus nerve, which runs between the brain and the stomach and increases acid at the thought of food or anticipation of stress. The final mediator working in the parietal cells to increase acid is the chemical histamine.

Peptic ulcer disease is usually seen in patients with high levels of acid, but acid production is not the only issue in ulcer, as people with duodenal ulcers can also have normal acid levels. We also know that genetic factors may play a part, as ulcer disease tends to run in certain families. This is poorly understood, but may be related to hormone or other chemical levels. Too, the stomach seems to empty more quickly in people with duodenal ulcer disease, presenting increased amounts of acid and pepsin to the duodenum. The ability of the tender lining of the duodenum to resist this acid may also be impaired. Less bicarbonated secretions from the pancreas have been observed in duodenal ulcer patients. Bicarbonate usually neutralizes acid;

impaired bicarbonate production would therefore allow an increase in acid.

Traditional ulcer therapy

The classic treatment for peptic ulcer was unchanged for many years. Bland diets heavy in milk products reduced the production of acid. Antacids were taken to neutralize the acid, while anticholinergic drugs such as belladonna worked on the nerves to the stomach to suppress acid production. When medical therapy failed, surgical procedures were employed, either to remove the acid-forming part of the stomach or to cut the vagus nerve and eliminate the nervous control of acid production. These treatments failed in many ways.

Despite what many still believe, diet does not play a major role in causing or treating ulcer disease. Whereas some highly seasoned or fibrous foods may aggravate symptoms in some patients, they make no difference in the amount of pain or the rate of ulcer healing in most. The traditional bland diet, which is high in both calcium and protein, may in fact stimulate

acid secretion and worsen ulcer symptoms. And from a nutritional standpoint, bland diets leave a lot to be desired. Hourly milk, another popular approach, may also be harmful, since large amounts of milk products can worsen arteriosclerosis and gallbladder disease. The use of baby foods or strained foods, popular several years ago, is archaic.

Belladonna and other anticholinergic drugs can reduce acid secretion by as much as 50 percent in the resting state, but are less effective when food stimulation increases the acid. Certainly these drugs don't offer as much acid relief as one would want, and complications often arise. The most severe complication is an acute attack of glaucoma in people with a tendency toward it. Men with enlarged prostates can develop complete urine retention. Similarly, antacids very effectively neutralize stomach acid, but they must be taken frequently—usually at one-, two-, or three-hour intervals after meals and at night—and many people develop diarrhea and other gastrointestinal symptoms as a result.

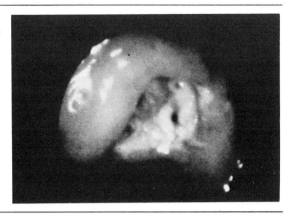

Photograph of an ulcer taken through a fiberoptic endoscope (see page 130). [Courtesy Olympus Corporation]

Surgical procedures for ulcer disease have saved many lives and have made other people more comfortable. But cutting a vital nerve or removing part or all of a vital digestive organ is at best a crude solution to what is essentially a chemical problem.

A more rational approach to ulcer therapy involves using a drug to stop the parietal cells from secreting acid without affecting the other functions of the body. This precise approach is now possible with a new medication called cimetidine.

CASE HISTORY

J. Y. is a fifty-five-year old schoolteacher. For years he had a nervous stomach. Butterflies, nausea, and heartburn were everyday occurrences; he kept antacid tablets in his classroom desk drawer. Several years ago, after he experienced severe pain and vomiting, he visited his doctor, who ordered a barium upper GI X ray and found a duodenal ulcer. From then on, J. Y. struggled with bland diets and antacids after meals. They helped for a while, but long, stress-filled periods of work would usually be followed by a flare-up of his ulcer symptoms. He stopped smoking and drinking, and periodically used tranquilizers. His ulcer symptoms controlled his life.

Several months ago, J. Y. visited his doctor again and was counseled anew about lifestyle and the avoidance of specific irritants. He began taking cimetidine and has been free of symptoms since.

How cimetidine works

Drugs work on the body in one of two ways. Some are nonspecific and exert their physical or chemical effect on any tissue or organ with which they come in contact. Because of this nonspecific relationship, high concentrations are often needed, and side effects are common. Other drugs act specifically and can be used in very low concentrations because only a small number of cells are involved. Cimetidine is such a drug. It belongs to a class of compounds called receptor antagonists.

The receptor theory of drug action means that certain drugs seek out a specific target or receptor on or within a cell. The receptor latches on to the drug molecule, and this bond then triggers a biological effect. Of course, the receptor itself must be able to attract the drug, and the cell in which the receptor is located must be able to react to the receptor-drug bond. One specialist compares this receptor-drug relationship to a lock and a key. Just as a key must fit a lock, so the receptor and drug must be compatible; and as the lock mechanism opens when the key is turned, so the cell responds to the drug-receptor bond. Some drugs act at the receptor site and stimulate the cell to do its work. Others are antagonists to the cell's work.

Histamine has been known for years to produce acid secretion in the stomach. In fact, it is the drug that stimulates the parietal cells to produce acid in response to the thought or presence of food. You might expect that classic antihistamines would reduce this effect just as they reduce histamine-mediated allergy symptoms, like runny nose and cough.

Classic antihistamines,

however, have no effect on acid secretion. In the 1960s one researcher speculated that the receptors on the gastric cells that attracted histamine and led to increased acid were structurally different from the receptors involved in histamine allergic symptoms. He named these receptors H2 receptors. He then systematically altered the structure of histamine and tested each new compound to see if it had the ability to attach to the H2 receptor and block histamine's effect.

Hundreds of compounds later, he found cimetidine. It is structurally related to histamine but prevents histamine interaction by being attracted specifically to the receptors that would ordinarily attract it. Cimetidine is, then, an H2 receptor antagonist to histamine.

Weighing the benefits

Cimetidine blocks acid production more effectively than any drug previously used. Many investigators have documented and reported their results in recent journals and medical symposia. Overall, cimetidine heals duodenal ulcer in more than 75 percent of patients within four to six weeks, a rate far superior to that of traditional methods. Its greater specificity notwithstanding, an important factor may be that patients accept cimetidine treatment so well. Traditional ulcer therapy was cumbersome; the frequent and large doses of antacids often interfered with other drugs the patient may have been taking. Fewer than 30 percent of ulcer patients followed traditional therapy as directed. Cimetidine, on the other hand, has infrequent side effects, few drug interactions, and is taken simply as one pill four times a day. It is no more expensive than antacid therapy.

Although cimetidine dramatically reduces stomach acid, it cannot be considered a cure because it doesn't alter any underlying factors. Stress, overstimulation of acid, or other factors may provoke recurrence of the ulcer after the patient finally stops taking cimetidine. But the reported studies show that ulcers recur far less often in patients treated with cimetidine than they do with other forms of treatment. In one study, for example, ulcer symptoms recurred in 13 percent of patients treated with cimetidine and in 47 percent of patients treated in the traditional way. In another study, the cimetidine group experienced 18 percent recurrence; the control group, 80 percent recurrence. Cimetidine appears to heal ulcers more quickly, relieves symptoms, and reduces the chances for recurrence.

What are the side effects?

Unfortunately, H2 receptors are not limited to the stomach; they occur in the heart, brain, blood vessels, and other places as well. Cimetidine also works in these sites and can lead to some side effects such as dizziness, diarrhea, and headache. However, these side reactions are rarely severe enough to necessitate stopping the cimetidine treatment.

The most controversy about cimetidine relates to its reported effect on male sexual functioning. Most men on the drug have a 40 percent reduction in sperm count (which is not enough, however, to reduce fertility), and a few cases of loss of libido and even impotence have been reported. Long-term use, for three months or more, has brought a few reports of male breast enlargement. Studies on animals have shown that cimetidine bonds to the receptors for testosterone, the male sex hormone, and this may be the basis of its sexual effects.

There is a tendency among both physicians and their patients to consider a drug with dramatic effects to be a panacea for all related conditions. Many experts, however, feel that cimetidine should not be used automatically on all patients whose symptoms merely suggest duodenal ulcer, but rather should be restricted to patients in whom the diagnosis of duodenal ulcer has been established by upper GI examination or endoscopy.

Yet should it be withheld from those patients who would benefit from it just because of potential side effects? Remember that antacid therapy, the alternative, has side effects too. Many people take ulcer disease lightly: ''I thought it was something serious, but my doctor told me it was just an ulcer.'' Yet ulcer disease ac-counts for 10,000 deaths and 40,000 disabilities each year. The estimated economic loss to the United States alone may be as high as $3 billion. Every drug in the doctor's bag for ulcer must therefore be considered. Today, at least, cimetidine remains a major treatment advance.

What the future holds

The United States Food and Drug Administration has approved cimetidine for treatment of an acute flare-up of the symptoms of duodenal ulcer. It is usually discontinued within nine to ten weeks. Maintenance therapy is usually not necessary because a large percentage of ulcer patients have pain-free periods anyway.

Cimetidine is being studied on stomach ulcer, and even though the results appear as promising as those for duodenal ulcer, its role there has not yet been established. A gastric or stomach ulcer is a much more complicated medical problem, not so clearly related to acid. Similar work is going on to assess cimetidine's role in several other medical conditions related to stomach acid. It has, for example, relieved the pain of reflux esophagitis, a condition in which a structural abnormality at the junction of the stomach and esophagus permits acid to seep into the esophagus, irritating its lining and causing pain. And it has been effective in helping people with severe injuries who often develop ulcers in response to the stress of those conditions.

Cimetidine may also be effective in other intestinal malabsorption problems. Clearly, the final chapters on cimetidine have not yet been written.

Resources

■ Your doctor should be able to provide further information and refer you to a gastroenterology specialist.

■ Cimetidine (Trade name Tagamet) is manufactured by:

Smith, Kline, and French Laboratories
1500 Spring Garden Street
P.O. Box 7929
Philadelphia, Pennsylvania
19101
215-854-4000

Vitamin A for acne

Zits, blackheads, blemishes, pimples—these are some of the unkind names used for mankind's most common skin disease, acne. Almost everyone has experienced some type of pimple or blemish on the face, back, or chest at some time and almost everyone has seen these sores finally regress. For others, however, acne is a real torment. Persistent, severe, usually unresponsive to treatment, acne often leaves large scars. The outlook has been bleak for these unfortunate individuals.

Now, however, a variant of vitamin A called retinoic acid is giving new hope.

CASE HISTORY

C. G. is a thirty-three-year-old woman who has had acne as long as she can remember. It began in her adolescent years when she noted a few pimples on her face. Abrasive skin cleansers, frequent scrubbing, and over-the-counter medicated lotions gave no relief. By age sixteen, the acne had spread to scattered areas on her chest and back. On the advice of friends she avoided chocolates and dairy products. On the advice of cosmetologists she avoided makeup of any kind. On the advice of her doctor she used topical products that burned her skin and caused it to peel. Plug extractors, surgical drainage, and antibiotics—she tried them all. All gave early but unfortunately temporary relief.

For years C. G. was told that she would eventually outgrow her acne, but by age thirty-two, that seemed frustratingly less likely. C. G.'s dermatologist eventually referred her to a study group using a capsule of retinoic acid. In four months the oiliness of her skin decreased, the redness, pain, and prominence of most areas were markedly reduced, and some areas had cleared completely. Six months after therapy began, her skin continues to improve.

13-cis-retinoic acid

Acne occurs when excess oiliness of the skin irritates the pores, obstructing them and causing infection. Although often called a disease of adolescence, acne is certainly not limited to that age group. Adolescents are more prone to acne, though, because the hormonal changes of puberty seem to trigger excess activity in the oil glands of the skin.

Many skin specialists have used vitamin A for acne for years. In some forms it has had little effect. In its most potent form it has provided many dramatic results. High doses of vitamin A, however, can lead to serious medical problems, and for many the vitamin A cure was worse than the original acne problem. Hypervitaminosis A syndrome involves rough, cracked skin, headache, vomiting, severe liver problems, and mental derangement that mimics schizophrenia.

The search for an effective but less toxic form of vitamin A led eventually to 13-cis-retinoic acid. It was used initially at the National Institutes of Health in Bethesda, Maryland, on fourteen patients with very severe acne that was progressive and resistant to all other forms of treatment. It was given in a capsule, the dosage based

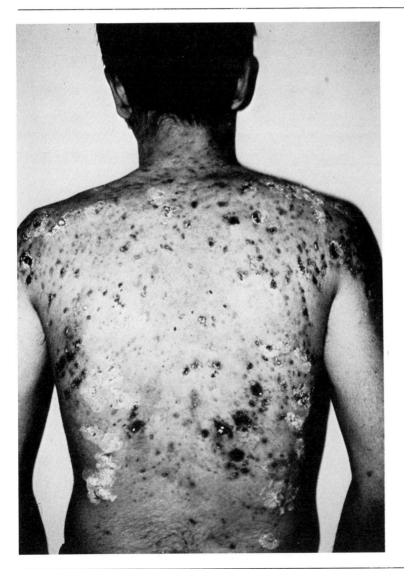

on the patient's weight. No other medications or treatments were used during the control period. Over four months, as reported in the *New England Journal of Medicine* in a highly acclaimed article, thirteen of the fourteen patients in the study had complete remission of their severe acne. The remaining patient had 75 percent clearing. Twenty months later, when the report was published, remission was still in effect. There were minor recurrences in three of the original fourteen, but traditional acne treatment cleared these flare-ups easily. Other investigators have since confirmed these results.

How 13-cis-retinoic acid works is not known, but researchers suspect it affects oil production in skin glands. After the NIH project was started, all the patients commented that their skin was less oily. Objectively, the secretions of the sebaceous glands, which provide some of the surface skin oil, were reduced by as much as

Specialists have had success with 13-cis-retinoic acid on severe acne such as this.

90 percent. Nothing used thus far had had so dramatically reduced sebaceous gland secretion.

Although 13-cis-retinoic acid has given the safest, most effective results for severe acne to date, its long-term effects are not yet known. Vitamin A is important in the formation of skin and cavity covering tissue, and it affects the eyes, liver, bones, nervous system, and reproductive organs. The possible effect of high doses of this form of vitamin A on those tissues must be considered. During the study, almost all of the patients noted some dryness of the skin and numbness of the nose and mouth. Some had nosebleeds. After the treatment was completed, however, their skin returned to normal, and in no case were the side effects severe enough to restrict therapy. The drug also apparently affects the way our bodies handle fats.

The researchers have carefully followed the patients with all these problems in mind. So far, no major complications have been noted, but for the time being, the use of 13-cis-retinoic acid is restricted to patients whose acne is severe and has not responded to traditional treatment.

Applying traditional therapy

Acne treatment is primarily directed at reducing the oiliness, obstruction, and infection of skin glands. Since 13-cis-retinoic acid is still in the testing stages, doctors suggest the following forms of treatment:

- Frequent washing helps reduce surface oils. Overly vigorous cleansing, however, may worsen the problem.

- No diet will cause or cure acne, but if some foods appear to aggravate the condition, avoid them. Foods high in iodine, such as shellfish, may be a problem for people prone to acne.

- Topical products that cause drying and peeling reduce the oils. Though there are many, look for those containing benzoyl peroxide, the most reliable and effective over-the-counter topical treatment for acne.

- If these methods don't work, see your doctor, who may use instruments called comedo extractors to drain persistent pimples, antibiotics, and other prescription products that are generally stronger than those you can buy over the counter.

- Oral contraceptives often help many women, but estrogen use may have its own problems over the long haul. In men, its feminizing effects eliminate it from consideration.

Beauty may be only skin deep, but that has provided little consolation to the scores of people who have had to live with the frequently disfiguring sores of acne. For people of all ages, dermatologists have a variety of prescription drugs available in their treatment arsenal for acne; 13-cis-retinoic acid promises to be the most effective of all of them if long-term results even approximate the excellent ones seen thus far.

Resources

- A dermatologist can provide the best counsel on acne problems

- 13-cis-retinoic acid is manufactured by:

Hoffmann-LaRoche, Inc.
Nutley, New Jersey 07110
201-235-5000

Alternatives to mastectomy

Conceptions from the past blind us to facts that almost slap us in the face.

Dr. William Stewart Halsted, 1896

One out of every fourteen women alive today will eventually develop breast cancer. Each year over 100,000 new cases are discovered.

It has been almost ninety years since Dr. W. S. Halsted of Johns Hopkins University in Baltimore performed the first mastectomy for breast cancer. Ironically, many surgeons today still use his theory of how cancer spreads to justify the radical procedure: surgery to remove the entire breast, the muscle, and the lymph system of the chest wall.

Based on a new theory of cancer spread, however, an expert panel of the National Institutes of Health recently recommended a less extensive operation as standard therapy for breast cancer. And at many medical centers in the United States, primary radiation therapy offers another alternative that seems to be just as effective as even radical mastectomy—and without such a profound effect on a woman's body image.

Standard breast cancer treatment

Dr. Halsted performed the first radical mastectomy in 1894 based on his concept that the tumor always spreads first into the muscle and lymph node system closest to it, then progressively outward. Surgical removal of the entire breast and the muscle and lymph system of the chest wall was considered essential to stop the progress and recurrence of the tumor.

Thousands of women are familiar with the one-stage operation that involved diagnosis and treatment at the same time. A suspicious lump was removed while the patient was under general anesthesia. Then, while the patient was still asleep, the tissue was sent to the pathology laboratory where it was analyzed as a "frozen section," a quick but accurate method of examining the tissue without the usual formal staining methods. If a malignancy was found in the surgical specimen, radical mastectomy was immediately performed, and the woman woke up to find a diagnosis of cancer and the loss

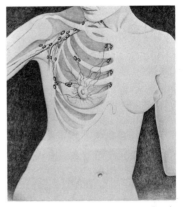

Each breast contains a network of lymphatic channels that drain toward lymph nodes along the breast bone and underarm area. Cancer cells in the lymph nodes indicate that the disease has spread to more distant parts of the body. (Courtesy National Cancer Institute)

of a breast at the same time. Radical mastectomy was considered an important treatment for breast cancer; it raised the survival rate for women with the condition from 20 to over 50 percent.

Large-scale comparisons of treatment programs in many different institutions, however, indicate that such extensive surgery may be unnecessary in most cases. In fact, radical mastectomy has now been all

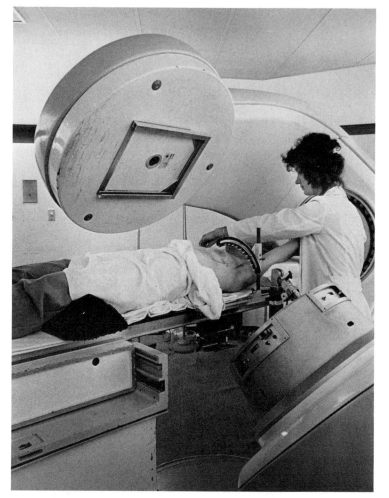

A lumpectomy is usually followed by one or two forms of radiation therapy. Here, a radiation technician adjusts the linear accelerator according to the radiation dose to be administered. [Photo by Michael J. Lutch, courtesy Beth Israel Hospital, Boston]

but abandoned, being reserved for only a few selected cases. Comparable results have been demonstrated with simpler operations.

In June 1979 the National Institutes of Health panel of experts repudiated the Halsted operation and recommended instead that a "modified radical mastectomy" be considered standard breast cancer therapy. In this operation the entire breast is removed, but the chest muscles are left in place. This results in greater use of the arm and less swelling than was common with the more radical procedure, and breast reconstruction to restore more normal contours is possible. The panel also recommended continued study of lumpectomy—removal of the tumor only—plus radiation, chemotherapy, and other procedures.

CASE HISTORY

J. S. is a forty-year-old news-reporter in a major eastern city. On routine physical examination a small lump was discovered in her right breast. Based on the way it felt, her physician told her that there *was an 80 percent chance of malignancy and suggested a "modified radical mastectomy." He explained that breast removal was the "treatment of choice" and offered the best chance for cure.*

Fearful of a mastectomy and what it would do to her physically and emotionally, J. S. asked about alternatives. While her physician acknowledged that certain medical centers in the United States and Europe were performing lumpectomy, he noted that success was not yet proven with this therapy, *and the radiation therapy leaves the breast worse-looking than after a mastectomy. J. S. pursued a second opinion from another respected surgeon, who assured her that the lesser surgical procedure was indeed a viable alternative for some people and referred her to a center that offered it. After consultation with the second physician, J. S. underwent lumpectomy and primary radiation and has done well for the past three years.*

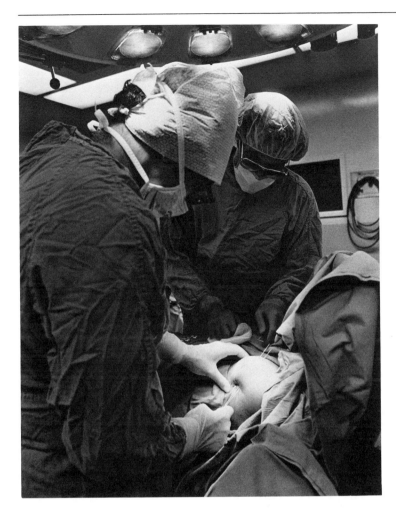

where the procedure has been performed longer confirms their expectations.

Radiation therapy is a well-accepted form of cancer treatment. It has been successfully and extensively used for years to treat cancers of the brain, lung, lymph organs, and many other parts of the body. Its use as a primary therapy for breast cancer is new, however.

In this method, the suspicious lump and a bit of surrounding breast tissue are removed through a small incision, leaving the breast normal in appearance, a so-called lumpectomy. If laboratory analysis confirms that the tissue is malignant, treatment options are discussed with the patient. Mastectomy may be one option; primary radiation therapy another. The lumpectomy alone is not sufficient treatment for breast cancer since all cancer cells may not have been removed with the limited surgery. Further, cancer can occur in other parts of the breast, and the aim is to prevent local recurrence, whether by surgery or radiation.

If the patient chooses primary radiation and her doctor agrees, no further surgery is

Radiation therapy and lumpectomy

Because of the high incidence of breast cancer and because many women choose not to accept mastectomy, doctors are searching for a safe alternative treatment for this frustrating problem. "Most sensible women want to preserve their life and their breast. I think it's possible to do both," says Dr. Leslie Botnick of Boston's Beth Israel Hospital. Dr. Botnick, who is chief of radiation therapy at the Harvard Medical School teaching hospital, and

others have had encouraging success with primary radiation therapy for early forms of breast cancer. Their five-year survival rates, one indicator of the success of cancer therapy, for stages I and II breast cancer (stages I and II include those breast cancers less than 2 inches in diameter and without evidence of spread to the lymph nodes under the arm), compare favorably with those of surgery, and they expect that the long-term ten- and fifteen-year figures will be comparable as well. Experience in countries performed. Instead, plans are made to treat the breast with radiation. The area to be treated is carefully measured, and an exact dose of radiation is administered with a linear accelerator. This 4-million-volt high-energy unit treats the tumor area specifically and does not burn or scar the skin, as was common with older radiation devices. The treatment is given daily for a month, until a total dose of 4,500 to 5,000 rads (the units of measure for radiation) is reached. Since linear accelerator therapy has few and minor side effects—slight itching and redness of the skin are common—it is usually given as an outpatient procedure. The women can continue normal work or home activities.

Because local recurrence of tumors has been seen with external radiation alone, a second, booster dose of radiation is administered. This time it is given internally by placing small seeds of the radioactive isotope iridium-192 directly into the tumor site through small tubes. The placement of these tubes requires a minor surgical procedure and a hospital stay of about three days.

During this time, the isotope remains in the breast to give an additional 2,500 rads. "The continuous radiation of the implant has a greater effect on cancer cells without affecting surrounding normal tissues as much as the external doses," says Dr. Botnick. When the iridium implant is removed, the treatment is complete.

After radiation therapy the breast becomes more firm and is unable to produce breast milk because of the damage to glandular structures. However, 80 percent of the women who have had the procedure rate the cosmetic result as "good to excellent."

There are many misconceptions about the hazards of radiation therapy; many fear that the therapy alone will cause cancer to appear years later. Radiation specialists feel that these fears are groundless. As one explains, "Whereas low doses of radiation given over a long period of time, or poorly controlled at the time of exposure, have been found to be carcinogenic, there is no evidence that modern high-dose controlled radiation therapy increases cancer risk." The former treatment was common years ago for acne and

other skin disorders, and to shrink the thymus gland.

Radiation therapy is not considered for all patients with breast cancer, even by the centers that have had increasing success with it. It is seen as an alternative rather than as standard therapy. The decision to choose this therapeutic option is a complicated one that requires the cooperation of radiotherapists, surgeons, and oncologists (who may recommend chemotherapy as well)—and the patient, who at last has an option other than life or breast.

Chemotherapy

When the National Institutes of Health panel repudiated the Halsted operation and recommended the study of other alternatives, they acknowledged a theory about the growth and spread of breast cancer different from that which Halsted originally proposed. Cancer cells have commonly been found in the bloodstream, so it is obvious that they can travel throughout the body as well as into the immediately surrounding tissues. Although surgery can successfully remove a tumor localized to the breast, no amount of surgery, no matter how extensive, can totally control a cancer that has gone beyond its boundaries. One of the difficulties in cancer diagnosis is determining when such spread has occurred. It may have happened before the tumor was large enough to be felt.

The use of drugs to attack cancer cells throughout the body has been an accepted form of cancer treatment—sometimes primarily, and sometimes as an adjunct to surgery and/or radiation. Previously, chemotherapy was begun only when there was evidence that the cancer had grown or spread. Now, however, many patients are being treated with chemotherapy at earlier stages, to attack tumor cells when their spread is suspected. In the case of breast cancer, certain clues suggest that distant spread may have occurred, even though it cannot be confirmed. One such clue is the presence of tumor cells in the lymph nodes under the armpit. The NIH panel recommended that a sample of underarm nodes be removed for study when a breast cancer is being evaluated. With any evidence of tumor in the nodes, many specialists recommend

the initiation of chemotherapy.

Anticancer drugs are not used without strong indications because they have frequent and sometimes serious side effects. They work by attacking rapidly growing cells, and they affect cancer cells, which are particularly rapidly growing, to a great degree. However, all body tissues are affected to some degree, and rapidly growing normal cells are more seriously affected—thus the toxic effects of chemotherapeutic agents on bone marrow, hair follicles, and intestinal organs. Patients on chemotherapy typically become anemic, lose their hair, and develop intestinal problems.

In the case of breast cancer, hormones can also be used as chemotherapy. An estrogen receptor test is now performed on many, if not most, breast cancer samples to determine whether the cancer cells still contain enough of the original character of breast cells to be dependent on estrogen for growth. If they are, it means the breast can be treated with hormones to suppress estrogen and therefore the cancer. "Estrogen receptor negative" implies a poorer prognosis and means that anticancer drugs may be

more effective than hormones in controlling tumor growth and spread.

The last recommendation of the NIH panel is perhaps the most important from the patient's point of view. Cancer diagnosis and treatment, they felt, should be a two-stage procedure. First, the diagnosis should be conclusively proven. Then, only after discussion of all the options with the patient, therapy should be started. The panel encouraged full and open discussions. Many states have gone further and passed patients' rights legislation that requires a physician to inform a woman of all the alternatives available for the treatment of breast cancer. (See the discussion of patients' rights on pages 242–246.)

Beth Israel's Dr. Botnick agrees. In fact, his hospital has consistently been one of the national leaders in patients' rights programs. "None of the currently available techniques for treating breast cancer is an absolute answer," he says, "but there are options. The patient should and must play a vital role in determining which of those options is eventually used."

Diabetes Diabetes Diabetes

Man may be the captain of his fate, but he is also the victim of his blood sugar.

Dr. Wilfred Oakley
Transactions of the Medical Society of London, 1962

Diabetes mellitus is a disease of worldwide proportion, affecting perhaps 200 million people. After obesity and thyroid disorders, it is the third most common metabolic problem in the world, affecting children, adults, and elderly people.

Diabetes is also an ancient disease. Imaginative descriptions of its symptoms can be found as early as the Ebers Papyrus of Egypt, dating to about 1500 B.C. Recognizing the extreme hunger and thirst, the copious urine flow, and the pronounced wasting of fat and muscle tissue culminating in coma which characterize the condition, Aretaeus of Cappadocia wrote in A.D. 70, "Diabetes is a strange condition which consists of the flesh and bones running together into the urine." Aretaeus also gave diabetes its name, from a Greek root meaning "to run through." In the 17th century, Thomas Willis described the urine "as if imbued with honey," and the word mellitus ("honey eyed") was added to the name.

Today, diabetes is seen as a disease different from what was recognized even a few years ago. New insights into the elevated blood sugar and relative insulin deficiency of the condition have established that diabetes has many varied causes. Heredity is a factor, as are viruses and the autoimmune phenomenon, but their relationships are still unclear.

Insulin therapy can treat diabetes but not cure it; there is no cure for diabetes, and the disease still takes its toll. Great strides have been made in treatment, however. Artificial pancreas systems, pancreas transplants, synthetic insulin, and other innovations (most not yet perfected) promise greater blood sugar control. Still, nagging questions haunt diabetologists and their patients. Will better control of blood sugar prevent the all too frequent complications of diabetes? Are other factors involved that are as yet unknown? How should we measure blood sugar control? Is standard blood sugar testing an accurate monitor of an individual's sugar control?

Early in the twentieth century, a child with diabetes mellitus simply didn't grow up. The baffling disease with unbridled blood sugar accumulation inevitably led to death within a year. The discovery of insulin in 1921 saved many lives and brought an appar-

Diabetes Diabetes Diabete

ent answer to the mystery of diabetes. Diabetes could be understood at last as one disease with one metabolic cause, insulin deficiency, and one treatment, insulin. And so, children with diabetes who take insulin now live into adulthood.

After many years, however, enthusiasm for insulin was tempered as it became clear that insulin wasn't the cure that it promised to be. Despite insulin treatment, diabetes is a chronic illness, and long-term complications have appeared: cardiac disease, blood vessel disorders and stroke, kidney failure, and blindness. All were unknown as complications of diabetes in the pre-insulin era.

Today, diabetes is the third leading killer in the United States, responsible for over 300,000 deaths per year. Ten million Americans have diabetes, and 6 percent more join the ranks annually. If current trends continue, an American child born this year has one chance in five of ultimately developing the disease. The number of diabetics is increasing because (1) diabetics now live longer; (2) their increased life expec-

---

Warning signals of diabetes

Insulin-dependent (juvenile) diabetes is characterized by the sudden appearance of:

C onstant urination
A bnormal thirst
U nusual hunger
T he rapid loss of weight
I rritability
O bvious weakness and fatigue
N ausea and vomiting

Any of these signals can mean diabetes. Children usually exhibit dramatic and sudden symptoms and must receive prompt treatment.

Non-insulin-dependent (maturity) diabetes may include any of the signs of juvenile diabetes, or:

D rowsiness
I tching
A family history of diabetes
B lurred vision
E xcessive weight
T ingling, numbness, pain in the extremities
E asy fatigue
S kin infections and slow healing of cuts and scratches, especially of the feet

Many adults may have diabetes with none of these symptoms, and the disease is often discovered during routine physical examinations.

tancy means they live long enough to have children, and their children inherit the diabetes gene; and (3) obesity, which precipitates diabetes in those predisposed to it, is increasing.

There are many complications of diabetes. It is the leading cause of blindness. Diabetics are seventeen times more prone to kidney disease than nondiabetics, twice as prone to stroke, five times as prone to gangrene, and have a greater risk at childbirth. According to the American Diabetes Association, the economic toll of diabetes mellitus is estimated at $5 billion per year.

About diabetes

In 1889 French pathologists Oskar Minkowski and Baron Joseph von Mering set out to determine if the pancreas gland was essential to life. In an experiment that would no doubt have riled today's antivivisectionists, they surgically removed the gland from several dogs to see what would happen. If the reported story is true, a remarkable bit of serendipity occurred the next day when a laboratory caretaker noticed that the dogs' urine was attracting an unusual number of flies. Minkowski and von Mering analyzed the urine and found in it a high concentration of sugar. They reasoned that removal of the pancreases had led to a disruption of sugar metabolism and a condition resembling diabetes.

Minkowski and von Mering tried to cure their surgically created diabetic dogs by administering extracts of the dogs' pancreas glands by mouth. Countless other researchers attempted the same experiment, and all were continually frustrated. Today we know why: insulin is a protein that is inactivated by enzymes in the mouth.

The breakthrough finally occurred on July 30, 1921. Canadian researchers Frederick Banting and Charles Best injected their insulin isolate in diabetic dogs, and the blood sugar levels fell. The news spread rapidly, and insulin was soon widely used in humans with good results.

Today we know more about the pancreas and its role in diabetes. The pancreas is a gland in the back of the abdominal cavity lying within the curve of the duodenum, or first part of the small intestine. It has an exocrine portion, which produces digestive juices and excretes them into the small intestine, and an endocrine portion, the islets of Langerhans, which produce insulin and other hormones that regulate the blood sugar.

Within the islets there are at least four different types of cells. Alpha cells secrete the hormone glucagon, which raises the level of glucose in the blood. Beta cells, which make up 75 percent of the islets, secrete insulin. Delta cells secrete the hormone somatostatin, which interferes with the secretion of both insulin and glucagon. Pancreatic polypeptide cells (F cells) produce another hormone, the function of which is not clear.

After a meal, the blood glucose levels begin to rise as glucose is absorbed from the stomach. In response to the rising sugar levels, beta cells secrete insulin, which travels throughout the bloodstream assisting various organs to convert the sugar into energy. Anything that disrupts this function at any stage can lead to increased blood sugar and diabetes. The beta cells can be interfered with in their production of insulin, or insulin may be produced normally but prevented from working at its targets.

Current understanding of diabetes has led to new terminology. Gone are the terms *juvenile diabetes* and *adult diabetes*. The new semantics recognize that the many causes of diabetes require different approaches. Diabetes is now classified in a spectrum ranging from potential or statistical risk to frank disease. Two major types, however, have been distinguished. Diabetes that requires insulin for therapy, so-called insulin-dependent diabetes mellitus (IDDM), is the disease formerly termed juvenile diabetes. The second major type is non-insulin-dependent diabetes (NIDDM), formerly called adult diabetes, which generally does not require insulin for therapy.

The research war on diabetes and its causes has many fronts. When all the evidence is put together, diabetes appears to be related to three factors: infection by one or more viruses, genetic tendency, and the body's ability to turn against itself—the so-called autoimmune mechanism.

Diabetes and virus infection

The relationship of virus infection to diabetes mellitus has been known for some time. In 1899 a case of diabetes following an attack of the mumps was reported by Dr. H. F. Harris, a Philadelphia physician, in the *Boston Medical and Surgical Journal* (forerunner to the *New England Journal of Medicine*). More recently, diabetes has been commonly observed to begin during or after attacks of viral infections such as hepatitis, mononucleosis, and coxsackie flu syndrome. The disease has also been seen in laboratory animals after they have been injected with coxsackie viruses. Furthermore, diabetes has a seasonal incidence, most often occurring during the winter flu season. The first proof that a virus could actually cause diabetes mellitus came in 1979.

CASE HISTORY

After two days of muscle aches, headaches, sore throat, and other flulike symptoms, a ten-year-old Washington, D.C., boy rapidly became lethargic and collapsed. He was taken to the hospital, where he was found to have diabetes, with a blood sugar level of 600 mg (the normal level is 120 mg or less). He was given insulin, but after an initial improvement he worsened, lapsed into a coma, and died seven days later. At autopsy, pathologist Dr. Marshall Austin of the National Naval Medical Center in Bethesda, Maryland, found that the insulin-secreting beta cells in the islets of Langerhans in the boy's pancreas had been destroyed by inflammation. Samples of the inflamed pancreas were taken to the National Institutes of Health laboratories of Dr. Abner Notkins, who had been doing research on viruses and diabetes in mice for some time.

Dr. Notkins and his associate virologist Ji-Won Yoon were able to isolate a virus known as coxsackie B4 from the boy's pancreas. They injected the virus into lab mice, which promptly developed diabetes with beta cell damage and increased blood sugar. Later, the same coxsackie B4 virus was isolated from the blood of the mice. Subsequent analysis of samples the boy's blood taken on admission and before death showed rising antibody titers to the same virus, proof that it was not a contaminant. He definitely had an infection by the coxsackie B4 virus.

This case was recently reported in the *New England Journal of Medicine* and was greeted with much fanfare in medical circles. In the same issue of the journal Dr. Allan Drash of Pittsburgh's Children's Hospital suggested that "this established as clearly as we can today that a virus can cause diabetes." This conclusion was reinforced by a report released in the July 1980 issue of the *British Medical Journal* documenting that 11 patients developed diabetes after a recent outbreak of infectious hepatitis.

Obviously there is more to the cause of diabetes than viral infection, or everyone with a viral infection would develop diabetes. Coxsackie B4 virus, for example, is found in the blood of half the population, yet only .5 percent develop diabetes. Other factors must clearly be involved. But a relationship between viral infection and diabetes might mean that a vaccine could someday be developed to prevent the disease in people who are at high risk to contract it.

Diabetes and heredity

Diabetes tends to run in families; the familial nature of the disease has been recognized for some time. Since members of the same family often share the same diet and environment, however, a high incidence of diabetes in a family does not necessarily mean that genetics are involved.

The study of identical twins has shed light on the diabetes inheritance question. Working at King's College Hospital in London, Dr. David Pyke studied 100 pairs of identical twins in the early 1970s and found that when one twin of a pair developed diabetes after age fifty (usually non-insulin-dependent diabetes), the other also developed the condition within several years. If one twin developed diabetes before age forty (usually insulin-dependent diabetes), the other one did in only 50 percent of the cases. The conclusion is that non-insulin dependent diabetes is primarily genetically determined, but additional factors are needed to trigger insulin-dependent diabetes. If insulin-dependent diabetes were entirely genetically determined, both twins should have developed the condition, since both share the same genes.

Tissue typing also gives strong evidence for the genetic role in diabetes. Everyone's tissue can be characterized by its HLA (for human leukocyte) antigens, proteins on the surfaces of body cells. Certain antigens are seen in patients with specific conditions and are therefore markers that the patient is predisposed to the disease (see "Update: Genetics," pages 224–239). The antigens are determined by genes on the sixth chromosome and an area on that chromosome called the HLA complex. Several genes in this area have been seen frequently enough in diabetic patients that researchers feel they may be important determinants of diabetes. How genes lead to diabetes is not yet known, but it is thought that they make the beta cells more susceptible to damage by other agents.

Diabetes and autoimmunity evidence

The human body has the ability to make

antibodies to fight off invading cells. This is called the immune response. Sometimes, in so-called autoimmune reactions, the immune response is deranged and the body manufactures antibodies against some of its own cells. In the mid-1970s three English researchers found evidence for the autoimmune phenomenon in diabetics. They found that 85 percent of children with newly discovered diabetes had antibodies to islet beta cells in their bloodstream. When all the beta cells disappeared, as the diabetes progressed, the antibodies vanished. Some have speculated that viruses act in diabetes by the autoimmune mechanism. Instead of affecting the pancreas directly, the virus may, they feel, produce an autoimmune reaction which in turn kills the beta cells.

Exactly how genetic factors, virus infections, and autoimmune phenomena fit together to produce diabetes is still a mystery. All may not be necessary in every case, or other as yet unknown factors may be at work. But all three are clearly involved, and we have certainly come far from the one disease–one cause concept of diabetes that existed just a few years ago.

Measuring blood sugar

Many years after their disease is discovered, a high percentage of diabetics develop nerve and blood vessel damage, kidney disease, and blindness, despite the insulin they take each day. Many researchers suggest, therefore, that blood sugar control has nothing to do with the development of these complications and that other factors may be involved. Most diabetic specialists, however, feel that there is a relationship between blood

sugar control and the long-term complications of diabetes, and that better control of blood sugar will result in fewer long-term problems. They further suggest that conventional insulin therapy does not really provide good blood sugar control, and that our current tests for blood sugar are not capable of demonstrating the long-term control.

The current blood sugar test measures the level of blood glucose at the time the blood was drawn. Hours earlier or later that value may be radically different. The only way to measure glucose control throughout the day with conventional methods would be to perform an unrealistic number of blood tests.

A new blood test developed by Dr. Kenneth Gabbay, at the Children's Hospital Medical Center in Boston, may provide information about long-term glucose control. The test, currently only a research tool because of its cost and difficulty, measures glucose buildup on hemoglobin molecules, called glycosolated hemoglobin or hemoglobin A_1C. Hemoglobin, the protein in red blood cells that carries oxygen, has a life span of 120 days in the bloodstream. After 120 days it is broken down, and new hemoglobin forms to take its place. During its life the hemoglobin takes up glucose molecules circulating in the blood and becomes hemoglobin A_1C. The higher the blood sugar over a long period, the more hemoglobin A_1C forms. Dr. Gabbay and his researchers have found that hemoglobin A_1C is about 5 to 7 percent of total hemoglobin in the nondiabetic patient. But in uncontrolled diabetics hemoglobin A_1C reaches 10 to 20 percent or more. The test developed by Dr. Gabbay is a long-term indicator; short-term fluctuations do not affect the

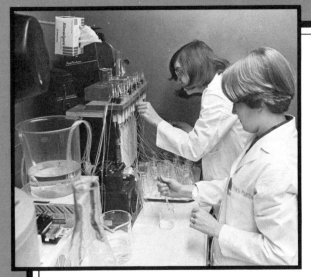

Original device developed in 1977 to conduct test for hemoglobin-A_1C, a new method of determining diabetes. (Photo by Bradford F. Herzog, courtesy Children's Hospital Medical Center, Boston)

results. According to Dr. Gabbay, "Glycosolated hemoglobin testing gives an average blood sugar level over the lifetime of the red blood cell." According to Dr. Arthur Rubenstein, a diabetes specialist in Chicago, "With glycosolated hemoglobin testing you can pick up in a minute the person who has had chronically poor control. Prior to this test you simply couldn't find that indi-

vidual." Some diabetologists question whether glycosolated hemoglobin testing will ultimately be a good monitor of glucose control. Further work is needed, but at least most specialists agree that the current blood glucose test is a poor monitor.

The artificial pancreas

Even though insulin therapy has been lifesaving, many specialists feel that insulin therapy as we know it today actually gives poor sugar control and that the difficulties this poor control causes patients is responsible for the long-term complications of diabetes that are so prevalent. One solution would be an artificial pancreas that mimics the action of the insulin-secreting beta cells. The normal pancreas keeps the blood sugar level within an acceptable range by a finely tuned balancing act. When blood sugar increases after a meal, insulin is released to help the body use that glucose. In hypoglycemic (low blood sugar) states such as fasting, other hormones are released to get more glucose into the bloodstream. Through this pro-

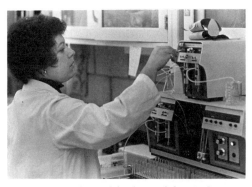

Device currently used for hemoglobin A_1C tests, now available at most major hospitals. (Photo by Bradford F. Herzog, courtesy Children's Hospital Medical Center, Boston)

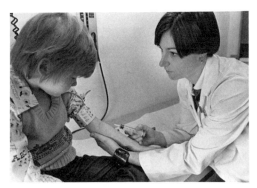

The new test for diabetes is performed with a simple blood sample. (Photo by Bradford F. Herzog, courtesy Children's Hospital Medical Center, Boston)

cess the level of blood glucose normally ranges from 70 to 120 mg. Because insulin is usually given to the diabetic only once or twice a day, however, the level of control can't approach that of the normal pancreas, and glucose swings as wide as 50 to 200 mg are common.

For years researchers have felt that an ideal artificial pancreas would have to provide both functions of the islet beta cells: producing and storing insulin; and monitoring the blood sugar and releasing insulin according to those glucose levels. At the University of Toronto, Drs. Albisser and Liebel have approached this idea with a device that continually withdraws blood, analyzes it for glucose, then triggers an appropriate amount of insulin to be released into the bloodstream. This feedback control, or closed-loop system, has kept the blood sugar of even brittle diabetics (those whose blood sugar is especially difficult to control) within a normal range. However, the system requires an array of instruments that literally fill a bedside area: an apparatus to withdraw blood, an analyzer to measure the glucose, a computer to correlate the insulin dose, and a portable pump to infuse the insulin. Further, it constantly bleeds the patient to sample the glucose concentration. If this state of the art in artificial pancreases is not ideal, perhaps the era of miniaturization will eventually provide a similar device that can be surgically implanted like today's cardiac pacemakers.

Many scientists now think that the continuous glucose-monitoring system, the most difficult part of an artificial pancreas to construct, may not really be necessary. Drs. William V. Tamborlane and Philip Felig at Yale University have successfully kept glucose under control with a pump that delivers a small or basal dose of insulin continuously, and larger amounts before meals, through a small needle implanted just under the skin and a portable pump that is attached to a belt. Their patients can go about their normal activities. Compared with the traditional once- or twice-daily insulin injection, this continuous infusion or open-loop system maintains glucose levels that approximate those provided by a normal pancreas. This system is different from the feedback or closed-loop artificial pancreas system of the Toronto researchers, in that blood sugar is not monitored. The insulin injections

Today's compact, portable insulin pump continuously injects a small amount of insulin through a needle implanted in skin. (Courtesy Joslin Clinic Diabetes Foundation)

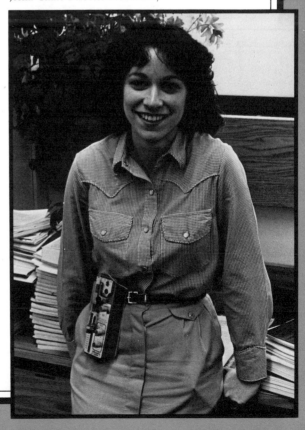

are preprogrammed but can be changed at any time with a manual override on the hip-held device.

Boston's Joslin Foundation and Clinic for diabetes, well known for its research on diabetes and treatment of diabetic patients, has also been using the portable insulin pump to regulate blood sugar. Doctors there hook their brittle patients up to a closed-loop artificial pancreas (similar to the one in Toronto, developed in conjunction with Miles Laboratories) to determine their insulin needs. With this information they program the portable insulin pump.

The Joslin physicians are extending the use of the portable pump to pregnant diabetics. "Women who are pregnant and diabetic have a particularly high incidence of babies with birth defects," notes Dr. Louis Vignoti. "Our preliminary studies show that the portable insulin pump may reduce that figure to compare with nondiabetic patients." The medical researchers hope to study 150 pregnant diabetics and as of this writing are looking for volunteers.

Dr. Vignoti reports that Joslin researchers are also working on an artificial pancreas that uses living cells. Insulin-producing beta cells from rats are placed inside a small sac, which is covered by a membrane that allows sugar molecules to pass in and insulin molecules to pass out. The sac is then implanted completely under the patient's skin. Large white blood cells, which would ordinarily respond to the rat beta cells and destroy them as foreign tissue, cannot pass through the membrane. The cells inside the membrane respond and react to the blood sugar level just like a normal pancreas. "The system works in rats and calves," Dr. Vignoti comments.

"Now we have to try it in people." This system has much promise, but it is not really an artificial pancreas; it is, rather, a form of pancreas transplantation.

Any of these systems will eventually supply the information needed to answer the persistent question of whether poor control of blood glucose is, in fact, the major factor in long-term complications. Commenting on artificial pancreas research in the *New England Journal of Medicine*, American Diabetes Association president Dr. Ronald Arky used a space-age metaphor: "Advancement toward an artificial pancreas is now beyond the 'stratosphere,' [and we] hope that, in a short time, the 'moon' will be reached."

Pancreas transplantation

With all the inherent difficulties in constructing and miniaturizing an artificial pancreas, there has been much interest in transplanting pancreas tissue or islet cells from one person to another. "If your own pancreas doesn't seem to work, why not get a bit of someone else's that does just fine?" said one prominent specialist. There is evidence that pancreas transplantation can prevent long-term complications. Dr. Mauer and his colleagues at the University of Minnesota have shown in laboratory animals that the kidney lesions of diabetes that develop after pancreas removal disappear when islet cells are transplanted, resulting in the return of blood sugar levels to normal.

Transplanting the whole pancreas is a very difficult surgical procedure. The location of the pancreas in the back of the abdominal cavity creates technical problems, and the digestive juices produced by the exocrine portion of the pancreas often interfere with healing. The transplanted pancreas literally eats away the protein and tissue of the recipient. However, islet beta cells alone have been transplanted by injecting them into veins near the liver. Dr. Paul E. Lacy and his colleagues at Washington University in St. Louis have shown that islet cells continue to function, even though removed from the pancreas, and restore blood sugar to normal levels. Therefore, they would make an ideal transplantation source.

As with the transplantation of any organ, rejection is the major problem (see "Update: Transplants," pages 172–185). The body rejects any tissue that isn't similar to it, and in the case of the pancreas, that rejection proceeds vigorously. Drugs can suppress rejection, but, at the moment anyway, the side effects of these drugs are a poor alternative to those of long-term insulin use. Until the rejection problem is solved, pancreas transplantation won't be practical.

Recently, Dr. Lacy seems to have solved the problem in rats by isolating the islet cells from healthy rats in a tissue culture at sub-normal temperatures for one week before injecting or transplanting them into diabetic rats. After only one dose of a drug to suppress rejection, the new rats began to make insulin with the transplanted cells, and they have continued to do so for several months. If this procedure can be demonstrated successfully in humans, pancreas transplantation without the complications of suppressive drugs might be a valuable treatment alternative, particularly if a way could be found to use donor tissue from animals. Certainly it solves the problems that the artificial

pancreas models have only attempted to do by providing both blood sugar level monitoring and insulin secreting.

Somatostatin

Any report on diabetes has to include a few words about somatostatin. This naturally occurring small protein (it is composed of only fourteen amino acids) affects blood sugar levels. Originally discovered in the brain as a growth hormone inhibitor by researchers at the Salk Institute in 1972, it has subsequently been found in other tissues, including pancreas islets. Work by Dr. John Gerich at the University of California and Dr. Roger Unger at the University of Texas Southwestern Medical School has suggested that somatostatin can improve sugar control in 25 percent of patients with insulin-dependent diabetes when used along with insulin. Apparently it works by suppressing glucagon, the hormone produced by the pancreas to increase blood sugar as part of its balancing act.

However, glucagon probably does not have an essential role in diabetes mellitus because large amounts of it do not cause sugar intolerance, in either non-diabetic or diabetic subjects. Even though further work is under way to clarify its actions, the ultimate role of somatostatin may be limited because it interferes with digestion and nutrient absorption.

Insulin synthesis

The exciting field of genetic engineering is making an impact across the spectrum of medicine. Many scientists feel that bacterial cells can eventually be made to produce large amounts of insulin in the laboratory. The procedure involves either making a copy of the DNA that produces insulin or putting genetic material from body tissues into bacterial cells which in turn produce the insulin (see "Update: Genetics," pages 224–239). In 1978 researchers at the City of Hope National Medical Center in Duarte, California, took the first step by chemically creating some fragments of the gene that produces insulin. Scientists at the San Francisco Genetic Engineering Laboratories of Genentech Incorporated assembled these fragments and inserted the synthetic genes for each of the two insulin chains into the bacteria *Escherichia coli*. The bacteria began turning out insulin chains, in effect becoming bacterial factories. Such production on a large scale would dramatically increase the supply of insulin, which currently is available only from pork or beef pancreases and is therefore limited. Genetic engineering could also produce insulin identical to that produced normally in the human body and would eliminate the adverse reactions to commercial insulin that are sometimes, although infrequently, seen.

One possible result of DNA research is learning exactly how human genes operate to make insulin. This information may make it possible to remove the beta cells of a diabetic, alter their DNA to improve their insulin-producing ability, then replant them in the body. This would, of course, be the ultimate in genetic or repair shop engineering.

The eye and diabetes

On the opthalmology front the war against diabetes has made exciting strides. After years of impaired sugar control, diabetics eventually develop a thickening of the small blood vessels and poor circulation. As a result, many new blood vessels develop to provide alternate paths of blood flow. In the eye, these new vessels are fragile, and can easily break and significantly reduce vision. So great is the problem with small vessel disease in the eye that diabetes is the number-one cause of blindness. Eighty percent of all insulin-dependent diabetics eventually progress toward blindness. The argon laser and xenon arc, by attacking new blood vessel growth, have reduced visual loss by over 50 percent in treated patients, according to the ongoing National Early-Treatment Diabetic Retinopathy Study.

Diabetics also develop visual difficulties because of cataracts. High blood sugar eventually finds its way to the lens, where it is converted to sorbitol, which causes clouding and cataracts. At the Massachusetts Eye and Ear Infirmary, experiments on aldose reductase, the enzyme that effects the change of glucose to sorbitol, are under way. If the action of the enzyme is inhibited, sorbitol and resulting cataracts do not form.

A cure for diabetes

Fifty years ago, Dr. Elliot P. Joslin, noted researcher and founder of Boston's famed Joslin Clinic for Diabetes, stated that the treatment of diabetes was a triad: "diet, insulin, and exercise." That is still true today. Insulin is the primary treatment for insulin-dependent diabetes, although diet and exercise may influence the dosage needed. In non-insulin-dependent diabetes, the body's sensitivity to insulin is impaired, so diet and exercise play a major role in treatment. Eighty percent of patients with maturity-onset diabetes are obese. Most can be treated by diet alone, according to the American Diabetes Association; the body's sensitivity to insulin improves with weight loss. Few patients follow diets for any extended period, though, and so the track record of dietary management of maturity-onset diabetes is understandably poor. Behavior modification is the obvious answer; only an altered life-style can ultimately regulate dietary intake.

Exercise helps control weight by increasing the number of calories used each day, but it may also improve the body's sensitivity to insulin. Too often medications are given to reduce insulin resistance in patients with maturity-onset diabetes at the expense of proper diet and exercise, which can have the same effect. Again, some patients may require drug therapy, but the potential impact of life-style, exercise, and diet should not be minimized.

The prospect of a life with diabetes mellitus is hard to accept, particularly in view of the long-term complications that seem inevitably to occur. If research on mechanical devices, transplants, genetic engineering, and eye surgery continues to be successful, the life expectancy of a diabetic, which has risen to one-third less than that of a nondiabetic person, will increase dramatically. Even more important, by reducing blindness and nerve and blood vessel disease, the quality of a diabetic's life will improve. All this, however, does not constitute a cure. Not until further research on diabetes enables scientists to understand its causes will excitement about a diabetes cure be real. And while that cure has yet to be found, it may be in sight today.

Resources

Referrals for diabetes treatment and diagnosis are best handled through your doctor, hospital, or state medical society. The best sources of reliable information are:

■ American Diabetes Association
National Office
600 5th Avenue
New York, New York 10020
212-541-4310

(American Diabetes Association state or regional offices are listed in your telephone directory.)

■ National Diabetes Information Clearinghouse
805 15th Street, N.W.
Suite 500
Washington, D.C. 20005
202-638-7620

■ Juvenile Diabetes Foundation
23 East 26th Street
New York, New York 10010
212-889-7575

(Juvenile Diabetes Association regional offices are listed in your telephone directory.)

■ Each United Way office is independent and may or may not have association with a local or regional diabetes society. Contact your local office of the United Way (listed in your telephone directory) or:

United Way
National Office
801 North Fairfax Street
Alexandria, Virginia 22314
703-836-7100

For the past few years, U.S. Senator George Proxmire and his staff have presented Golden Fleece Awards to obscure research projects which seem to lack any apparent value.

If these awards were given earlier in this century, research that eventually led to major medical breakthroughs might well have earned Golden Fleece distinction. For major medical breakthroughs—those discoveries that have altered the shape of medicine—most often result from basic research in related fields—physics, chemistry, optics, biology—and the initial work may seem trivial to the ignorant eye.

Genetic research, for example, began with studies of plants and fruit flies. Fiber optic techniques, today used to observe and treat the body's inner recesses, were originally developed for use in the communications industry. The CAT scan's development stems from radiation technology experiments conducted by physicists; today the CAT is virtually irreplaceable for specific kinds of head and body X-ray examination. And the sonar techniques used to track submarines in war led to the subsequent use of ultrasound in medicine.

Planned research seldom produces breakthroughs. The potential application of a specific finding must be recognized by a perceptive and foresighted scientist. As Albert Einstein once observed: "Do not stop to think about the reasons for what you are doing, about why you are questioning. Curiosity has its own reasons for existence."

BREAKTHROUGHS

Microsurgery

The natives came by degrees to be less apprehensive of any danger from me. I would sometimes lie down and let five or six of them dance on my hand.

Jonathan Swift
"A Voyage to Lilliput,"
Gulliver's Travels, 1726

Imagine being Gulliver on the island of Lilliput and being asked to perform even a simple task, and you will have some idea of the problems today's microsurgeons face. These specialists concentrate on parts of the body barely visible to the naked eye—tissues as thin as paper, blood vessels and nerves no thicker than a pin. The gateway to their miniature world is the operating microscope, which greatly magnifies the surgeon's field and has opened new vistas for reconstructive surgeons.

Microsurgery is the use of a microscope to see and repair tissues too small to work on with the eye alone. Its development has been gradual, aided by the continuing invention of more delicate instruments and finer sutures (stitches) and by the expanding imagination of its practitioners.

Surgeons have used magnification to see small objects since the 1890s, when jeweler's loupes were first used. In 1921 Swedish physician Dr. Carl-Olaf Nylen first used a microscope to correct chronic ear infections, and for many years thereafter operating microscopes were used almost exclusively for conditions involving the ear. Today, however, microsurgery has applications in virtually every field of medicine. Microsurgeons can rebuild faces ravaged by cancer, prevent strokes, restore fertility, renew vision, and reattach extremities that have been severed.

From surgery to microsurgery

In a recent Palestinian excavation, the bones of a Paleolithic Neanderthal man were found with one arm skillfully amputated at the elbow. Rocks and flints were the only instruments when this young man lived 40,000 years ago, but it is the earliest known case of successful surgery. Flints eventually gave way to bronze tooth saws, and they to the elaborate ebony- and ivory-handled instruments of the barber surgeon, whose striped barber pole symbolizes the white of gauze against a blood-red background.

Today's delicate stainless steel scalpels, probes, and forceps reflect the range of operations in the surgical battery. Each surgical specialty has equipment designed specifically for the problems at hand, from the saws, screwdrivers, and plates of the orthopedist to the long narrow clamps of the vascular surgeon. Similarly, microsurgeons have equipment unique to their field—instruments and sutures that reflect the fragility and size of the tissues they encounter.

The operating microscope, a $20,000 unit, magnifies the field and the body tissues and organs up to forty times while providing bright, clear viewing. Foot pedals move, adjust, and focus the microscope, freeing the surgeon's hands for the delicate work of the operation. Two viewing scopes permit both a chief surgeon and a first assistant to work together, and a television screen can often be connected so that other members of a surgical team can follow the procedure.

Connecting the ends of blood vessels that are as narrow as paper clip wires re-

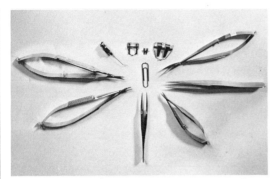

Tiny and delicate microsurgical instruments reflect the size of the body structures on which they are used. (Courtesy Rush-Presbyterian St. Luke's Hospital, Chicago)

quires sutures that are finer than human hair. The needles themselves are .003 inch in diameter, about the breadth of a baby's eyelash, small enough to pass through the eye of a sewing needle. Up to twenty sutures must be precisely and evenly placed around the circumference of a typical 1/16-inch-diameter blood vessel so that blood flow can be restored without leaking through the suture site. (Imagine two marks on a piece of paper 1/16 inch apart and trying to put 8 to 10 dots between these two marks.) The sutures must be tied with exactly the right amount of tension. If they are too tight, a clot forms and the junction is useless. If they are too loose, blood leaks through the opening.

Surgeons who specialize in microsurgery must learn a new approach to surgery. The tissues cannot be touched or handled directly lest they tear. All tissue handling is done with fine instruments.

Over the years, surgeons have designed instruments when those commonly available were inadequate for their needs. Similarly, microsurgeons have developed their own tools for working with these delicate sutures. Tiny forceps, scissors, and clamps made of the lightweight metal titanium were patterned after jeweler's instruments. Handling instruments this small requires skill and an obviously steady hand. Any movement or twitch can destroy the paper-

thin tissue. Magnified thirty to forty times by the microscope, "such a twitch looks like an explosion on the viewing screen," says one microsurgeon.

It takes three to four years to master microsurgical skills. Surgeons in training practice placing sutures in fine rubber or plastic sheets or tubing. Only when proficient with handling the small instruments do they graduate to living tissue—first on the tiny light blood vessels of small laboratory animals (which approximate the size of an artery in the finger), then at last to human tissue in clinical situations. Microsurgeons must have patience and endurance and be able to work for hours at a time looking through the microscope. During long operations surgeons frequently spell each other to relax their weary muscles and relieve the intense pressure.

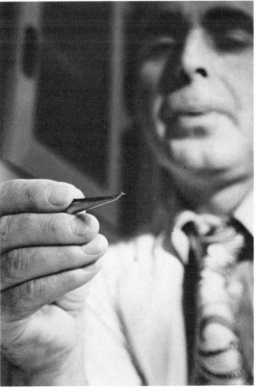

A microsurgical needle is only .003 inch in diameter, barely visible to the human eye. (Courtesy Rush-Presbyterian St. Luke's Hospital, Chicago)

Microsurgery and replantation

CASE HISTORY

R. K. is a seventeen-year-old music student in New York City and a serious flutist with a promising classical career. While returning from school one evening she was pushed by a stranger into the path of an oncoming subway train, and her right hand was cut completely off. Coming quickly to the scene, alert policemen put the severed hand into a bag of ice from a nearby restaurant. R. K. was rushed to Bellevue Hospital, where surgeons began an operation to reattach the hand to her arm, an operation that took fifteen hours to complete and was successful. Several months have passed since then. Though much rehabilitation is necessary, there is hope that R. K. may use her hand to play her music again.

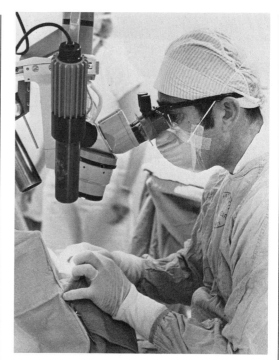

Today's microsurgeon uses an operating microscope to magnify the operating field. (Courtesy Rush-Presbyterian St. Luke's Hospital, Chicago)

This dramatic story made headlines in the spring of 1979. But this was not the first time that surgeons had successfully reattached a severed limb. Chinese surgeons pioneered replantation as early as the 1960s. The landmark event involving limb replantation in the United States took place in Boston in 1972, when Massachusetts General Hospital surgeons performed the operation on a young man whose arm had been severed in a freak accident. Since then, replantation of fingers, arms, and legs has been successfully accomplished hundreds of times all across the country.

Reattaching a severed body part involves more than simply putting the parts back together, however. Beneath the smooth covering of skin is a complicated array of blood vessels, nerves, tendons, bones, and muscles. Each has its own specific and exact function, and each must be intact if brain signals are to be properly translated into motion.

A replantation operation can be performed only if the severed body part has been protected in ice immediately after the injury to prevent deterioration of its tissues. The operation itself must be performed as soon as possible after the injury.

In replantation surgery, severed ends of each of the interior structures must be located, carefully matched to their mates, and delicately reconnected. Bone ends are pinned together. Muscle bodies, coverings, and tendons are sutured together. Blood vessels must be carefully reconnected so that their interiors remain open to restore their function as a conduit for blood.

Perhaps the most delicate part of a replantation operation is reattaching the severed ends of nerves, which must be done if the reconnected part is to feel pain and touch, hot and cold, and move again. Within each nerve are many bundles of individual fibers. Unless those bundles are exactly matched, messages from the brain can never reach the right areas of skin or the right muscle.

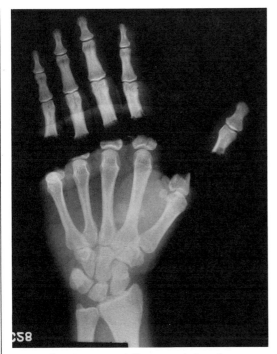

X ray showing severed fingers and thumb, the result of an electric saw injury. This type of damage is typical of the challenge faced in replantation surgery.

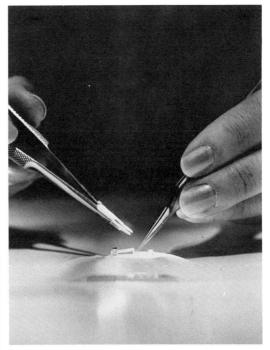

All microsurgical ties must be placed using instruments; direct use of hands would tear delicate sutures and body structures.

Not every person with a traumatic amputation is a candidate for replantation. Sometimes the severed body part is too crushed or mangled to be of any use to the patient—provided that surgeons could even reattach it successfully. If too many nerve ends have been destroyed, the limb may never regain the proper sensation or function.

Ingenuity becomes a key tool in treating cases that don't qualify for replantation. Restoring proper function often requires "rearranging" body parts, as the following case from the Children's Hospital Medical Center in Boston demonstrates.

CASE HISTORY

Sixteen-year-old New Hampshire student C. R. was on vacation in Florida when he lost the thumb and index finger of his right hand in a band saw accident. Surgeons at *the local hospital were unsuccessful in an attempt to reattach the thumb. Sometime later he consulted plastic and reconstructive surgeons at the Children's Hospital Medical Center in Boston, who proposed an operation to transfer one of his large toes to replace the missing thumb. A team of surgeons operating for twelve hours was successful in giving C. R. a new thumb. He now has good mobility and feeling, and is doing well.*

"We call it a 'thoe,' " comments Dr. Joseph Upton, a plastic surgeon who was a member of the Children's Hospital team that operated on C. R. "It's a toe replanted on the hand to replace the missing thumb. The thumb is the most important digit on the hand and must be replaced if the hand is going to have anything more than minimal movement. The great toe is the closest we can get to a thumb. Transferring it restores much of the function that was lost in the accident." Microsurgical techniques and the operating microscope have made such innovations possible. The first toe-to-thumb transfer was reported in 1968, and toe-thumb transfers are now performed in many medical centers with a high rate of success.

After a replantation or substitute transplantation, it takes about ten days before surgeons know whether the replanted part will survive. "If it survives for ten days, the chances are it will survive permanently," one surgeon comments.

Rehabilitation after a replantation is a lengthy process. Circulation is restored during the operation, but function and sensation do not return immediately. Tendons take one month to heal; bones take two to three months; nerves regenerate at a rate of one inch per month. It can take six months before sensation and function are restored in a replanted finger, and even longer when a limb is involved.

Surgeons have had the most success with the replantation of digits—fingers and toes. Dr. Robert Schenck, director of hand

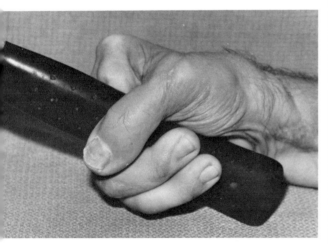

A "thoe." This patient's thumb was lost in a tractor accident. The new "thumb" is actually the patient's big toe, which has been replanted on his hand to restore grasp. (Courtesy Rush-Presbyterian St. Luke's Hospital, Chicago)

surgery at Rush-Presbyterian-St. Luke's Medical Center in Chicago, and one of the pioneer microsurgeons in the United States, puts the replantation operation into perspective: "Although the success rate for replantation of digits is excellent, major limb replantation is still 'frontier surgery.' It still involves some of the best and some of the worst results." And, cautions Dr. Schenck, "the replanted part is never as good as it was originally." A replanted arm may be shorter, a replanted finger stiff. To patients who have undergone replantations, however, these limitations are minor compared with the advantage of having the part in place again.

Microsurgery and plastic surgery

One of the most radical advances made possible by the techniques of microsurgery is called free flap transfer. "In this plastic surgical procedure," explains Dr. John Curtin, director of plastic surgery at the Rush-Presbyterian-St. Luke's Hospital in Chicago, "a large portion of skin and its underlying tissue are transferred to another part of the body to cover a skin defect at that site." Arteries and veins in the free flap are connected to similar vessels at the new site. The procedure of reattaching severed hollow organs such as blood vessels is called anastomosis. Without this attachment, such a large skin piece would die because of lack of circulation.

Free flaps are frequently performed on patients who have lost a large piece of skin in an accident or who have had major surgical resections (skin removals) for cancer. "In the past," notes Dr. Curtin, "it was the practice of many cancer surgeons after removing the tumor to leave the wound open for approximately a year to make sure that there was no recurrence of the cancer." This was particularly prevalent in head and neck cancers. Such a situation could be devastating to the patient's morale. In fact, "there has been a very high incidence of suicide among these pa-

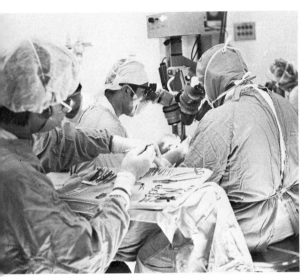

The operating microscope has two sets of eyepieces so a second surgeon or assistant can also view the operating field. (Courtesy Rush-Presbyterian St. Luke's Hospital, Chicago)

tients," says Dr. Curtin. Now free flaps can be used to reconstruct the mouth or repair a ravaged face, to rebuild an esophagus or to cover major skin defects. In all these circumstances and more, new thick skin covering is a must for healing to take place.

The free flap procedure replaces a technique called pedicle flap, which was also used to cover skin defects. In this older procedure, which was done in several steps over many months (many of which were spent in the hospital), patients often were forced to assume grotesque and tortuous positions with one arm attached to a stomach or face, or both legs attached together, while the transfer of skin from one location to another was being accomplished. Microsurgeons can now do the same thing in one step in a few hours.

Restoring fertility with microsurgery

The leading method of birth control around the world is neither the oral contraceptive nor the diaphragm nor the IUD. It is voluntary sterilization. In the United States alone, 10 million people have chosen vasectomy or tubal ligation for contracep-

tion. Recognizing its "permanence," many hospitals require consent forms signed by both husband and wife before the procedure is perfomed. All too often, though, the permanence of sterilization creates a later crisis for many people when unforeseen circumstances lead them to change their mind about not having more children.

In a sterilization operation, the tubes of the reproductive organs (vas deferens in men, Fallopian tubes in women) are cut in half and the ends tied. It is a short operation, lasting a half-hour or less, but the results are permanent. The reproductive cells cannot pass through the surgically created block, and the person is functionally sterile. Attempts to reconnect these tubes have been unsuccessful because of their small size. The male spermatic tube is ⅛ inch or less in diameter, but the inner opening barely permits a fine pin to pass through. The Fallopian tube is slightly larger in diameter but also extremely narrow inside.

Twenty-five to thirty thousand patients visit obstetricians and urologists each year hoping to undo a sterilization procedure. Using microsurgical techniques, physicians are now able to restore fertility and reverse sterilization with dramatic success in men and women alike. In several hundred cases, success rates ranging from 70 to 100 percent have been recorded. Pregnancies have followed in a high percentage of cases, usually within the first year after sterilization reversal, and no problems have been reported with either the pregnancies or the babies.

With microsurgery, Fallopian and spermatic tubes can be reconnected with great precision, ensuring an opening for the passage of ova or sperm. The operation is much more involved and expensive than the original sterilization—it may take three or four hours and cost $3,000 or more. Urologists who are reversing vasectomies with microsurgery report success rates as high as 95 percent. "Sperm begin to appear within a few weeks, and the sperm counts are normal within three to six months," comments St. Louis urologist Dr. Sherman Silver. University of British Columbia obstetrician Dr. Victor Gord has a success rate of nearly 90 percent in restoring fertility to women.

Surgeons who attempt sterilization reversals can't guarantee results. The operations are very delicate, and if much damage occurred during the original sterilization, subsequent attempts to reconnect the tubes may be very difficult. Patients who are about to undergo voluntary sterilization are cautioned not to take the procedure lightly, and to ask that their physicians remove as small a piece as possible from the spermatic or Fallopian tubes and to avoid using electrical cautery. This makes reconstruction easier should the patient want it later. "No one can predict the future," cites one urologist, "and what seems like a firm decision for sterilization now may be regretted in the future."

Microsurgery and the brain and nervous system

The brain has been recognized as one of the most complex organs since its microstructure was first studied by Bolognese anatomist Marcello Malpighi in the 1650s. Even in the past fifty years, despite the evolution of medical techniques, neurosurgical advances have come slowly. But today in this area of the body where anatomical structures are small and intricate and where one wrong move can mean death or a lifetime impairment, microsurgery is having a tremendous impact.

CASE HISTORY

R. T. is a fifty-five-year-old nurse. Other than a past history of diabetes she has had no significant medical problems. Three months ago she had a brief episode of right-sided weakness lasting less than three minutes, and since this experience took place on a stressful day, she ascribed it to nerves. But some weeks later, while eating dinner with her family, she suddenly became unable to speak, muttered in unintelligible phrases, and collapsed with extreme right-side weakness. En route to the hospital in the ambulance she regained her speech, and in the hospital her strength returned after several hours. A diagnosis of TIA (transient ischemic attack) was made. X-ray studies demonstrated a partial block in the left middle cerebral artery. A microsurgical operation restored blood flow, and she is doing well now, three years later.

TIA is a warning that blood flow to important brain structures is restricted. Further restriction could lead to stroke and a permanent loss of function. Partial or complete blockage of the blood vessels supply-

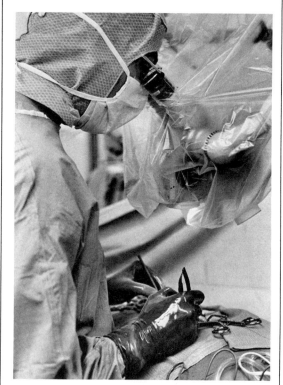

A neurosurgeon restores brain circulation to prevent a stroke. (Courtesy Rush-Presbyterian St. Luke's Hospital, Chicago)

ing the brain is one of the major causes of stroke. Of the half million new stroke cases that occur each year, one-third die within a month, and one-half of the rest become permanent invalids. Microsurgery has been highly successful in preventing strokes in susceptible patients by rerouting blood into an unobstructed artery, an operation that was impossible with traditional techniques.

In this operation, the surgeon locates a healthy, free-flowing artery on the scalp (usually the temporal artery, located just in front of and above the ear) and frees it from its attachments. Next, a one-inch hole is made in the skull and a section of the blocked artery is isolated. Using microsurgical techniques, the scalp artery is attached to the blocked brain artery, restoring its blood flow. A large percentage of strokes occur in this area, so the operation has great potential for preventing disability. Dr. Duke Samson, a neurosurgeon at the University of Texas Health Sciences Center, recently published a survey of arterial bypasses for stroke prevention. He found that it is more effective than medications in preventing strokes.

Elsewhere in the nervous system, neurosurgeons use miniature clamps and instruments to "clip off" aneurysms, small weaknesses in brain vessels that can and frequently do rupture, causing sudden death. Fifty percent of all patients with ruptured brain aneurysms die before they reach the hospital, and many more die shortly thereafter. Before microsurgery, the operation to repair this problem was dangerous. Johns Hopkins University neurosurgeon Dr. Melvin Apstein and his colleagues recently completed a survey comparing microsurgical and traditional surgical techniques for aneurysms. They found that with traditional operations as many as 70 percent of the patients died on the operating table, and as many as 50 percent of those for whom the operation is successful left the hospital with neurologic defects as a result of the operation. With microsurgery, 90 percent of the patients studied left the hospital normally. "Few things in medicine have had that kind of impact," the authors noted. The increased success in dealing with small structures through microsurgery has drastically reduced the operation's mortality rate.

Nerve and spinal cord injuries are also benefiting from the new surgical skills. Sections of nerve can be grafted when the severed ends of a damaged nerve are too far apart to pull together. Eventually, long-nerve grafts in patients with spinal cord injuries may restore at least partial feeling. In a spectacular case attempted recently at New York University Medical Center by its renowned microsurgical team, nerve grafts were attempted to restore function in a baby suffering from meningomyelocele, a condition of paralysis below the waist resulting from a poorly developed spinal cord. Unfortunately the results won't be known until the baby is old enough to begin walking.

In a report to the American Pain Society, Las Vegas and Virginia neurosurgeons described microsurgery for ruptured herniated lower back discs. They report decreased disability time, less blood loss, and fewer complications when the more accurate and meticulous operation is performed. Dr. Pat Williams of the University of Nevada at Las Vegas has operated on over 1,000 patients with disc problems and reports in *Medical World News* a 98 percent cure rate with microsurgical techniques: "By cure, I mean patients who are economically productive and comfortable with pain medication." With Williams's technique, his patients' hospital stays dropped from an average of nine days to three days.

Neurosurgeons are also now able to operate through the nose to remove pituitary tumors, which can cause acromegaly (gigantism) or Cushing's syndrome, which is rapidly fatal. Without the microscope,

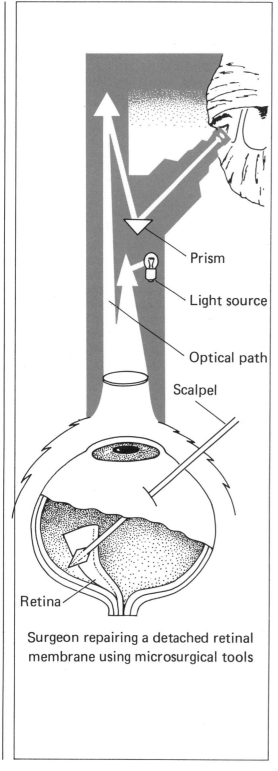

Prism

Light source

Optical path

Scalpel

Retina

Surgeon repairing a detached retinal membrane using microsurgical tools

surgeons previously had to go through the top of the head, risking damage to the optic nerve and perhaps blindness.

The range of microsurgery

Virtually every area of medicine has benefited from microsurgery, though not always as dramatically as in the preceding examples.

■ The ear, nose, and throat specialist relies on the operating microscope to correct middle ear problems and to operate on the vocal cords through the endoscope (see "Breakthroughs," pages 126–135).

■ Orthopedists have been able to transfer sections of bone with its blood vessels intact to repair or replace bone damaged by cancer or severe infections.

■ Plastic and general surgeons can reconstruct a breast after biopsy or cancer surgery.

■ Ophthalmologists can more easily remove cataracts, and in a procedure called vitrectomy they can restore vision by clearing away the bloody debris from rupture of blood vessels inside the eye, a problem that often affects diabetics in their later years. Microsurgical techniques in ophthalmology have also been used in repairing retinal detachments.

The future

The unique ability of microsurgery to permit the precise attachment of small blood vessels and nerves has made possible a procedure called "bench surgery." Primarily used in urology, bench surgery involves removing the organ, say, a kidney; repairing it while out of the body, "at the bench," as it were; and returning it to the body. Bench operations have been performed for kidney or ureteral stones, in reconstruction of kidney and blood vessels to reduce hypertension, and in repairing organs sustaining massive damage in an accident. The procedure was developed by microsurgeons at University Hospital in Boston.

New York University's Dr. William Shaw, the microsurgeon involved in R. K.'s hand reattachment, feels that bench surgery may someday offer a different approach to cancer management. "If cancer occurs in a specific organ or extremity, that part can be removed surgically, repaired 'at the bench,' given any appropriate chemotherapeutic drugs, then replanted back in the body," he notes. This would spare the rest of the body the unnecessary effects of chemotherapy, and stronger drugs could therefore be given. In laboratory studies experimenters have determined that a surgically amputated leg could remain unattached to the body for two to three days, if proper attention to cooling and preservation is maintained. This would obviously result in decreased function, "but that is certainly better than losing the leg and perhaps the life to cancer," Shaw concludes.

The technology of microsurgery makes it theoretically possible to work on structures that are smaller and more delicate than those being attempted today. But the human hand has limitations that the operating microscope, sutures, and instru-

Cataract operations and other delicate eye surgery require an operating microscope. (Courtesy Rush-Presbyterian St. Luke's Hospital, Chicago)

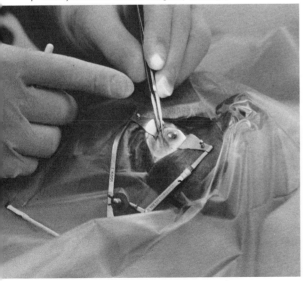

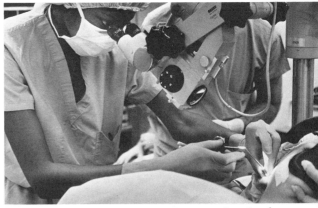

Delicate middle ear structures can be repaired with the aid of the operating microscope. (Courtesy Rush-Presbyterian St. Luke's Hospital, Chicago)

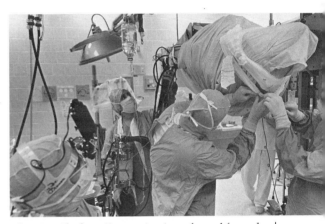

This "upside-down" operation is performed for sudden loss of vision due to retinal detachment. The surgeon at lower left monitors the operation through the magnifying device. (Photo by Bradford F. Herzog, courtesy Massachusetts Eye and Ear Infirmary, Boston)

ments do not. Instruments are now being designed to transfer the surgeon's movements to more precise mechanized ones.

The advancement of instrumentation as typified by the burgeoning specialty of microsurgery has enabled medicine to enter a new age of precision and to meet new challenges. "Where the telescope ends the microscope begins," wrote Victor Hugo in *Les Misérables*, "which of the two has the grander vision." For the many people who have benefited by microsurgery, the microscope has grand vision indeed.

CAT scanning

Come, come, and sit you down. You shall not budge! You go not till I set you up a glass Where you may see the inmost part of you.

William Shakespeare
Hamlet, ca. 1601

In 1963 a South African physicist, Dr. Allan McLeod Cormack of Tufts University, published a paper in the *Journal of Applied Physics* detailing a mathematical formula for reconstructing images using various X-ray projections. The paper was received with little or no fanfare in the medical community, and the author received only two or three requests for reprints.

Sixteen years later the fanfare was distinctly larger as Cormack was awarded a share of the Nobel Prize in medicine. His 1963 work, along with that of electronics engineer Godfrey Neubold Hounsfield in England and others, led to the development of the CAT scanner, now regarded as a revolutionary innovation in diagnosis.

CAT stands for *c*omputerized *a*xial *t*omography. It is a form of X-ray study that obtains a 360-degree picture of a small area of a patient's body—in effect, a slice image which one could say resembles a slice of ham. The X-ray device is called a CAT or CT scanner.

The award of the Nobel Prize to Cormack and Hounsfield was an unusual one for a variety of reasons: neither man was in medicine or had a doctoral degree; they worked independently—in fact, they had never met; and, interestingly, CAT theories were not their primary interest. Cormack considered his work a ''sideline,'' a respite from his major interest in subatomic particles.

Hounsfield developed the first CAT prototype in 1971, in the central research laboratory of London-based EMI, Incorporated. (Formerly Electronics and Musical Industries Limited, the company was best known previously for bringing the Beatles recording group to worldwide popularity.) EMI is now a giant in CAT scanner manufacture, and along with five other companies has produced the 2,000 or more units in worldwide use.

Computerized axial tomography often yields information not available by other techniques; it replaces other studies that are painful and sometimes dangerous; and it spares many patients unnecessary surgery. The most spectacular early innovation in CAT scanning was in brain and head diagnosis. Subsequent use in other areas of the body promises similar success.

The introduction of CAT scanning into radiologic diagnosis has also produced reverberations in the socioeconomic theater. The instrument is very expensive, perhaps more so than any other diagnostic tool. A hospital pays well over $1 million to install and begin operation of a CAT scanner, making the device too expensive to be purchased by every community hospital. Yet there has been a mad rush across the country to buy the equipment, spurred on no doubt by its overwhelming acceptance by the radiology community and vindicated perhaps by the Nobel Prize.

Another factor in the eyes of many is what has been called the ''technological imperative''—the desire to have the latest, most complex gadget. (In the case of CAT scanners this enthusiasm has been called ''CAT fever.'') To control the purchase of

CAT equipment and other similarly expensive paraphernalia, many state and federal agencies require certificate of need (CON) requests to be submitted by hospitals, and then they approve only a limited number, based upon utilization and a "state perceived need." Professional consumerists such as the Ralph Nader–affiliated health research group have supported these efforts. Critics of government regulation say such restriction reduces the quality of medical care available to the public, particularly when it applies to "state of the art technology." In many cases when health systems agencies have turned down CON requests for CAT scanners, physician groups have purchased the unit privately and installed it off hospital premises. California has thirty such private units, Florida twenty-five, and other states are catching up quickly. Estimates suggest that 20 percent of all CAT scanners in the country are in doctors' offices. Regardless of the eventual distribution of CAT scanning equipment, few would disagree with its intrinsic value.

What is CAT scanning?

German physicist Wilhelm Roentgen discovered X rays in 1895, and X-ray procedures have changed little since then. In traditional X-ray studies a cathode tube produces a wide beam of electrical energy (X rays) which is directed at photographic film. The patient stands between the tube and the film plate so that the radiation must pass through his or her body to reach the film. An image is produced on the film based on the property that radiation passes through objects at different rates depending on their densities. In the case of human tissue, bone, which has the highest density, restricts the passage of radiation and produces the least exposure, appearing white on the X-ray film. Similarly, air, with the lowest density, produces the highest exposure and appears black on the film. Muscles, organs, and other soft tissues fall somewhere in between as shades of gray. Traditional X rays are taken of only front or side views of the body.

The CAT scanner, on the other hand, uses a beam of X rays to provide a cross-sectional view of a part of the body. The X-ray tube is similar to that used in traditional X-ray units and the radiation is identical; however, lead shields with small holes called collimators narrow the X ray to a fine beam, which is then scanned across the body. An electrical detector on the opposite side of the patient replaces the film and receives the radiation, while another lead shield in front of the detector eliminates any radiation scattering. The X-ray tube and detector scan across the body and are rotated 360 degrees around the patient, repeating the scan from many different angles. A computer analyzes the information from each of the angles and produces a clear cross-sectional image on a

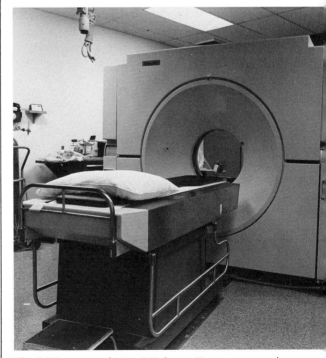

The CAT scanner obtains 360-degree X-ray views, resulting in a cross-sectional study. The X-ray tubes are located in the large circular device shown here.
(Courtesy Brigham and Women's Hospital, Boston)

screen, which can be photographed for storage. Several cross sections, one after the other, can be studied to re-create the whole body or organ part. Anatomical parts and their relationship to each other can be viewed with astonishing clarity in a way never before possible with conventional X rays.

The initial CAT prototype unit obtained 360 separate images for each slide, one for each degree as it rotated around the patient. A single cross-sectional view took as long as five minutes to complete and was restricted to areas such as the head, where no organ movement occurs to blur the photographic image. Subsequent generations of CAT scanners have a narrower cross section providing greater accuracy, and a wider beam, so that fewer individual images or passes need be made for each slice. In the latest version, detectors completely surround the patient and only the X-ray tube moves. Each slice can be completed in just a few seconds, which permits the study of all body areas, even those with moving parts. Just as a fast-action camera can "stop the action," so the new rapid CAT scan can stop bowel and organ activity to produce a clear image.

CAT vs. traditional X rays

As the traditional X ray passes through tissue, the beam casts an impression or shadow on photographic film. Such a two-dimensional view superimposes one organ onto another and makes discrimination between them nearly impossible.

With CAT scanning an X ray passes through tissue in the same manner, but an electrical detector replaces the X-ray film. The detector permits the precise computer analysis of tissue densities so that tissues may be clearly distinguished from one another. The CAT scan, then, provides a three-dimensional view of organs and allows a cross-sectional study of the body interior that was previously revealed only through surgery or autopsy.

Radiation and CAT scanning

In a time when most citizens are cautioned to avoid unnecessary exposure to X rays because of their harmful long-term effects, it is necessary to evaluate every diagnostic study involving X rays in terms of its radiation risk. CAT scanning involves multiple radiation exposures to produce one image, but the actual dose of radiation received is equal to or less than that of many conventional studies.

When a traditional X ray is taken, every area penetrated by the X-ray beam and appearing on the film gets the same amount of radiation, measured in rads. (A rad is a unit of X-ray exposure and a measure of radiation intensity.) In the case of a skull X ray, if radiation equal to ½ rad is used, every area in the head is exposed to ½ rad of radiation. Multiple views compound this exposure. In the traditional skull series four different views are taken, so the patient's head and every cell within it will then have received four times ½ rad, or 2 rads total exposure. With CAT scanning, each cross-sectional view requires 2 rads of exposure, but the cross sections are narrow

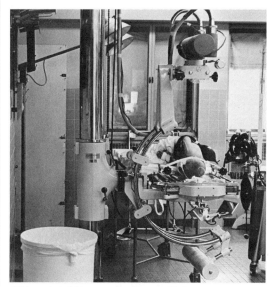

This painful X-ray procedure, called a pneumo-encephalogram, was the only means of scanning the head for years. (Photo by Daniel Bernstein)

and do not overlap, so the amount of radiation received by any cell in this example is the same with either technique, namely, 2 rads. In the case of kidney evaluation, many X rays are necessary in the standard IVP (intravenous pyelogram) X ray. The total radiation exposure may then be 3 or 4 rads or more. With CAT scanning of the kidney, narrow individual slice views limit the total radiation of the kidney to 2 rads, less than the standard.

CAT scanning and the head

The accurate diagnosis of intracranial medical problems such as brain tumors, abscesses and infections, hemorrhage or bleeding into the brain, and various congenital or developmental disorders has always been difficult. Standard skull X rays are valuably only in limited circumstances, and other studies are painful and often dangerous. For example, so-called pneumoencephalograms which involve injection of air into the chambers of the brain, and angiograms, which involve injection of contrast material that will appear on X-ray film into blood vessels, have mor-

tality rates of less than 1 percent. Up to 10 percent of these patients, however, can have complications or additional symptoms afterward. CAT scanning requires no invasive or surgical procedure and is therefore much less risky than these traditional studies. "With CAT scanning," says Dr. Howard Abrams, chairman of radiology at Boston's Peter Bent Brigham Hospital, "there has been a drastic fall in the number of more hazardous diagnostic procedures." Recent published studies show a 20 to 80 percent drop in pneumoencephalogram studies and 20 to 70 percent drop in angiogram studies since the advent of CAT.

Because of its high sensitivity, CAT scanning has increased the accuracy of neurologic diagnosis. In tumor diagnosis it is 96 percent accurate, in infections 95 percent accurate, and in demyelinating disease (which destroys nerve tissue, such as multiple sclerosis) up to 50 percent accurate. All surpass conventional techniques in this regard. In the diagnosis of brain hemorrhage due to stroke or trauma the superiority of CAT is perhaps most evident: accuracy rates approach 100 percent.

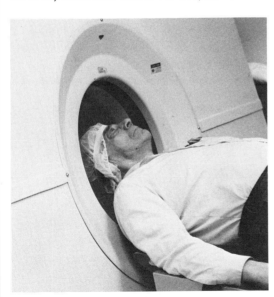

CAT scanning now permits painless and thorough head examination.

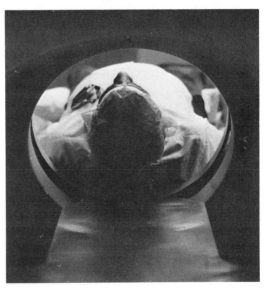

The CAT unit literally surrounds the patient's head. (Photos by Joseph Murphy)

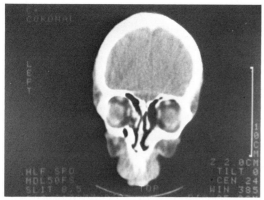

Coronal CAT scan of the head showing facial bones and sinuses, indicated by dark areas in center. Eye sockets and muscles can also be seen here. (Photo by Joseph Murphy)

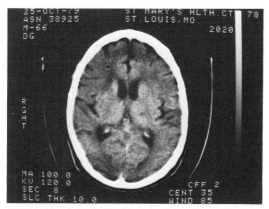

CAT scan of the brain. The skull is indicated by white area surrounding scan. Dark areas are cerebrospinal fluid which surrounds the brain, outlines the convolutions on its surface, and fills the spaces or ventricles in the interior. (Courtesy Ohio Nuclear)

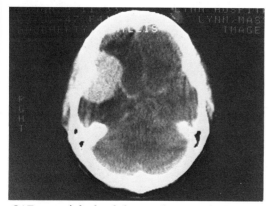

CAT scan of the head showing large tumor (light-colored area at upper left) with blood vessels leading into it. (Photo by Joseph Murphy)

CASE HISTORY

A. Y. is a nineteen-year-old college student without a past history of any significant medical problem. On a midsummer weekend evening he was driving home from a movie when his automobile was suddenly struck from the side by another. When the paramedical rescue unit arrived, they found him pinned in the wreckage, unconscious and unresponsive but still alive. Using the powerful extricating tool the Jaws of Life, A. Y. was removed from his car and transported to the local hospital emergency room within thirty minutes of the accident. He remained unconscious, was breathing poorly, and had changes in neurological signs suggesting hemorrhage and pressure on the brain. While plans were being made for possible emergency neurosurgery to relieve the pressure, a CAT scan demonstrated no bleeding, suggesting that the pressure would subside on its own, and cerebral or brain contusion was diagnosed. Surgical plans were canceled, and the patient was observed in the intensive care unit. Over several days, A. Y. gradually reawakened and has done well since. Now, three months later, he has returned to school and has no apparent complications from the accident.

Prior to CAT scanning, an unconscious patient with neurological changes might have been subjected to emergency surgery to clarify the diagnosis. The symptoms of bleeding and swelling are similar and difficult to distinguish. CAT scanning has become a benchmark of truth in head trauma; in A. Y.'s case it showed that bleeding did not occur and that surgery was not necessary. If bleeding had occurred, however, CAT would have demonstrated its exact location, the size of the clot, and its effect on adjacent brain structures, giving an excellent prognosis and lending direction to therapy. Other tests are no more than 50 percent effective in this regard. A study comparing therapy for head injuries before and after CAT was available showed the number of exploratory surgical procedures to be reduced by 94 percent with the advent of CAT.

As to the question of long-range disease outcome, CAT scanning has had major impact in a few areas, limited necessarily because effective treatment for cancer, stroke, and many neurologic problems is not yet available. But early and accurate diagnosis can improve the quality of life even if it doesn't necessarily lengthen it. As Dr. Abrams comments in a recent issue of the *Medical Tribune*, "The business of medicine is not necessarily to cure disease. Ninety percent of the time it is to resolve uncertainty . . . that is an enormous contribution to the quality of a patient's life." That CAT scanning has dramatically altered neurology and neurosurgical practice is confirmed by Boston University neurosurgeon Dr. Edward Spatz: "Knowing what we do now, neurosurgery before CAT was available was like practicing medicine in the Dark Ages."

CAT scanning and the body

The original use of CAT was for head scanning, and most certificates of need still restrict its use to this part of the body. Body scanning is quite different. Many physicians argue that CON restrictions lead to second-class care where medical diagnosis is concerned. Highly accurate and safe imaging studies are already available for the chest and abdominal organs and the extremities, and CAT will not replace them. Radiologists generally agree that it isn't enough for a new procedure to provide accurate information; it must add to, surpass, or give different information from what we already have, or be cheaper or safer. CAT is not an appropriate examination tool for the inside of the bowel, for example, to look for ulcers, polyps, bleeding, and so forth. Contrast studies such as

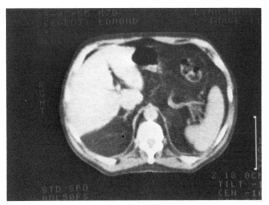

CAT body scan showing the liver at left and spleen at right, with blood vessels leading into the spleen. The spinal column, diaphragm, and aorta can also be seen. [Photo by Joseph Murphy]

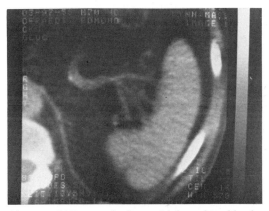

Close-up CAT scan of spleen with branching blood vessels. [Photo by Joseph Murphy]

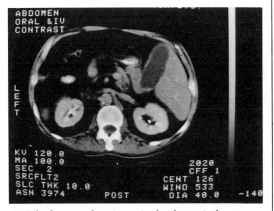

CAT body scan showing spinal column in lower center, kidneys on either side of spinal column, and liver at upper right. Ribs are shown by small white patches. A liver tumor is shown by dark area. [Courtesy Ohio Nuclear]

upper gastrointestinal and barium enema X rays, supplemented by direct visualization by endoscopy (see "Breakthroughs," pages 129–133), are already nearly 100 percent accurate. Angiography is still needed for the study of blood vessels. Ultrasound is preferred in studying medical problems in pregnant women (see "Breakthroughs," pages 118–120); and, because it is directed at a narrow slice of tissue, CAT is certainly not a substitute for films that provide a general screening of large organs or body regions or for nuclear medicine studies such as bone scans. Each CAT slice is less than ½ inch thick. It would take too many slices to scan completely a large organ or body part.

But CAT is highly effective in evaluating the precise anatomical location of solid masses and of their relationship to abdominal organs. CAT scanning is most useful when used in conjunction with information from other studies. If, for example, a tumor is noted in the kidney on IVP examination, CAT scanning makes it possible to plan therapy for that tumor. The tumor location can be exactly noted with respect to other organs, and its exact size and distance from the skin can be measured. Dr. Harold Weintraub, a CAT specialist at the Lynn Hospital, a community hospital north of Boston, states, "Therapy planning with CAT permits the radiotherapist to direct the X-ray therapy so that it strikes only the tumor and misses other organs. Because the study is so safe, the tumor can be evaluated and studied at frequent intervals, thereby assessing its response to therapy."

Many radiologists feel that CAT is now the method of choice to evaluate solid organs such as the liver, spleen, and pancreas, and areas of the body such as the pelvis where many different types of tissues and organs lie adjacent to one another. Such areas and organs have been notoriously difficult to evaluate, but using differences in water content and densities,

CAT can readily delineate organ and tumor boundaries and resolve anatomical detail to a degree not before possible. The CAT can determine tissue density differences as small as .5 percent, and identify tumors or masses as small as ¼ inch. Fine discrimination of areas even smaller than this is theoretically possible with CAT techniques, but it would require much larger doses and exposure of X rays than is desirable.

At the University of Kansas and other medical centers the effect of a CAT breast scan is being compared with traditional mammography and physical examination to diagnose breast cancer. In initial reports on over 1,000 patients, CAT scanning was 20 to 30 percent more accurate than mammography and up to two times more accurate than physical examination in identifying tumors as small as 1/16 inch in diameter. Traditional mammography cannot reveal a tumor less than ¼ inch in diameter.

Because of its precision in mapping various parts of the body, the CAT scan is now used as a guide for surgeons to obtain biopsies or perform delicate needle injections or aspirations. Most radiologists feel that CAT body scanning is in its infancy and that its continued use will extend or at least further define the limits of its potential.

Is it worth the cost?

If only it were free, there would be no debate about the uses of CAT scanning in medical practice. The CAT safely provides accurate and sensitive information. It has altered traditional treatments and made an impact on long-term survival. But CAT scanning is also expensive. There will be nearly 2,500 CAT units in the United States within the next few years, and the annual cost to the public is estimated at $1.5 billion per year—.7 percent of the total health care cost. When this much public money is involved, any tool must be evaluated carefully.

Not every hospital can afford to buy a CAT scanner. Many hospitals, however, cannot afford to be without one. "Every 400-bed hospital that has an active emergency room with patients who have head trauma or with an active neurosurgical staff needs a CAT scanner," notes Dr. Abrams.

A hospital pays about $750,000 to buy a CAT scanner. Repair and maintenance contracts, facility construction, operating staff, and physicians to interpret its work add considerably to that figure. To amortize this cost, hospitals charge between $150 and $500 per examination. Dr. Weintraub, whose CAT scanner is located in a 350-bed community hospital, is convinced it is worth the price. "The cost is coming down," he states. "The first scans three years ago cost about $400; now that we are using it more and for a greater variety of medical problems the cost has come down to $160." Weintraub's community-based department currently performs 6,000 scans per year—twice the recommended minimum number for proper utilization established by the Department of Health, Education, and Welfare.

While admitting that the examination is expensive, other radiologists point out that CAT scanning is actually saving money. "It isn't merely an additional health care expense," cites Dr. Carl Larson of Boston's Lahey Clinic Radiology Department. "Rather it replaces tests which were costly in their own right. In contrast to those tests which were often painful, hazardous, and required a hospital stay to perform, CAT scanning can safely be done on an outpatient basis." Furthermore, the many accurate diagnoses of CAT scanning often eliminate unnecessary operations and reduce patient days in the hospital. Several published studies have shown that the average length of stay for patients with neurological problems has diminished

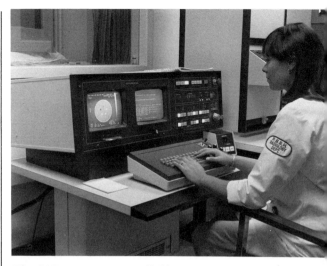

The CAT scanner is controlled by a computer console. The image appears on the viewing screen and may be photographed for permanent inclusion in the patient's records. (Courtesy Brigham and Women's Hospital, Boston)

since CAT diagnosis and the alternatives in therapy that it provides have become available. Cynics would undoubtedly point out that all hospital beds are full anyway—so that discharging a patient with a neurological problem two days earlier would only result in that bed's being filled by another patient with another problem, and therefore give no ultimate saving. According to health planners, though, alternatives to surgery and diagnostic procedures that do not require hospitalization will eventually reduce the inpatient load a community generates. The result can be smaller hospitals performing more efficient work with less staffing and expense—the long-term goal of health planning. Taking these factors into account, at least two studies, at the Toronto General Hospital in 1975 and by the Arthur D. Little Company in 1977, show no projected increase in health care costs from CAT scanning, even when anticipated 1980 figures are considered.

CAT has come a long way from the mathematical calculations of Professor Cormack in Medford, Massachusetts. While only recently found in major teaching hospitals, CAT units are now in demand by large and small hospitals alike. Those CAT scanners have given a new accuracy to diagnosis and a new perspective on treatment, but the examination requires sophisticated training and knowledge to interpret. According to Lynn Hospital's Dr. Weintraub, "There simply aren't enough [doctors] trained in CAT diagnosis to put one in every hospital and still be confident about their readings, even if those hospitals could afford to buy one." Cost notwithstanding, radiologists experienced in CAT diagnosis feel that at least 2,000 scans a year are the minimum to provide the necessary experience for reliable interpretation.

To overcome this problem, one company, American Medical Incorporated (AMI), which operates several hospitals throughout the United States has a novel approach. It has a fleet of twenty-one mobile CAT scanners, each mounted in a large truck and trailer, which make rounds to selected AMI-operated and other participating hospitals to provide CAT "curb service" to institutions that otherwise could not meet certificate of need volume requirements to buy a unit for themselves. Regardless of which approach is used, sharing facilities and regionalization efforts have proved effective.

In the final analysis, rigid government regulations for distribution of CAT units are not the answer. While attempting to serve the pubic interest, they often restrict the best medical care available. Medical science must take a greater role in its own policing. Physicians must continue to be critical of CAT scanning. Strict indications must accompany each order for CAT examination. An uncontrolled distribution of CAT units must not be allowed. If CAT scanning is to confer "the greatest benefit on mankind" per Cormack's Nobel Prize criteria, medical enthusiasm must be tempered with sound clinical judgment and proper attention to costs and benefits.

Ultrasound

... What surprised me was the clarity and force of the ASDIC indication. I had imagined something almost imperceptible, certainly vague and doubtful. I never imagined that I should hear one of the creatures asking to be destroyed. ... The ASDIC did not conquer the U-boat; but without the ASDIC the U-boat would not have been conquered.

Sir Winston Churchill
from The Second World War, vol. 1,
The Gathering Storm, 1948

The Allied Submarine Detection Investigation Committee (ASDIC) device Churchill noted and praised was actually sonar. Widely used for oceanographic depth recordings in the 1920s and 1930s and for submarine detection in the two world wars, sonar employs a pulse echo technique to bounce sound waves off the ocean floor and chart the echoes of the return of the waves. Mankind cannot, of course, exclusively claim sonar as a human invention; bats and other animals use similar internal systems to guide their travels and hunts.

Today, the principle behind sonar is one of the most rapidly expanding diagnostic techniques in medicine. Ultrasound (sonography or ultrasonography), which uses high-frequency sound waves to diagnose disease, has been around in one form or another for thirty years. But ultrasound's potential has been realized only in the past few years as the procedure to transform ultrasound waves into images has been developed.

Modern ultrasound technology has applications throughout general medicine and in many diverse medical specialties —from cardiology, where ultrasound can detect heart attacks and congenital or developed structural defects, to neurology, where the technique is used to predict strokes. Ultrasound has probably been greeted most enthusiastically in obstetrics, where it has special value because of its safety. Because no X rays or invasive devices are involved, ultrasound cannot harm or complicate reproductive structures or the developing baby. Ultrasound also has direct applications to therapy, often allowing doctors to perform lifesaving procedures that were impossible only a few years ago.

How ultrasound works

Sound waves of different frequencies are all around us. Ordinary speech, for example, is composed of waves between 100 and 400 cycles per second (hertz). A car's idling engine may be around 20 hertz. Your fine stereo receiver should be able to reproduce sounds over the frequency range of 16,000 to 18,000 hertz. These are the limits of human hearing. But although sound waves either above or below the frequency of human hearing can't be heard, they still exist. One example is the training whistle used to call dogs which is inaudible to humans yet can be heard by the animal. Sound waves used for medical purposes have frequencies ranging from 1 to 10 million hertz, far beyond the human ear's normal limits.

Medical ultrasonography had its beginnings in the late 1940s when three investigators reported that high-frequency sound waves could be directed into the body and reflected or echoed off internal organs. Drs. John Wild, Douglass Hawry, and Karl Dussek, using navy sonar equipment, made observations that formed the base of today's technology.

Ultrasound waves can be produced in many ways. In medical diagnostic instruments, the wave originates in a small crystal that vibrates when an electrical current is passed through it. The crystal is contained within a probe about the size of a hand-held microphone. When the probe is placed in contact with the skin, it transmits the ultrasound waves through the body in a straight line. As high-frequency sound waves pass through the body, they encounter the different densities of various organs and reflect back toward the probe like an echo. For example, sound waves reflect the difference between the rib cage and a lung and the lung and the heart. Therefore ultrasound is able to demonstrate the size, shape, and position of most of the organs in the body. The greater the difference in density between the two tissues, the greater the echo as the sound wave encounters the boundary between those tissues.

The sound waves in medical ultrasound

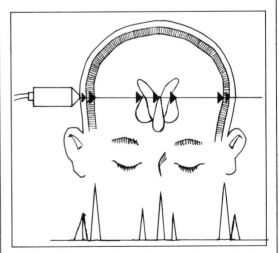

Ultrasound wave originates in a small probe that is placed against the skin. Sound waves bounce off tissue and reflect back to the probe, which doubles as a receiver. Every echo is recorded as a deflection on an oscilloscope screen. (Courtesy Children's Hospital Medical Center, Boston)

occur in regular and frequent pulses, usually between 500 to 1,000 times per second. Between each pulse the transmitting probe acts as a receiver of the sound wave echoes as they return from the various tissue boundaries. The returned sound waves are then converted to electrical energy by the equipment and displayed on the screen as an image of the structures they encounter.

The development of ultrasound

Much progress has been made in the display of ultrasound images. With the earliest ultrasound, the so-called A-mode (A for amplitude) units transmitted a single straight-line ultrasound wave so that distances between various organs' boundaries were identified and recorded as simple deflections or "blips" on an oscilloscope screen. The most common use of this early ultrasound was a study called the echo encephalogram, an ultrasound brain study. The soft tissues of the brain (not visible on standard skull X rays which show only the bony skull) had presented a diagnostic challenge for years. It was only natural that ultrasonography first turned in that direction.

The echo study was based on the principle that midline brain structures would be shifted by bleeding or pressure within the skull. Ultrasound could pick up that shift and record it on the oscilloscope screen as a deflection. Measurement of the deflection was difficult, however, and the resulting diagnosis often unreliable. Ultrasound studies have now been largely abandoned in brain diagnosis because of the extraordinary accuracy of CAT scanning, but A-mode tracings are still valuable in other areas, as we shall see.

Ultrasound images have markedly improved through subsequent generations of ultrasound machines. The second generation, or B-mode (B for brightness), sends out a fan of ultrasound waves, resulting in a cross-sectional image that enables ana-

tomical features to be recognized. This is the type of unit most used in hospitals. The image on the screen is a static frozen-motion study of the area, much like a photograph. It has wide application in the evaluation of organs and tumors in the abdominal cavity and particularly in the pelvic area, which is notoriously difficult to evaluate.

The latest ultrasound generation, called real-time, is similar to fluoroscopy but uses no X rays. It permits movements such as heartbeats and flowing blood to be presented as they occur in motion. This technique has made possible the amazing fetal treatments that are just being developed.

Ultrasound and obstetrics

Ultrasonography is the procedure of choice for the obstetrician because high-frequency sound waves are harmless to mother and developing child. Besides the spectacular innovations in fetal treatment, more common routine obstetrical care is made easier. Ultrasound is used to monitor half of all pregnancies and deliveries today.

With ultrasound, the obstetrician can measure the size of the fetal head, an important factor in determining the stage of gestation. The placenta can be located

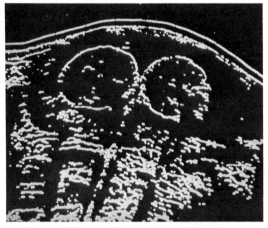

An ultrasound image of a pregnant uterus showing twins. Both heads are visible as outlines in center of photo. (Courtesy Brigham and Women's Hospital, Boston)

safely, providing vital information in the evaluation of bleeding during pregnancy and for reducing the complications of amniocentesis, the procedure for withdrawing amniotic fluid for genetic studies (see "Update: Genetics," pages 227–230). The existence of breech or other unusual birth presentations can be easily and quickly determined. And, for the mother whose abdomen seems larger than it should be for her stage of pregnancy, ultrasound can demonstrate the number of babies she is carrying.

Ultrasound has also been used to diagnose critical problems in pregnancy, as the following case history illustrates.

CASE HISTORY

For the first half of her pregnancy everything was going well for C. G., but at the twenty-sixth-week checkup her physician felt that her womb was larger than normal. An ultrasound exam was performed, revealing that the developing fetus had hydrocephalus, a buildup of fluid in the chambers of the brain making the head larger than usual. After consultation with several specialists and the parents, C. G.'s doctors decided to attempt to relieve the pressure in the developing baby's head by draining off the fluid. The procedure was risky, but without it there was no chance of the child being born without brain damage and severe retardation, since hydrocephalus does not permit the brain to develop normally.

Using ultrasound equipment to fix the proper locations, the doctor inserted a needle through the mother's abdominal wall and guided it into the fetal brain, to remove fluid. Since that initial attempt, the procedure was repeated several times. The hope was to continue the procedure until the baby's birth, when an operation to "shunt" the fluid into the circulation permanently could be performed.

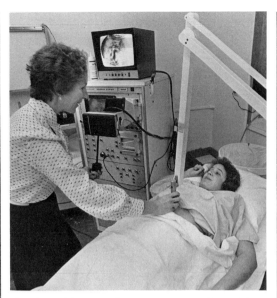

An obstetrician examines a pregnant patient with ultrasound. The image of the baby is transmitted to the television screen at upper left. (Photo by Bradford F. Herzog, courtesy Children's Hospital Medical Center, Boston)

Hydrocephalus in the developing fetus presents an extraordinary medical challenge. It progresses relentlessly and without relief of the inevitable pressure buildup, and the brain is slowly destroyed. Children born with undetected hydrocephalus have little functioning brain tissue and are severely retarded. Operations to relieve the fluid buildup by shunting it into the circulation are common after birth, but by then much damage has already occurred. Dr. Jason Birnholz, an expert in ultrasound diagnosis and director of ultrasound at the Boston Hospital for Women, commented on C. G.'s treatment: "Since we knew the fluid buildup was already there at twenty-six weeks, drainage of the fluid before birth was the only chance this baby had to develop normally." The baby eventually died, but Dr. Birnholz feels this may be because the treatment was started too late.

Before now, the protective environment of the uterus was a barrier to diagnosis and treatment of the developing fetus. Along with such other innovations as fetal monitoring (see "High Tech," pages 160–163), ultrasound is overcoming the barrier between the fetus and the outside world and aiding obstetricians in administering life-saving treatments. While C. G.'s case was the first attempt at controlling fetal hydrocephalus, ultrasound is used regularly to aid blood transfusions to correct Rh blood factor incompatibility, performed on the fetus while in utero.

Many ultrasonographers have recently reported success with the diagnosis of fetal heart malformations in utero. In one case at Yale University Medical School, a fetus in the thirty-fourth week of gestation was found by ultrasound study to have a defect in the right ventricle of the heart and the pulmonary arteries (the chamber that pumps blood to the lungs). Alerted to the problem by ultrasound diagnosis, surgeons saved the child at birth with an immediate heart operation. A twenty-eight-week-old fetus was found by ultrasound to have abnormal motion of a heart valve. At delivery, the child was in congestive heart failure and had an abnormal heart rhythm. Again, alerted to the problem, pediatricians corrected the rhythm and the baby has done well since. Birnholz's Boston group has had similar success with prenatal ultrasound heart diagnoses.

Dr. Birnholz feels that the coming years will bring several more firsts in fetal diagnosis and treatment. Drugs may be given directly to the fetus, a technique that is clearly more efficient than the current method of giving the drugs to the mother in hopes that they will cross the placenta to reach the fetus's bloodstream. More advanced surgical procedures may also be performed.

"Every week I find something new to look at," Birnholz comments. He has a new ultrasound unit that enables him to examine tiny fetal anatomical parts. The results of his research may shed new light on sudden infant death syndrome, a tragic condition that has recently been found to be related to eye movements (see "Discoveries," pages 31–34).

Since ultrasound imaging provides a reasonably clear indication of how a fetus is doing, Dr. Birnholz feels that every pregnant woman may soon be monitored by ultrasound. "We must do it more quickly and with less cost than we do now, though," he notes. "The future will surely bring low-cost units than can be used right in the doctor's office for screening."

CASE HISTORY

"Women want the security of knowing that their baby is healthy," Dr. Birnholz noted as he walked into the examining room. A little over a year before, the woman on the table had had a stillborn child with numerous congenital problems, including deformed limbs. This was her fourth pregnancy; two other children were normal and healthy. She was going to deliver in less than a month. "This baby looks just great," stated Dr. Birnholz as he pointed at the ultrasound screen and showed the mother her baby's arms, legs, and fingers. Her grin showed her obvious delight. "By the way," he said, "would you like to know if your baby is a boy or girl? I can tell you if you'd like." The woman thought for an instant, then smiled more deeply. "I'd rather be surprised," she said.

Predicting strokes

According to the Surgeon General's office, nearly 10 percent of all deaths in the United States each year occur from stroke, a medical condition in which blood flow to a part of the brain is severely restricted or cut off. Another 200,000 people survive strokes but remain disabled by paralysis, speech difficulties, and memory loss. Although most strokes occur in people over sixty-five, early deaths are common, particularly among blacks, who have a stroke death rate of two and a half times that of whites between the ages of twenty-five and sixty-five.

Although strokes can be caused by rupture or obstruction of small blood vessels and blood clots in the brain, 40 percent of all strokes are caused by narrowing of the carotid artery, the major blood vessel in the neck that delivers blood from the heart to the brain. The narrowing is usually caused by atherosclerosis, the progressive deposit of fatty and cholesterol material on the blood vessel wall.

The medical, social, and personal implications of stroke are enormous. Dr. Alfred Persson, a surgeon who heads the Vascular Laboratory of the Lahey Clinic in Boston, has seen many patients with atherosclerosis and is concerned. "Once stroke occurs," he emphasizes, "there is no treatment other than rehabilitation. It is therefore important to find the people prone to stroke in order to correct the condition before circulation is completely shut off." This means diagnosing blood vessel narrowing before it reaches a critical level.

Dr. Persson's laboratory is one of the first in the nation to use an ultrasound device called echo flow to help prevent strokes due to carotid artery narrowing by early diagnosis. Echo flow is based on the Doppler effect, a basic principle of physics which states that the frequency of sound reflected from a moving object (in this case the flow of blood through the arteries) varies with the speed of the object. When the carotid artery becomes narrowed, the velocity of blood flowing through the narrowed segment is increased. By locating the area of more rapid blood flow, echo flow locates any area of artery narrowing.

In the echo flow system, a small probe containing an ultrasound transducer is placed on the neck over the carotid artery. The sound waves are reflected from the moving blood back into the probe and are

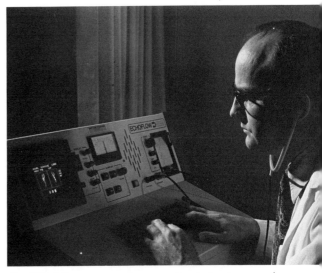

Dr. Alfred Persson examines an echo study of carotid arteries that supply the brain with blood. Computerized image of the arteries appears on the screen at far left. (Courtesy Lahey Clinic, Boston)

analyzed by a computer. As the probe is moved along the artery, the computer displays the information on a screen in a color-coded system. Red means normal blood flow; yellow, restricted flow; and blue, severely restricted flow—at least 75 percent. People with 75 percent restriction in blood flow are those prone to stroke.

Prior to echo flow, the only way of estimating carotid artery circulation was with an angiogram, a sometime dangerous X-ray study in which a contrast material is injected directly into the artery. Angiogram requires hospitalization, a small incision in the artery, and a small but real risk to the patient. Besides, angiograms only give static photographs of the artery's anatomy.

"The ultrasound study," says Dr. Persson, "gives more important information. It tells how much blood is actually flowing through the blood vessel, and it can be done right in the doctor's office in twenty minutes with no risk, harm, or pain to the patient."

Ultrasound carotid scanning will certainly not replace angiograms altogether. In a person with severe narrowing, an angiogram is important before surgery to define accurately the narrow segment for the surgeon. But ultrasound eliminates the need for angiograms in people whose symptoms only suggest carotid disease: patients with dizzy spells, temporary loss of nerve function (so-called transient ischemic attack or small strokes), physical examination findings of narrowing, or those with evidence of arteriosclerosis elsewhere. Such patients can often be spared the needless expense and pain of an angiogram while still being reassured by an accurate diagnosis.

Atherosclerotic blood vessel disease is not limited to the carotid artery. Circulatory restriction in the legs, for example, is very common. Doppler ultrasound probes have been in use for several years to evaluate the flow of blood in the leg when arterial or venous restriction is suspected. Modification of the echo flow system will undoubtedly be available soon to permit visual identification of the trouble spots in those vessels as well.

Ultrasound and the heart

In the cardiac catheterization laboratory, long tubes, or catheters, are inserted into a patient's arms and threaded slowly toward the heart, where they measure pressure, record electrical activity, and inject contrast material for X-ray study. While cardiac catheterization provides a wide range of essential data about the heart, there is some information it cannot provide. Cardiac catheterization cannot measure the thickness of the heart muscle, for example, and even more important, it cannot study the timing and motion of the heart valves and heart muscle as they act in concert during each beat or pumping cycle.

Echo cardiography, the ultrasound study of the heart, is the only test that can provide that information. Although it often complements cardiac catheterization, the echo cardiogram in many cases has made the more expensive ($1,500 and up for a cardiac catheterization) and clearly more dangerous procedure unnecessary.

CASE HISTORY

E. M. is a fifty-three-year-old woman in good health except for hypertension, which is managed by medication and is in good control. For one week she had been at home in bed with a flulike illness, suffering from fever, weakness, and generalized muscle aches. On the eighth day of the illness she experienced sharp chest pain, clearly worsened by deep breathing, sudden movements, or cough. The pains were similar to a pleurisy she had experienced with flu two years earlier. In two days her pain and fever were improved, but she was still quite short of breath and unable to walk up one flight of stairs to her room without stopping to rest.

On the eleventh day of her illness the shortness of breath was worse and breathing was difficult even while lying down. She did get relief, however, by sitting up. Her physician found signs of heart failure, a rapid weak pulse, and an enlarged heart on a chest X ray and admitted her to the hospital. An echo cardiogram study demonstrated a pericardial effusion—fluid in the sac surrounding the heart. On the same day, a needle was inserted through her chest wall and 360 cc (12 ounces) of fluid were removed. E. M. felt immediately better and was able to breath normally. She was started on cortisone, rapidly improved, and was discharged one week later. Subsequent ultrasound studies showed no recurrence of the fluid buildup.

Pericardial effusion is a life-threatening condition because it restricts the ability of the heart to receive and pump blood. It can follow infection (as in E. M.'s case), chest wall injury, or a variety of other medical problems. Pericardial effusion is often difficult to diagnose. The enlarged cardiac silhouette caused by the fluid around the heart can be confused with heart muscle enlargement on a traditional X ray.

Echo cardiography is the most effective way of making the diagnosis because of its ability to recognize different tissue densities and the anatomical relationship of one tissue to another. The test is easy and quick to perform on those patients who are quite ill. Portable units allow physicians to perform the study right at the patient's bedside or in the office—and since the echo cardiogram is conducted outside the body, no tubes, needles, dyes, or medications are needed.

Echo cardiography uses a type of ultrasound called time-motion study. It plots the cardiac echoes against time and depicts internal heart structures as undulating lines on a moving strip of paper. Each of the heart's internal structures—the muscle wall, the valves between the chambers, and the septum between the chambers —has specific echo tracings. Because the strip records the motion of all the cardiac structures together, the internal relationship of each of the structures can be examined in detail for the first time. Most important, these relationships are observed when the heart is beating. Echo cardiography, therefore, studies not only physical anatomy but its function as well.

Besides pericardial fluid problems, echo cardiography provides important diagnostic information on abnormal heart valves (such as mitral stenosis, a frequent rheumatic condition in which blood is restricted from passage into the left ventricle and backed up into the lungs), holes between the chambers (such as atrial septal defect, in which blood flow is shunted abnormally between the chambers), and various congenital problems. It can also be used to monitor patients after cardiac surgery. Its role in these areas often exceeds any other diagnostic study available.

Will echo cardiography replace cardiac catheterization? "Definitely not," stated Indiana University echo cardiography pioneer Dr. Harvey Feigenbaum at a recent meeting of the American Heart Association. "With the rapidly increasing use of echo cardiography, it is important to remember what the ultrasound study cannot do." Along with a panel of ultrasound experts, Dr. Fiegenbaum commented that cardiac catheterization is important for the study of pressure within the heart and blood vessels and to outline the flow of blood with contrast studies. Echo cardiography cannot give that information. Similarly, the current state of ultrasound technology cannot study heart muscle defects and viability and blood flow as nuclear medicine can.

The best advice most cardiac experts would have for patients, then, is to choose a physician who is well respected and knowledgeable in cardiac disease. The indication for an echo cardiogram must be well defined, and it should be performed by individuals well trained in skill and interpretation. It is considered as one of several important diagnostic options when studying the heart—but not as the complete answer.

Ultrasound and other organs

Offering little discomfort and few negligible risks, sonography is accurate, versatile, and comparatively inexpensive in evaluating many organs that were previously difficult to visualize with other imaging techniques. The ability to transfer reflected ultrasound echoes to an image displayed on a viewing screen has undoubtedly been the crucial factor. A technique called gray scale processing enables displays of the echoes in a variety of shades of gray (eight to sixteen different shades in current machines), according to the intensity of the echo. With gray scale, remarkable views of the shape and location of abdominal organs, masses, or tumors within the organs can be seen. The images can also be photographed for permanent inclusion in the patient's records.

Perhaps the most remarkable success in abdominal diagnosis is with the gallbladder. Ultrasound can diagnose gallstones with up to 98 percent accuracy, easily the equal of X-ray studies and without the radiation exposure. Many institutions feel ultrasound will eventually replace the X-ray study. University of Virginia radiologist Dr. A. Norman A. G. Brenbridge reports that "sonography of the gallbladder is so accurate that our surgeons have been willing to operate without [traditional] gallbladder X rays." Ultrasound gallbladder studies have been particularly valuable in a patient with acute pain in the right upper quadrant of the abdomen, demonstrating the offending gallbladder problem without the one- or two-day delays common to the X-ray study.

It is also helpful in evaluating patients with jaundice and liver and pancreatic disease. For example, studies report that using ultrasound and gray scale imaging, it is possible to detect pancreatic cancer (an insidious problem) with 70 to 95 percent accuracy. Continued use of the technique is important in kidney and adrenal gland tumors and cysts as well. Other organs such as the spleen are best visualized by other techniques.

CASE HISTORY

M. O. was a fifty-eight-year-old accountant in good health except for poorly controlled hypertension. He admitted to taking his prescription medication infrequently. At a routine checkup he complained of vague mid-abdominal pain but he had no history of heartburn, nausea, vomiting, or diarrhea. On examination, his physician felt a four-inch-diameter pulsating, slightly tender abdominal mass. M. O.'s blood pressure was 190/110 and the physician was concerned about an aortic aneurysm, a "bubble" or weakness in the wall of a

major blood vessel. Such an expanding weakness frequently can rupture, leading to immediate death. Ultrasound studies, however, showed a solid mass in front of the blood vessel, which itself was normal. The mass was biopsied and turned out to be a lymphoma, a type of cancer. Treatment was begun and two years later the man is doing well.

Before ultrasound, an angiogram, a complicated, painful, and sometimes troublesome X-ray contrast study, would have had to be performed to rule out the blood vessel problem.

Fluoroscopy by ultrasound and the real-time study have specific value to abdominal ultrasound for pediatric and adult patients alike. They permit instant evaluation of moving structures, and the probe can be passed rapidly over large body areas for survey scanning. An important use of real-time is to guide a needle tip passed through the abdominal skin to biopsy the liver, kidney, and other organs and to drain cysts or abscesses, procedures that inevita-

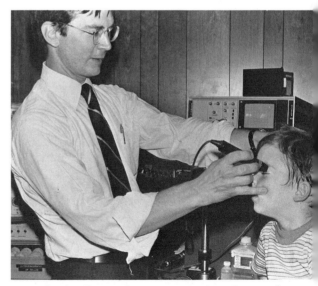

Dr. Richard Dallow performs one part of an ultrasound examination on a young patient's eye.

bly required surgery in the years before ultrasound.

Ultrasound and the eyes

The inside of the eyeball can be the site of many serious problems, often leading to loss of vision, and sometimes to loss of life. Tumors, foreign bodies, and retinal detachments, in which the visual cells are pulled away from the back of the eyeball, are just a few examples. A doctor usually examines the eyeball's interior through the pupil with an ophthalmoscope. Often the physician's vision is obscured by a cloudy lens called a cataract, or by bleeding or scarring of the eye. Ultrasound echoes, by outlining all the soft tissues in and around the eye, are now an indispensable part of the eye examination. The specially trained ophthalmologist can manipulate the ultrasound probe to study most of the eye features, completing a simple ultrasound measurement of the eye structures (necessary in any lens implant procedure) in five minutes, and the evaluation of more complicated cases of tumors or detachments in a half-hour or more.

Dr. Richard Dallow, an ophthalmologic surgeon at the Massachusetts Eye and Ear Infirmary in Boston, has handled ultrasonography for approximately 10,000 patients to date, probably as many as anyone else in the world. "Ultrasound is so important now because other developments in ophthalmology have made it important," says Dr. Dallow. "The artificial lens implantation and many other operations developed within the past ten years could not be performed as effectively without ultrasound as a diagnostic aid." In Dr. Dallow's opinion, "Ultrasonography is the most versatile technique currently available for soft tissue evaluation of the eye."

Ultrasound and mammography

The controversy over radiation hazards has led to much confusing information about the use of X-ray mammography (images of the breast) to screen for breast cancer. Many articles have appeared in the press pointing out the value of X-ray mammography for the early discovery of breast tumors. Others have warned that the radiation exposure involved increases the risk of cancer. The same debate in the medical community has led to the study of ultrasound mammography because the procedure uses no X rays and therefore presents no radiation hazard.

Several medical centers are now experimenting with ultrasound mammography. Doctors at the Mount Sinai Medical Center in Miami Beach reported at a recent national conference on ultrasound medicine that their experience with ultrasound mammography on 200 patients compared so favorably with standard procedures that they speculate that ultrasound mammography could become important as a screening device. Ultrasonographers at the Massachusetts General Hospital in Boston, who are also studying ultrasound mammography, had another opinion. "It should be stated that we do not recommend ultrasound as a screening procedure in the way X-ray mammography is used," commented a radiologist there. He pointed out that the ultrasound test is expensive (the machine alone costs $150,000, about three times as much as a conventional mammogram instrument) and requires many individual images and lengthy interpretation time. Nor has it been performed on enough patients to give a significant clinical basis for judgment. Most investigators do agree, however, that ultrasound is valuable in evaluating masses already found by X ray or thermography (an imaging test based on the relative temperature of body masses and organs), by evaluating whether the tumor is solid or cystic and perhaps even benign or malignant.

While many surgeons prefer to biopsy all breast masses, this is sometimes impractical. In *The Female Patient*, Albert Einstein College of Medicine professor Dr.

Gilbert Baum notes that some patients are not appropriate candidates for biopsy of the breast mass, particularly if they have had several previous biopsies. "Ultrasound combined with X-ray mammography can frequently resolve the nature of the lesion, thus obviating the need for repeated biopsies." Ultrasound seems to be complementary to other studies for evaluating the breast, but only time and lengthy research will determine its ultimate value.

A revolution in body imaging

From its nineteenth-century industrial beginnings, ultrasound has dramatically changed the concept of medical diagnosis in a variety of clinical situations. The relatively low unit cost (approximately $60,000 per machine) makes it a less expensive diagnostic tool—about $75 to $150 per examination—than many innovations such as computerized tomography (CAT scanning). The safety of ultrasound and its ability to peek into previously hidden body recesses gives it a distinct advantage over traditional X-ray studies. Of course, it is not always the best or final answer in many conditions, and so the modern hospital radiology department offers it along with other studies to be used when clinical judgment deems it most appropriate.

Massachusetts General Hospital radiologist Joseph T. Ferruchi, Jr., feels that continuing electronic advances will improve ultrasound images even more in the years to come and that the clinical usefulness of the tool will undoubtedly advance still further. Currently, ultrasound testing is performed with a hand-held ultrasound probe. Automated and computerized systems are now being tested which will increase the diagnostic accuracy and speed of sonography.

Fiber optics

Anonymous Doctor: "And tell us Dr. Franklin, what is the use of this thing you call electricity?" Dr. Benjamin Franklin: "May I ask you, sir, what is the use of a newborn baby?"

Transactions of the Philadelphia Academy of Science, 1927

When scientists first recognized in the 1950s that a thin glass rod could confine light within its center and transmit that light over the length of the tube, the science of fiber optics was born. Like any newborn, this discovery seemed to hold great potential. But exactly where would the future take that development?

With all their vision scientists of those years could not possibly have foreseen the profound maturing of their concept. The simultaneous development of narrow intense light beams called lasers (see "High Tech," pages 166–171) and ultrathin and pure glass fibers in the past fifteen years has led to incredible progress in the science of transmitting light. Fiber optics now has applications in diverse areas ranging from communications and business machines to fire detection and, most significantly for this volume, medicine.

Physicians have always been keenly aware of the importance of direct observation. Along with palpation (touching), auscultation (listening), and percussion (examination using a sound), observation is one of the keys to successful examination and diagnosis. Observation of the skin and external body structures has always been easy enough, but internal observations presented more of a challenge. The need to see into body orifices, however, has been keen at least since Roman times. A thirteen-inch bronze vaginal speculum was excavated at Pompeii.

The first endoscopic device was constructed with mirrors and optics and enabled German physician Philip Bezzini to see deep into the throat in 1807. Mirrors were still used to reflect light fifty years later when Polish physiologist Johann Czerniac demonstrated an endoscopic invention on vocal cords before interested audiences. And in 1868, Austrian physician Adolph Kussmaul observed the lining of the stomach by inserting an open tube into the gullet. The reflected light from a gasoline lamp provided the illumination for this recorded endoscopy (*endo* = inner; *scopy* = witness).

For 100 years thereafter, endoscopy equipment remained remarkably similar to Kussmaul's lamp and straight tube. Electric light eventually replaced the gasoline one, and lenses were added to the open tube to magnify the image. But the narrowed body orifices, the twistings and turnings of the intestines, and the inability to transmit light efficiently made images poor at best.

Fiber optics provided a breakthrough in endoscopic diagnosis, the ramifications of which are still being appreciated and discussed. Fiber optics made possible flexible endoscopes with controllable tips that can be steered around any number of interior body contours while under visual control of the operator. When used to study the gastrointestinal system, the procedure is performed by inserting the endoscope into the patient's mouth and advancing it slowly into the esophagus and thereafter into the stomach and beyond as necessary. Local anesthetic sprays and intravenous sedation make the procedure easily tolerable

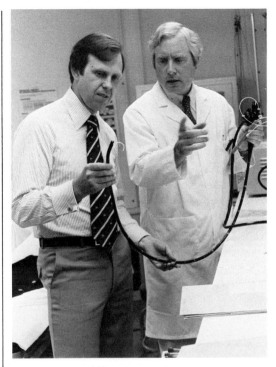

Dr. John Shea of Boston's Lahey Clinic demonstrates use of fiberoptic endoscope to the author. (Courtesy Lahey Clinic, Boston)

by most people. The interiors of joints, intestines, bronchial tubes, bladders, and abdominal cavities can thus be examined and studied (and even photographed) with this "anatomical periscope."

The principles of fiber optics

Fiber optics technology is based on the transmission of light through fibers or strands of glass or plastic. The idea is over a century old, perhaps beginning in the late nineteenth century when British physician John Tyndall made the observation that "part of the light illuminating the inside of a container of water was guided through a hole in the side of the vessel." His presentation before the Royal Society in England in 1870 was the first recorded demonstration that glass could transmit light by internal reflection. The following years produced many experiments with light transmission through glass rods. However,

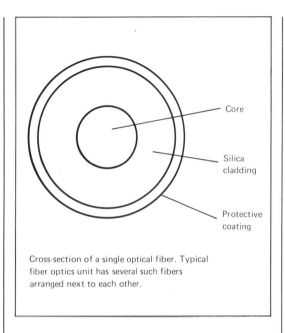

Cross-section of a single optical fiber. Typical fiber optics unit has several such fibers arranged next to each other.

Core

Silica cladding

Protective coating

there was little significance to this work because glass was so impure that light intensity diminished rapidly after entering it. Finally in 1970, Corning Glass developed a glass fiber so pure that light could be transmitted nearly one mile without losing significant intensity.

Optical fibers are made of the same minerals as regular glass: silica, soda, and lime. However, special processes must be used to ensure that the glass is flawless enough to transmit light over distances. The process begins with a glass tube the diameter of a half dollar and three feet long. The tube is filled with a chemical vapor and heated to 3,000 degrees Fahrenheit (1,600 degrees Celsius). When suction is applied to the heated tube it collapses into a solid glass core with an outer silica layer or cladding. While still hot, the three-foot rod is drawn into a hair-thin fiber nearly three and a half miles long. As the fibers are drawn up, they are coated with a thin plastic laminate to protect them from injury. A newly drawn fiber contains no impurities to diffuse or diminish light and is as strong as stainless steel.

The astonishingly thin glass fiber still

has the outer silica cladding. As light enters the interior core of the fiber it bounces off the outer layers in zigzag fashion, constantly being reflected back into the center. Since light cannot escape from the fiber, it follows the fiber to its end, even bending and twisting back and forth. Today, pure optical fibers transmit over 95 percent of the light they receive.

The stimulus to the development of flawless optical fibers came from the communications industry, whose scientists hoped to use the fibers for light wave communications. Today's ultrathin, ultrapure fibers are being installed in place of standard metal telephone wires. Using pulses of light, they can carry many times the information in much smaller wires. (This development would no doubt have pleased Alexander Graham Bell, who tried to transmit sound on a sunbeam as early as 1880.)

Fiber optic endoscopes use coherent bundles of optical fibers to transmit an image. A coherent bundle contains many optical fibers which are sorted and arranged carefully so that each fiber has the same relationship to all the other fibers at both ends of the bundle. An intact image is then transmitted from one end of the bundle to the viewer at the other. If the fibers do not have this precise relationship to each other (so-called incoherent bundles) the image would be distorted, even though the fibers would still transmit light. Fiber optic endoscopes contain both coherent and incoherent bundles. The incoherent bundle transmits light from a source outside the patient to illuminate the field inside the organ being examined. The coherent bundle transmits the image of the organ's interior back to the viewer.

Besides the fiber optic bundles, endoscopes have remote-control cords to steer and position the tip as it passes along its organ road. Many units also have side channels that permit a variety of tools to be used for diagnosis and therapy: suction de-

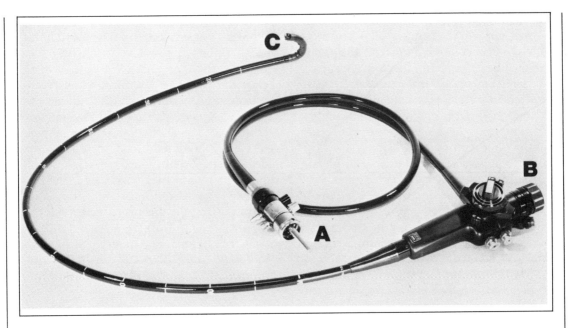

Fiberoptic gastroscope for stomach examination: (A) attaches to light source; (B) physician looks through eyepiece; (C) end enters stomach through patient's mouth. (Courtesy Olympus Corporation)

vices, biopsy instruments, brushes, snares and knives, and electrical cautery tips.

Gastrointestinal endoscopy

Digestive diseases are one of the largest public health problems confronting Americans, according to the final report of the National Commission on Digestive Diseases published in 1979. Illnesses of this sort account for 43 million hospital days each year, the major cause of hospitalization in the United States. Countless additional individuals also experience belching, heartburn, nausea, constipation, diarrhea, and abdominal pain and have not yet been diagnosed. As such the true incidence of digestive problems is really unknown.

Radiology has played the traditional central role in gastrointestinal diagnosis for years. Hundreds of thousands of Americans have undergone upper GI, barium enema, and gallbladder X rays for evaluation of their gastrointestinal symptoms. These studies use a contrast material resistant to the passage of X rays that provides shadows of the studied organs on the X-ray film. Endoscopy is challenging radiology's time-honored role in GI diagnosis because it provides direct visualization and promises to be more accurate. In the stomach and small intestine, for example, upper GIs can miss from 20 to 40 percent of all diseases. Endoscopy, on the other hand, is accurate at least 90 percent of the time.

CASE HISTORY

M. P. is a fifty-seven-year-old bank executive who had a long history of indigestion and heartburn. She would frequently become uncomfortable two to three hours after a meal. The discomfort would persist until she ate again or took antacids. Often she would wake up in the early morning hours with pain. She used alcohol only occasionally and took no aspirin or other drugs. Her problem was such that she kept antacids in every purse and desk drawer.

After a particularly severe episode of pain not relieved by antacids and lasting nearly two days, she visited her physician, who suspected peptic ulcer disease and ordered upper GI X rays. The contrast study showed a one-inch ulcer on the upper border of her stomach. She was advised to eat frequent small, nonirritating meals; avoid coffee, cigarettes, and alcohol; and use antacids. After six weeks of therapy, her symptoms were improved but still present and annoying. Repeat X rays showed no change in the ulcer. Her physician suspected that the ulcer was malignant and performed endoscopy to confirm the diagnosis. During endoscopy, the ulcer was identified and appeared to be benign. With the biopsy instrument, small pieces were snipped away for study in the laboratory. With another instrument, cells from the ulcer base were brushed off, again for laboratory analysis. No evidence of malignancy was found.

M. P. was placed on an intensive and closely followed medical program with cimetidine (see "Discoveries," pages 71–75), antacids, diet, and avoidance of irritants. Repeat X rays and endoscopy six weeks later showed complete ulcer healing. Now, two years later, M. P. feels fine.

The gastric ulcer presents a dilemma to the practicing physician. While often caused by irritants such as aspirin, acid secretion, or "peptic" causes, ulcers can be cancerous as well. With standard radiographic studies, it is sometimes difficult to distinguish malignant from benign gastric ulcers. If a patient did not respond to medical therapy, the physician often suspected malignancy and performed surgery to diagnose and probably remove the offending ulcer. Endoscopy can now eliminate the exploratory surgery. The ulcer can be looked at directly and samples taken to confirm or disprove malignancy. With negative studies, there remains good evidence that more intensive medical management is the answer.

Endoscopy is also used as a primary diag-

nostic tool to diagnose stomach bleeding. According to gastroenterologist Dr. Thomas Lieberman, in a review article on endoscopy in the *Surgical Clinics of North America:* "In acute gastrointestinal bleeding endoscopy is more accurate than conventional X rays, particularly for bleeding due to gastric or duodenal ulcer or esophageal varices [dialated blood vessels]. Some bleeding sites such as gastritis [an irritation of the stomach] can only be identified by endoscopy." By localizing the exact bleeding site, physicians can assess the possible need for surgery without a diagnostic operation. If surgery is needed, endoscopy guides the surgeon to the precise spot, making the operation easier. GI

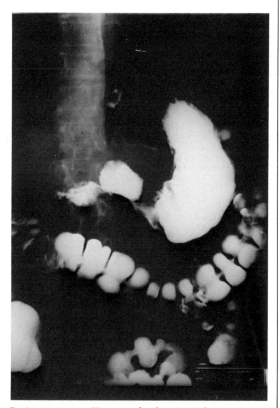

Barium contrast X-ray study showing a large stomach (gastric) ulcer, seen as white rectangular structure in the center of the photo. [Photo by Joseph Murphy]

specialists find that endoscopy accurately locates the bleeding site 95 percent of the time when performed in the first twenty-four to forty-eight hours. Endoscopy for GI bleeding is limited to diagnosis thus far, but exciting research indicates that bleeding may soon be treated through the endoscope with lasers, heat probes, or electrical cautery methods.

In addition to upper GI conditions, endoscopy may someday play a major role in gallstone treatment through an innovative technique called endoscopic papillotomy, or EPT. The experimental procedure attracted considerable attention in the fall of 1979 when the deposed Shah of Iran successfully underwent EPT treatment for

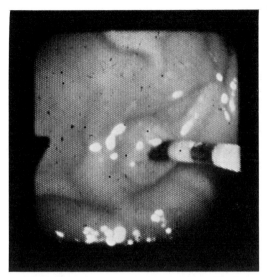

In photo taken through an endoscope, small tube is seen entering opening for common bile duct. (Courtesy Olympus Corporation)

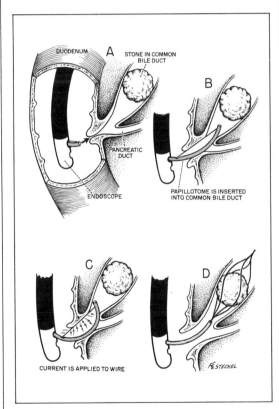

To remove a gallstone using EPT, the bile duct opening is enlarged by applying an electrical current to the cutting wire (A, B, C). A small wire snare is then passed around the gallstone (D) to pull it loose. (Courtesy Lahey Clinic, Boston)

removal of gallstones in New York Hospital. Researchers in Europe have studied the procedure since 1974, but EPT has generated much controversy in this country and has yet to be adopted for widespread use. Many doctors, however, feel that EPT holds considerable promise.

Gallstones often remain in a patient's common bile duct after he or she has had the gallbladder removed. Traditionally, these gallstones are removed with a second operation called a choledocholithotomy, a major operation requiring general anesthesia. With EPT, no operation is necessary. Instead, the endoscope is guided to the opening of the common bile duct. A thin catheter is advanced into the opening, and a small wire in the catheter tip forms a "bowlike knife." Electrical current passed through the wire cuts the opening until it is large enough for the gallstone to pass through. If the stone doesn't pass into the intestine and out of the body of its own accord, it can sometimes be retrieved with a wire basket.

In several reported studies, EPT has a success rate of close to 80 percent for re-

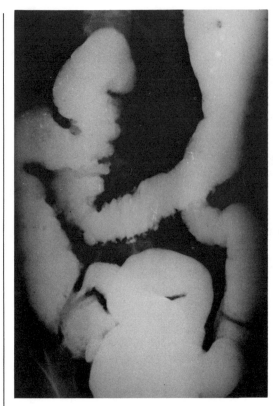

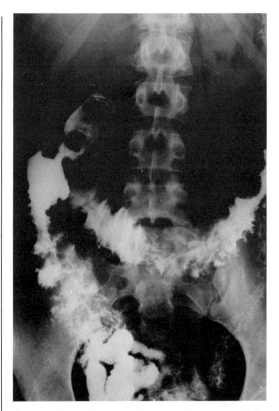

Fiberoptic instruments have become valuable in diagnosing ulcerative colitis, an inflammatory disease of the colon shown here by barium enema X-ray contrast study. When the colon is filled with *barium, the walls appear fragmented (center of left photo). After barium is evacuated, the inflamed colon is readily apparent (right).* (Photos by Joseph Murphy)

moving gallstones from the common bile duct, only failing when the retained stones were too large to be removed. Few complications are reported, and the procedure is performed without anesthesia, requiring only two to three days in the hospital. (The operation EPT replaces requires seven to ten days of hospitalization.) As Dr. John Shea of Boston's Lahey Clinic concludes: "EPT is an effective and safe management for common bile duct stones. When compared to surgery, EPT's benefits make it the procedure of choice in an increasing number of patients."

Fiberoptic evaluation has also allowed an access to the large intestine (colon) not previously possible. According to Dr. Timothy Talbott of the Ferguson-Droste-Ferguson Hospital in Grand Rapids,

Michigan, many polyps can be removed with the colonoscope instead of surgery. The colonoscope also aids in diagnosing inflammatory conditions such as ulcerative colitis.

Endoscopy is more expensive than X-ray evaluation. Although prices may vary around the country, upper GI and barium enema X rays usually cost $90 to $100, whereas endoscopy varies from $200 to $500.

Accuracy is the primary consideration in diagnosis. With symptoms like upper GI bleeding, when endoscopy is clearly more accurate than X rays in finding the site, the more expensive procedure should be done. If the two forms of diagnosis are comparable, however, cost benefits should be analyzed before one chooses between them.

Often both are performed and are complementary in terms of the information received.

Arthroscopy—endoscopy of the knee joint

Sports medicine specialist Dr. Gabe Mirkin has described the knee as "the most famous joint in sports." Bobby Orr, Joe Namath, Gale Sayers, and many other professional athletes have been sidelined during their careers from knee injuries. Athletes are not alone, however, in experiencing frustration, disability, and agony over this major joint. Countless housewives, executives, blue- and white-collar workers, retired citizens, students, young and old, men and women alike are familiar with the pain, swelling, and instability resulting from illness or injury to the knee.

One of the body's more complicated joints, the knee often presents a diagnostic enigma to the physician. Pain and disability can result from damage or inflammation in the bone, joint lining, cartilage, tendon, ligaments, or any combination of them. After examination, a frequent preliminary diagnosis of knee pain is "internal derrangement of the knee (IDK)," a term that indicates that the diagnosis is not definite. (Facetiously, one orthopedic specialist suggested this diagnosis should read simply, "I don't know.") Making a definite diagnosis is rarely easy, because thorough examination is difficult. X rays can be revealing but often are not, so any instrument capable of solving such dilemmas is an obvious asset. The arthroscope is one such instrument. Like its GI counterpart, it permits direct visualization of the inner surface of a body part, in this case the knee. Arthroscopy is performed under local anesthesia through a small incision over the knee. When surgery is inevitable and imminent, arthroscopy is performed under general anesthesia to guide the surgeon's incision.

The principal reason for arthroscopy is persistent knee discomfort without known cause. It is not used in the evaluation or treatment of any other joint.

CASE HISTORY

M. S. is a thirty-two-year-old schoolteacher with chronic knee pain. As a teenager she had taken ballet lessons and hurt her knee in a fall at age fifteen. X rays had been negative, and she was treated with rest and strapping. Thereafter, climbing stairs and kneeling down caused her frequent pain, and she eventually gave up her interest in ballet. In recent years, even social dancing and household and work chores caused pain. X rays continued to be negative. Arthroscopy was recommended, and a small band of tissue (adhesion) was found. It was cut through the arthroscope. Three months later her symptoms were gone, and three years later, despite active athletic and dancing interests, she has had no recurrence.

CASE HISTORY

P. W. is a forty-five-year-old bank vice-president. He had an active young life and is currently a country club tennis player. Frequently he developed acute pain while playing tennis. Occasionally his joint would "stick" or "click" when he tried to straighten it out. When his knee locked in a flexed position, he went to a hospital emergency room and was admitted and prepared for surgery. Arthroscopy demonstrated a small loose bone fragment, undoubtedly from an old injury, wedged under a small cartilage tear. The foreign body and cartilage tear were removed through the arthroscope, and P. W. is playing tennis and working without pain one year later.

In these typical cases, arthroscopy enabled a diagnosis that was not evident before and permitted treatment without surgery and its accompanying disability. Removal of small cartilage tears and loose bodies, cutting adhesions, biopsies of a variety of disorders such as rheumatoid arthritis, and irrigations are among the increasing number of procedures that can be performed through the arthroscope. When the procedure is performed by a skilled arthroscopic specialist, complications are rare. Accessory devices attached to and passing through the arthroscope permit these techniques to be carried out. One doctor estimated that 75 percent of all cartilage removal operations could be performed through the arthroscope. Other orthopedists think that figure is too generous and that the technique is used too frequently on patients who will ultimately need operations any way. Although only about 200 of the nearly 13,000 orthopedic surgeons in the United States perform surgery through arthroscopy, the number is clearly increasing. "It's like the difference between carpentry and watch making," says Dr. Robert Metcalf, assistant professor of orthopedics at the University of Utah College of Medicine. With arthroscopy the wound heals swiftly and leg muscles do not deteriorate because the patient is inactive. Rehabilitation is therefore rapid.

The future of arthroscopy is assured even though most orthopedists do not now use it routinely. In addition to the diagnostic and therapeutic uses, the implications of use of the arthroscope from a research and educational standpoint are many. Study of the natural history of joint disease, verifying diagnostic accuracy, and explaining the mechanics of injury are a few of the advantages of directly visualizing the interior of the knee joint. Photographs can be made to use in court cases to prove injury and to educate patients and students. In Dr. Minkoff's words, arthroscopy "accelerates the acquisition of knowledge about joint symptoms by relating clinical examination to the visual picture obtained."

Bronchoscopy—endoscopy of the lungs

Major advances in the diagnostic approach to lung disease are now possible because of the fiber optic bronchoscope. Like its gastroscopic and arthroscopic counterparts, the instrument contains fiber optic bundles which provide illumination to the field and visualization to the operator, and a small channel for the introduction of variety of biopsy, suction, and irrigation tools.

CASE HISTORY

K. M. is a three-year-old child who suddenly developed a repeated and persistent cough. His mother took him to the local hospital, where chest X rays showed a small closed safety pin in one of the bronchial tubes. K. M. was taken to the operating room, where the pin was removed using a telescopic bronchoscope. The child went home after waking from the anesthesia later that evening. He has done well and there were no complications.

Without the telescopic bronchoscope, surgery might have been required to remove the pin that K. M. swallowed. Fiber optics, however, have made possible this very tiny instrument that can reach deep into the bronchial tree of young children. The fiber optic telescopic bronchoscope is smaller than 1/8 inch in diameter. Yet a miniature telescope and lenses give a clear, wide-angle view with a magnified sharp image. Its small diameter permits the child to breathe without impairment during the procedure. It is inserted directly through the child's mouth and into the bronchial tubes. Besides foreign body removal, this incredibly thin yet effective instrument has been used to wash out and suction bronchial tubes plugged by mucus and leading to partial collapse of the lungs; surgically open up narrowed segments of bronchi; and diagnose a variety of problems from congenital abnormal connections between the esophagus and trachea to chemical burns and trauma. Diagnosis is quick, safe, and accurate.

Larger-diameter flexible fiber optic bronchoscopes have similarly altered the approach to adult lung disease. Bronchoscopy has been performed for many years, but until recently the instruments were large, rigid, and restricted in their use. The previous rigid instruments could only be advanced to the major bronchial tube openings, limiting the diagnostic and treatment possibilities. The flexible tip of the newer units can be flexed to 140 degrees from the vertical and can therefore safely be guided deeply into the small bronchi of the lung tree. Biopsies can even be taken in many instances from the lung tissue itself. Prior to fiber optic bronchoscopy, because of the limitations of the rigid instrument, a chest operation was often required for many of these problems. Now bronchial exam and biopsy and, in some cases, treatment, can

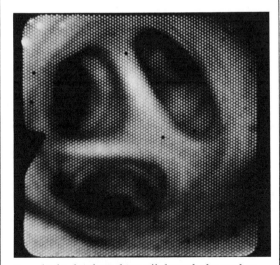

Bronchial tubes branching off through the trachea, as seen by fiberoptic bronchoscope.

be carried out safely on hospital wards or special diagnostic rooms.

Laparoscopy—endoscopy of the abdominal cavity

The differential diagnosis of acute and chronic abdominal pain is not an easy task. When the diagnosis is elusive, the clinician must call in all the diagnostic tools available—X rays of varying types, lab tests, and frequently repeated examinations. If the eventual result of these efforts is negative and the pain persists, the traditional next step has been a surgical procedure called laparotomy. Performed under general anesthesia, this "look and see" operation enables the surgeon to examine and feel all the abdominal organs for evidence of disease.

Now, in many cases, laparoscopy eliminates the need for this operation. Through a tiny abdominal wall "stab incision" the exterior of the liver, gallbladder, spleen, pelvic organs, and parts of the bowel can be seen and examined. Biopsies can be taken under direct visualization, as can surgical procedures such as "tube tying," a sterilization procedure in which the Fallopian tubes are tied to prohibit the passage of the ovum from ovary to uterus. In wide use across the world for many years, laparoscopy is gaining wider usage in the United States. Gynecologists have found particular value in elucidating the cause of pelvic pain, often a very elusive problem.

Endoscopes have become extraordinary diagnostic and therapeutic tools, affecting patients across the various medical specialties. Once only research tools, endoscopic techniques are now or should be in every general hospital. They are, however, not casual procedures and require distinct and extensive training to ensure safety and accurate results. Endoscopy has improved patient care but has also increased knowledge and deepened the awareness of many medical problems.

Glaucoma Glaucoma Glaucom

It is not now as it hath been of yore—
  Turn wheresoe'er I may,
  By night or day,
The things which I have seen I can
now see no more.

William Wordsworth
"Ode: Intimations of Immortality from
Recollections of Early Childhood,"
1803–6

Glaucoma has been called the "sneak thief of sight" because it destroys vision gradually and with few symptoms or warnings. Because of the insidious nature of glaucoma, its actual incidence is not known, but it is estimated to affect between 1 and 4 percent of the world's population over forty years of age. For the most part, glaucoma is genetically determined. Individuals with a family history of the condition have a three times greater risk of developing it than the rest of the population. Diabetics have twice the risk; blacks have three times the risk. The rate of glaucoma incidence rises with the age of the individual.

Methods for treating glaucoma changed little for many years. The most widely used medication was introduced over 100 years ago and is still in use—not because it is the ideal medica-tion, but because there have been few alternatives.

Recently there have been many breakthroughs in the understanding and subsequent therapy of this ravaging condition. Biochemical and electron microscope studies have provided more information about how the condition develops. A new medication, timolol maleate, promises more effective control of the problem with less frequent and milder side effects than those that often accompany traditional drugs. Finally, laser technology and microsurgery (see "High Tech," page 168, and "Breakthroughs," page 106) have made possible surgical corrections that were only dreamed about a few years ago.

About glaucoma

Glaucoma is a name given to several medical conditions that have one common factor—elevated pressure inside the eyeball sufficient to interfere with vision. Glaucoma does not take the same form in everyone. There are, in fact, at least forty recognized types.

In order to understand how glaucoma develops, you must understand the anatomy of the eye. The skin overlying the front of the eye is called the cornea. It is clear and colorless to permit the

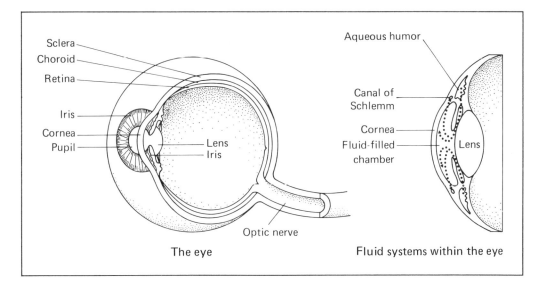

Labels (left diagram): Sclera, Choroid, Retina, Iris, Cornea, Pupil, Lens, Iris, Optic nerve

The eye

Labels (right diagram): Aqueous humor, Canal of Schlemm, Cornea, Fluid-filled chamber, Lens

Fluid systems within the eye

passage of light to the lens. The lens focuses light on the back of the eyeball, where millions of vision cells are located. These cells are connected to the optic nerve, which transmits the information to the brain. Between the cornea and the lens is the iris, the colored part of the eye, which contains a system of muscles that open and close the pupil. The spaces in front of and behind the iris are called the anterior and posterior chambers, respectively.

Normally the anterior and posterior chambers are filled with a fluid that bathes and nourishes the internal eye tissues. This aqueous humor, as it is called, is produced in the ciliary body, a structure in the posterior chamber. The fluid circulates and passes around the iris, through the pupil, and into the anterior chamber. From there it leaves the eye by passing through a sievelike structure called the trabecular meshwork, which surrounds the eye in a circle, and into the canal of Schlemm, which ultimately drains the fluid into the bloodstream. Pressure of the fluid within the eyeball, called intra-ocular pressure, is kept within a normal range by a balance between the formation of aqueous humor and its drainage. The system resembles a faucet and sink: the faucet is the ciliary body, the sink is composed of the anterior and posterior chambers, and the drain is the trabecular meshwork and canal of Schlemm.

Glaucoma is an imbalance between the production and drainage of aqueous humor. In rare instances, production exceeds drainage. In most cases, however, production is normal but drainage is blocked. In both kinds of glaucoma, fluid builds up in front of the lens, increasing the intra-ocular pressure in the anterior and posterior chambers. Eventually this increased pressure damages the optic nerve and destroys vision.

Intra-ocular pressure can be measured with a device called a tonometer. Pressure over 21 mm of mercury is considered abnormally high. Many people with glaucoma have lower pressures, however, and others have higher pressures without developing decrease or loss of vision.

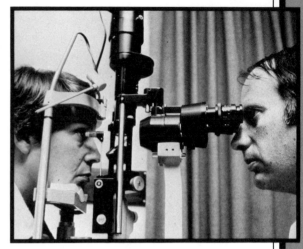

Doctor tests intra-ocular pressure with a tonometer, a standard exam for glaucoma.

CASE HISTORY

J. T., a fifty-eight-year-old black machinist, has always been fairly healthy. In a routine pre-employment physical examination four years ago, he was found to have high blood pressure and a slightly elevated blood sugar level, indicating an early case of diabetes. On a follow-up visit to the doctor he was given prescriptions for medications to lower his blood pressure and blood sugar level. He felt fine, however, and despite the warning that these conditions could eventually become more serious, he rarely took the medications. In fact, he took the blood pressure tablet only when he felt tense or had a headache and

thought that his blood pressure might be rising. Since the doctor had not given him insulin, he reasoned that the diabetes was not too serious. He didn't keep any of the appointments for return visits.

But eventually J. T. noticed that his vision was decreasing. He had difficulty describing the change; he just wasn't seeing as well. In the previous three years he had been to four different optometrists, but was never satisfied with the eyeglass prescriptions they gave him. His vision was slightly blurred, and he had trouble adjusting in a darkened room. In the past year he was involved in an auto accident, which occurred when he pulled out into the street without seeing a car approaching him from the side. During a visit to his company's health office because of a minor accident, he complained about his visual problems. The company nurse referred him to an opthalmologist, who found that he had glaucoma.

Although there are at least forty recognized types of glaucoma, over 90 percent are open-angle glaucoma. The angle refers to the junction where the trabecular meshwork and canal of Schlemm meet the cornea and iris. In open-angle glaucoma, the aqueous humor has free access to the drainage sites but the sites themselves are obstructed. Most cases of open-angle glaucoma are chronic, grow slowly, and lack early symptoms.

A small percentage of glaucomas are of the closed-angle variety, in which the angle between the cornea and iris is narrowed or completely closed, and the aqueous humor has no access to the drainage sites. Many cases of closed-angle glaucoma have acute, or sudden, symptoms. The most common symptoms are severe pain in one eye, blurred vision, nausea and vomiting, and seeing bright haloes or rings around lights because of tension and stretching in the cornea. The white of the eye may have prominent blood vessels and the cornea appear hazy. Closed-angle glaucoma is seen in the following cases:

■ *Enlarged iris:* If a congenital condition makes the iris too large, it can bow forward toward the cornea, thereby narrowing the angle.

■ *Increased lens size:* The lens normally grows larger with respect to the eye as a person gets older. If the lens is larger to begin with, it pushes the iris forward as a person gets older, narrowing the opening. This problem most often becomes symptomatic between the ages of sixty and seventy.

■ *Neovascular glaucoma:* This problem is seen in long-standing diabetics and hypertensives. Small blood vessels grow into the angle between the iris and the cornea. Eventually these blood vessels bring the two layers together, obliterating the angle.

There are also several other, rarer conditions resulting in the narrowing of the iris-cornea angle. Glaucoma may develop as a primary condition or as a condition secondary to other problems such as injury to the eye, diabetes, or high blood pressure.

In most cases, the progress of glaucoma is slow and painless. It follows a sequence of increased intra-ocular pressure; pressure on the optic nerve; loss of peripheral (side) vision early, and frontal vision later. The first two stages can be observed during an examination of the eye but are not noticed by the patient. The last is noticeable to the patient, but by then vision loss is permanent. It becomes important, therefore, to diagnose glaucoma during the first two stages, before much or any loss of vision has occurred.

As with blood pressure, it is necessary to take several readings of intra-ocular pressure with the tonometer. For one thing, the pressure fluctuates; it is influenced by certain medications and even by the time of day. Caffeine, for example, raises intra-ocular pressure; alcohol lowers it. The greater the intra-ocular pressure, the firmer the eyeball. All tonometers measure this firmness, some by applying pressure to the eyeball directly and others with a puff of air. Measuring intra-ocular pressure is a screening test that makes a good deal of sense. Since glaucoma has no symptoms in its early stages, and since the result—loss of vision—is irreversible, tonometry should be a part of every physical examination and preventive

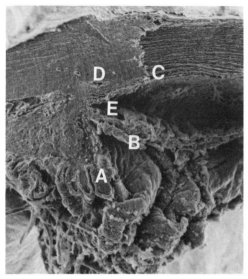

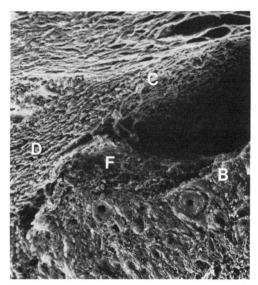

Normal eye, magnified 100x: Fluid is produced in ciliary body cells (A) and passes around iris (B) to the angle formed by iris and cornea (C). Fluid ultimately travels through Canal of Schlemm (D) by passing through the trabecular meshwork (E). (Photo by Thomas M. Richardson, M.D.)

Eye with glaucoma, 290x: In glaucoma, the angle between the cornea (C) and the iris (B) is obstructed by a growth of blood vessels (F), which prevents the passage of fluid to the Canal of Schlemm (D). (Photo by Thomas M. Richardson, M.D.)

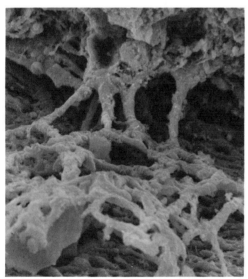

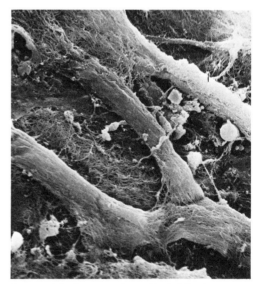

Close-up of trabecular meshwork in normal eye. Openings allow free passage of fluid to Canal of Schlemm. (Photo by Thomas M. Richardson, M.D.)

In eye with glaucoma (magnified 4000x), trabecular meshwork is obstructed by growth of many small blood vessels. (Photo by Thomas M. Richardson, M.D.)

medicine program. Everyone over forty should have a tonometry test every three to four years, or, if there is a family history of glaucoma, every year after age thirty.

Other commonly used examinations can also aid in the diagnosis of glaucoma. By measuring the visual fields, an opthalmologist can detect the loss of sight at the edges of vision—so-called tunnel vision, common in glaucoma as it progresses. With instruments such as the opthalmoscope and gonioscope, which enable a doctor to look through the cornea, an opthalmologist can see the interior of the eye and witness the structural changes that accompany an increase in pressure.

Treating glaucoma with medication

Traditionally, glaucoma is treated with medications that affect the nerves controlling the various functions within the eyeball. These nerves are part of the autonomic nervous system, an involuntary system that also controls many of the other body organs, such as the intestines, heart, and lungs. The autonomic nervous system has two components that work in opposition to each other to achieve stable organ functioning. The sympathetic component prepares the body for "fight or flight" in response to challenging stimuli; the parasympathetic component enables the body to rest. In the eye, the sympathetic system causes the pupil to dilate, or enlarge; the parasympathetic system causes it to constrict, or become smaller.

Both components of the nervous system transmit their messages to the tissues in the eyeball by chemicals called neurotransmitters. These chemicals affect both the production of aqueous humor by the ciliary body and its drainage into the trabecular meshwork and canal of Schlemm. Medications traditionally used for glaucoma work by affecting these neurotransmitters.

■ *Pilocarpine:* This, the most widely used medication for glaucoma, was introduced in 1877. It is administered topically as eye drops and mimics the parasympathetic neurotransmitter; the drug makes the pupil smaller and thereby facilitates the drainage of aqueous humor into the canal of Schlemm. Pilocarpine does lower the intra-ocular pressure, but it has disadvantages. The constricted pupil reduces the amount of light entering the eye, altering focus, night vision, and general visual acuity.

■ *Physostigmine:* This orally administered medication is similar to pilocarpine in that it constricts the pupil and increases the outflow of aqueous humor. It works by inhibiting an enzyme that would normally break down the neurotransmitter. But physostigmine causes severe visual difficulties, and prolonged use may lead to cataracts.

■ *Epinephrine:* This topical medication mimics the sympathetic neurotransmitter by decreasing aqueous humor production and increasing its outflow. Unfortunately, up to 15 percent of people cannot tolerate it because of the rapid heartbeat, red eyes, and headaches that are its side effects.

■ *Acetazolamide:* Introduced in 1954, this medication, taken by mouth, inhibits the enzyme carbonic anhydrase, which is found in many tissues and is important in the formation of aqueous humor. It can reduce intra-ocular pressure; but 50 percent of the people who take it become severely depressed and tired, and lose weight. They may also develop kidney stones because of its diuretic effect.

Although these medications have been effective through the years in controlling the progression of glaucoma by reducing the intra-ocular pressure, their accompanying side effects have often been annoying and, in some cases, debilitating.

What's new in the treatment of glaucoma?

In 1978 the U.S. Food and Drug Administration (FDA) approved timolol maleate (trade name Timoptic), a new drug that promises to be a dramatic advance in glaucoma therapy. Timolol maleate is a member of a class of drugs called beta blockers. Although the exact mechanism is not fully understood, timolol has been extensively studied and found to lower the intra-ocular pressure markedly. Animal studies with the drug were conducted at the Yale University School of Medicine and in France by a subsidiary of the Merck, Sharp and Dohme Pharmaceutical Company, which developed and produces the drug. Later, clinical researchers at more than twenty-five medical centers in the United States confirmed the results on humans.

Timolol reduces intra-ocular pressure with only twice-daily use, whereas existing medications often need to be used four times daily. It has an extremely low incidence of side effects. It does not affect the pupil; therefore, it does not lead to visual disturbances or decrease night vision. Because of its high degree of effectiveness, infrequent dosage, and few side effects, it will undoubtedly be more acceptable than the traditional drugs.

On the other hand, beta blockers are commonly used to control many heart problems and have the effect of slowing the heart rate. Patients taking other beta blockers for heart problems need to be watched more closely if they are also given timolol. Occasionally, minor eye irritation has been reported.

To date there is no perfect medication for glaucoma, and certainly no cure. But for thousands of people with glaucoma, timolol maleate may make the condition more tolerable.

Laser treatment for glaucoma

"Every one of you hath his particular plague," wrote Pittacus in 600 B.C., and for many people with diabetes and high blood pressure, that plague is the almost certain prospect of losing their sight to a condition called neovascular glaucoma. In its early stages, neovascular glaucoma is characterized by the growth of abnormal blood vessels in the angle of the eye's anterior chamber. These blood vessels obstruct the drainage system and inevitably cause a rise in the intra-ocular pressure. If left untreated, the rise in pressure relentlessly destroys the delicate nerves in the back of the eye and causes substantial vision loss and eventually blindness. Until now the treatment for neovascular glaucoma has been a dilemma for opthalmologists. Conventional medications and surgery were rarely successful in halting the disease. For many patients with the condition, however, the laser is changing all that and blindness is no longer inevitable.

"It's much like weeding a garden,"

explains Dr. Richard Simmons of the Massachusetts Eye and Ear Infirmary, the originator of a laser treatment for neovascular glaucoma. Dr. Simmons's treatment has an elaborate name —goniophotocoagulation—but the procedure itself is ingeniously simple. A laser beam focused on each of the blood vessels that grows to obstruct the angle and restrict fluid drainage burns and destroys them, and drainage is restored to normal. Several treatments may be necessary. "There are hundreds of blood vessels growing there," says Dr. Simmons, "but you just keep going back and clearing them out one by one until the growth of new blood vessels stops."

The laser is an intense beam of light that can be focused with such precision that little or no normal tissue is destroyed in the process (see "High Tech," pages 166–171). The laser beam is attached to a slit lamp, a magnifying device that enables the ophthalmologist to look through the cornea and into the angle where the abnormal blood vessel growth occurs. Performed as an outpatient procedure, the laser treatment requires one drop of topical anesthetic to "freeze" the cornea and is painless. Overall, laser treatment is remarkably free of complications.

Since its development at the Boston hospital in 1976, goniophotocoagulation is now well established at many medical centers across the country. "The laser treatment is actually a preventive measure," Dr. Simmons states. Destroying the abnormal blood vessels keeps the drainage angle open; the intra-ocular pressure does not go up and glaucoma does not develop. In 50 percent of neovascular glaucoma cases, laser treatment successfully prevents pressure

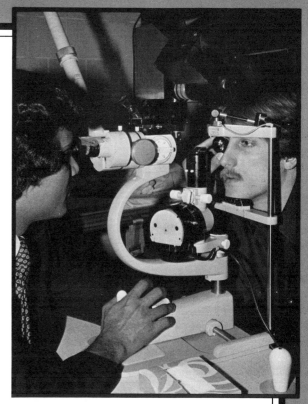

Laser treatment for neovascular glaucoma is performed painlessly in an outpatient setting. (Courtesy Massachusetts Eye and Ear Infirmary, Boston)

buildup. In another 25 percent, the condition is partially remedied with the laser, and medications can then control fluid drainage. In the remaining cases, the disease is so far advanced that the laser is ineffective; pressure continues to increase and irreversible glaucoma results. The condition must be diagnosed in its infancy, when the blood vessel growth is small enough to deal with. Opthalmologists who specialize in laser treatment recommend that people who are prone to develop neovascular glaucoma, such as those with high blood pressure and diabetes, should be examined frequently for early changes in intra-ocular pressure or in the appearance of the angle.

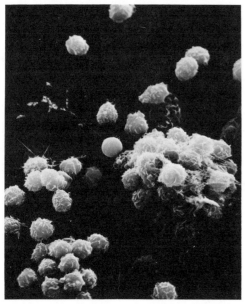

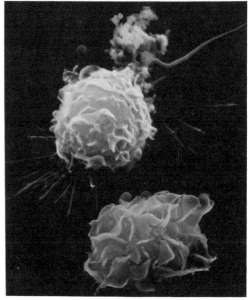

Isolated endothelial cells (magnified 2200x) that line the meshwork secrete G-A-G protein, which researchers feel may be responsible for the development of glaucoma. (Photo by Thomas M. Richardson, M.D.)

Same endothelial cells, magnified 8800x. (Photo by Thomas M. Richardson, M.D.)

In the future

Even though new medications like timolol maleate and the technological advance of the laser have done much to control glaucoma, they are not the ultimate answer to this condition. In order to "cure" the second leading cause of blindness, medical researchers will first have to find its cause. They are therefore studying the eye with the electron microscope, using high-level magnification and a biochemical approach. (Biochemistry is the study of the chemistry that takes place inside living cells.)

Determining the exact nature of the obstruction in the trabecular meshwork, for example, is one of the major challenges in glaucoma research today. The meshwork is very small, much narrower than a cotton thread, and is therefore difficult to study. Dr. Thomas Richardson of the Massachusetts Eye and Ear Infirmary is conducting detailed studies of the meshwork with the electron microscope, an instrument that permits tissues to be magnified several hundred thousand times, using human eyes donated to his laboratory. Dr. Richardson thinks that the clue to glaucoma may lie in the cells lining the meshwork and drainage system, the so-called endothelial cells, which may themselves produce a substance that impedes the drainage of aqueous humor. He explains his research: "We know that in glaucoma the meshwork is filled with a thick, almost gelatinous substance called G-A-G [glyco-amino-glycan]. Since the meshwork seems to be the site of

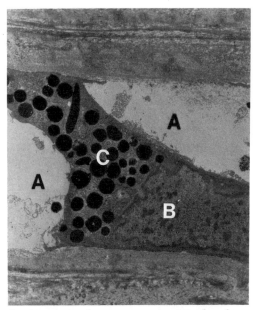

In pigmentary glaucoma, opening in trabecular meshwork (A) is blocked by an endothelial cell (B) that has been swelled by the absorption of granules of pigment. (Photo by Thomas M. Richardson, M.D.)

surrounding structures, actually clog up the trabecular meshwork. The cells lining the meshwork pick up the pigment particles, eventually break down, and physically obstruct the drainage system.

There is no cure for glaucoma yet, but scientific technology has shed new light on its causes and provided more effective therapy. The results are encouraging enough to promise hope for future control of this debilitating problem.

Resources

■ Information about glaucoma is best obtained from an opthalmologist, a medical doctor specializing in diseases of the eye.

■ Resource information is also available from:

National Eye Institute
9000 Rockville Pike
Bethesda, Maryland 20014
301-496-4000

National Society to Prevent Blindness
79 Madison Avenue
New York, New York 10016
212-684-3505

Better Vision Institute
230 Park Avenue
New York, New York 10017
212-682-1731

■ Local chapters of Lions Clubs, International, often sponsor glaucoma screening programs:

Lions Clubs International
York–Cermac Road
Oak Brook, Illinois 60521
312-986-1700

obstruction, this carbohydrate may be responsible.'' By isolating individual cells and growing them in tissue culture, Dr. Richardson and his colleagues hope to determine whether the endothelial cells are responsible for producing G-A-G. If their research is fruitful, a major breakthrough in the understanding of this complicated condition will have been made.

If it has not solved the mystery of glaucoma, the work in the Boston laboratories has already provided important information about the nature of many types of glaucoma. One example is pigmentary glaucoma, a particularly serious form of the condition that primarily affects young white males. The electron microscope has shown that pigment granules, which flake off the iris and its

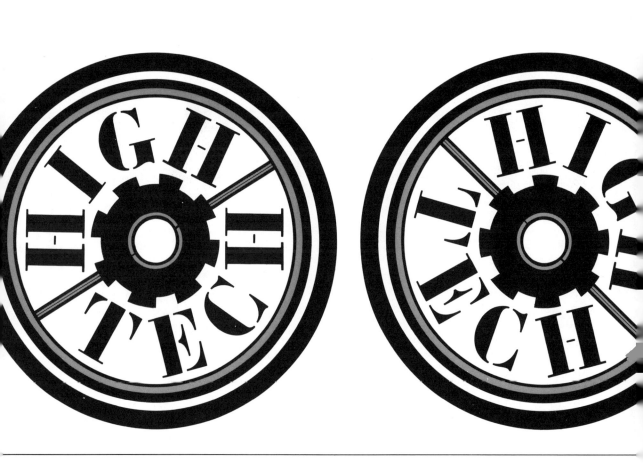

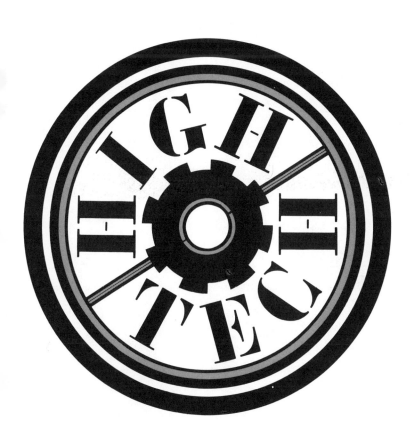

The past decade has produced a technological revolution in medicine. New instruments and techniques arising from space-age inventions have drastically affected the diagnosis and treatment of countless medical disorders. A Reading machine, for example, now enables blind individuals to "read" books. Laser technology has drastically shaped eye surgical procedures; and drug therapy and medical monitoring permit precise evaluation of drug dosage and gauge the body's reaction to treatment second by second.

But technology can represent a two-edged sword. Its benefits are evident throughout medicine; yet many blame technology for dehumanizing medical practices today and driving health-care costs to all-time highs. Too often technology *replaces*—rather than *supplements*—basic medical skills such as communication with patients and treatment based on observation and examination.

While astonishing new life-sustaining devices have raised technology to the level of art, today's medical world must keep technology in perspective. After all, technological advances must benefit the patient to play any effective role in medicine. The ultimate value of technology lies in the expansion and cultivation of current medical knowledge— without creating enslavement to technology for its own sake.

Kurzweil Reading Machine

I was eyes to the blind . . .

Job 29:15

Frenchh educator Louis Braille was sightless himself when he developed the system of raised dots that enables the blind to read with their fingers. Braille's system became the only method of written communication for sightless people, though not during his lifetime. And so it remained for a century and a half until 1972, when the brainchild of computer professional Raymond Kurzweil became the next major breakthrough in reading for the blind. In use for only five years, the Kurzweil Reading Machine (KRM) is expanding job and educational opportunities and opening the covers of books, magazines, and periodicals to the blind for the first time.

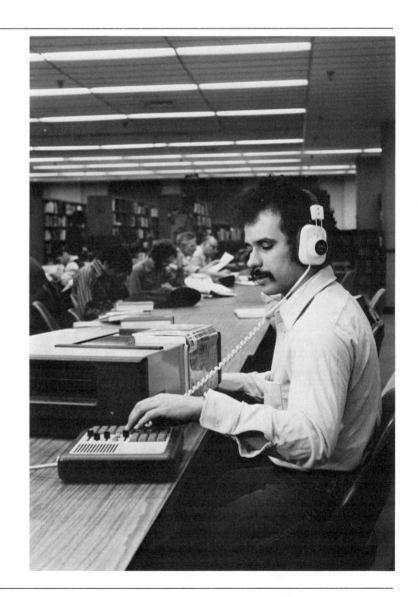

"Miracle on West 53rd Street"—Sightless man reads a book from the Mid-Manhattan Library in New York with the KRM. Sound is played back through earphones. (Courtesy Kurzweil Computer Products)

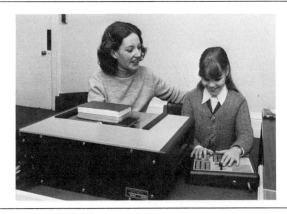

Sightless child is instructed in use of KRM at St. Dunstan's School in London, England. (Courtesy St. Dunstan's School)

CASE HISTORY

P. B. is a twenty-four-year-old government employee who has been blind since birth. Having attended a school for the blind, she has mastered braille and works full time in the Department of Handicapped Services in New York State. P. B. has a rather unusual hobby for a blind person—she is an avid reader. Each evening on her way home from work she stops at the Mid-Manhattan Library and reads best-sellers, biographies, and her favorite periodicals. Since she moved to New York one year ago, her parents send her letters three times a week; reading them keeps her up to date on her native Boston. Until she moved to New York, P. B.'s reading was limited to braille materials. Now she reads books off the general shelves.

The KRM

Even for those of us who take libraries for granted, the thought of a blind person going to a library to read sounds a bit unusual. The Mid-Man-hattan Library, however, is not the usual library. As a service to blind individuals of New York City, Mid-Manhattan has four Kurzweil Reading Machines, all available for public use.

Except for the usually sparse braille and talking book sections, a library might just as well have empty shelves as far as the blind are concerned. In many libraries, the Kurzweil Reading Machine is changing all that. The KRM provides sightless library users access to virtually any book on the shelves, as well as to most typewritten and printed material.

A machine that reads, the KRM converts printed material into spoken English. It reads several hundred styles and most sizes of type, as long as it is printed and not in script. Although it was one of the first to obtain the reading machine, the Mid-Manhattan Library is not unique. As of 1980, 200 desk-top units are located throughout the country in special schools for the handicapped, public schools, and libraries. The Smithsonian's Museum of History and Technology exhibits the Kurzweil Reading Machine in its Hall of Medicine and gives regular demonstrations of its capabilities. The Boston Children's Museum, committed to raising public consciousness about handicaps, also exhibits one of the latest models to show its visitors that physical problems can be overcome.

How does it work?

The KRM is an outgrowth of computer technology. The machine was the result of New Yorker Raymond Kurzweil's attempts to teach a computer to recognize printed characters and letters. The latest version of the unit fits comfortably on a desk top and resembles a small duplicating machine. You simply place printed material face down over a glass plate on the machine's upper surface. You then activate a small control box, and a scanning mechanism under the glass plate automatically locates the first line of type and begins interpreting it. Within a few seconds, an electronic voice is heard reading the material.

The Kurzweil Reading Machine contains four parts: the reading scanner, the computer,

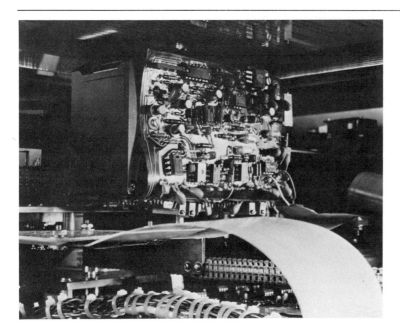

The KRM contains an optical scanner that reads printed material. Printed material can be seen through glass plate at top of photo. (Courtesy Kurzweil Computer Products)

the control box, and the speaker.

The heart of the KRM is an "optical character recognition system." A high-resolution camera, many times more sensitive than the human eye, scans each line, converts the images into electrical form, and transmits the data to a small computer contained within the machine. The computer is able to recognize individual letters and numbers, groupings of letters, spaces, and punctuation marks, based on the geometrical shape of each letter and its parts as viewed by the camera.

Stored within the computer's memory are over 1,000 linguistic rules and 2,000 exceptions to the rules, enabling it to compute the pronunciation of each word. Because it is programmed to recognize rules of syntax and punctuation marks, the computer can also compute stress contours

of an entire sentence and provide appropriate inflections.

English speech is made up of sixty or so basic units of sound called phonemes. The KRM has a voice synthesizer which translates the computer information into phonemes to produce understandable speech. The computer controls the electronic sound, producing circuits in the same way the human brain controls the jaw, throat, and tongue muscles to shape the vocal tract in generating human speech. Different from many voice synthesizers which have mechanical, monotonic sounds, the KRM has a resonant, almost baritone voice that captures effectively many of the nuances of human speech. Though it has a slightly artificial sound, it is easy and pleasant to listen to, even over long periods of time.

The control box of the KRM is compact and physically

separate from the reading unit and enables the user to make a wide range of choices about how the material is read. On the most basic level, the reading rate can be varied up to a high of 300 words per minute; the tone can also be varied to make it more understandable. To further increase comprehension, previously read words, phrases, and sentences can be repeated via memory circuits, and individual words can be spelled. A hand-tracking format on the controls enables the user to scan or browse a page optically, find out the overall layout, the number of columns, and the location of pictures and diagrams. In three or four hours, a blind person can be taught to use the machine and be comfortable with its operation.

The promise of KRM

The electronic data that determine how words are pronounced are contained on small cartridge tapes which can easily be changed. Tapes are now being developed with the phonemes of foreign languages; soon the KRM will speak to sightless people in many countries.

Another change of cartridge tape permits the unit to speak the language of mathematics and become an advanced talking calculator. It can be programmed to provide trigonometric and exponential functions and logarithms, as well as to solve complicated scientific and business problems. The tape cartridge permits storage of material for later recall. A new speech output system converts the latest version of the KRM to a talking computer terminal at the touch of a button. With this system, blind employees and students can now have the same access as their sighted colleagues to computer information normally displayed on video terminals or printed out on paper. The KRM is compatible with most standard computers and is opening up whole new vocational possibilities for sightless people in data processing departments, credit offices, and customer service departments.

For those who prefer the permanence of Braille material, the new Kurzweil Print to Braille system can convert textbooks, hard- and soft-cover books, magazine and journal articles, and most typewritten pages to Braille. It is less expensive—and much quicker—than previous conversion units. Using the Kurzweil system, a 500-page book can be converted to braille in three days, instead of the three to six months currently required using conventional hand-transcribing methods. The Library of Congress recently purchased a Kurzweil Print to Braille system to facilitate conversion of much of its stack material. In the past only about 300 of the 40,000 books and titles published each year were converted. Now that is expected to be greatly increased.

The promise of KRM has only begun to be realized. Rayond Kurzweil and his team of phonetics experts, design and systems analysts, and engineers are continuing to refine the KRM, which has already had an extraordinary impact on the lives of people with visual handicaps. Each model is easier and more pleasant to use. The latest, KRM 3, has three separate computer voice controls, enabling the listener

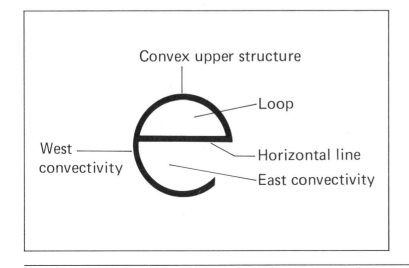

The KRM recognizes each letter by its geometric shapes. (Courtesy Kurzweil Computer Products)

to adjust the intensity of the *s* or hiss sound, voice quality or resonance, and high or low pitch. No two people have the same listening preferences; now the KRM can be controlled to the user's liking, played back on the speaker or privately through headphones, and adjusted for the noise level in a room, much as a person would do in a normal conversation.

In the past, there were never enough readers, never enough braille or talking publications, never enough academic and professional stimulation, and never enough privacy for the blind individual. Now, by having access to professional and reference materials, magazine and journal articles, and personal correspondence, sight-handicapped people can have independence, privacy, and the chance to live up to their intellectual capabilities.

As one blind KRM user in Lawrence, Massachusetts, said, "I'm saving my money to buy a KRM. I don't need a big house; a fancy car would be of no value to me. But the KRM would bring me the world."

Resources

In October 1979, international recording artist Stevie Wonder became the first individual to own a Kurzweil Reading Machine. Its price tag of $20,000 makes it more appropriate for libraries, schools, and other public facilities where many people can use it. Included in the price is the instructional material and personal demonstration necessary to become competent and comfortable with its use. Information on the KRM is generally available from state library commission offices, divisions for the blind, or directly from Kurzweil Computer Products, 32 Cambridge Parkway, Cambridge, Massachusetts 02142.

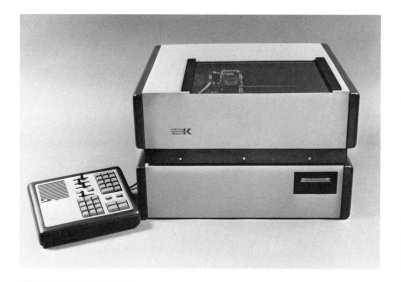

The Kurzweil Reading Machine conveniently fits on a desktop. Printed material is placed on the glass plate. Control box for the unit is at left. (Courtesy Kurzweil Computer Products)

Telemetry in miniature

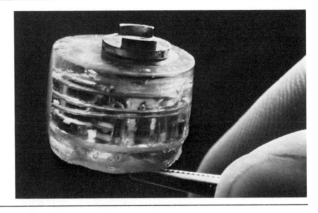

In the Psychology Department of the Massachusetts Institute of Technology, "Squeaky" was making its way through a maze, sniffing the food pellets that will be its eventual reward. Elsewhere in the laboratory, a research associate was watching a computer screen and recording the activity in the rat's limbic system, a part of the brain involved in decision making. The laboratory animal in this 1977 study of brain anatomy was being tracked by a tiny monitor/transmitter attached to its head.

Originally developed by M.I.T. researcher David Pettijohn for laboratory research use, this unit may soon have quite an impact on the world of medical monitoring. Weighing only 4 g (less than ⅛ ounce), it permits the study of many body systems at rest and activity without the need for wires or other restrictive devices. This miniature monitoring device is already in use in over 200 settings.

CASE HISTORY

Tethered by wires to the electrical equipment that monitors and records his heartbeat, M. N. is uncomfortable and restricted in the cardiac care unit. As he stretches his arms to relieve the tension, an alarm sounds in the nursing station. The nurse quickly scans the bank of monitor screens and notices what appears to be an irregular heart rhythm on M. N.'s monitor. She rushes to his side, realizing that only ten hours have elapsed since his heart attack and that rhythm abnormalities are a frequent complication. She is relieved to find M. N. comfortable, with normal blood pressure and pulse. A loose wire caused the monitor pattern. "Ah, technology," she sighs, and tightens the wire, restoring a normal pattern on the screen.

The Monitronix

Monitoring is widely used in medical practice, from the rather simple measurements of temperature, weight, and blood pressure to the more

The Monitronix is about as high as a thumbnail and weighs only four grams. (Courtesy Midgard Electronics)

complicated analysis of heart and brain wave activity. More sophisticated monitoring systems are able to measure the electrical currents generated by the chemicals that make up our organs as they interact. The major problem with today's monitoring systems is the cumbersome equipment necessary to detect and transmit electrical signals. Attached by wires to bedside recording devices, monitored patients traditionally have been restricted to bed or a very short radius of activities; or they wear portable devices about the size of a cigarette pack that are fragile and limiting, since they are worn on a belt or strapped to the body. Current monitoring systems also have the deficiency of long electrode wires, which cause movement artifact (distortions on the screen) and interference with transmission.

The Monitronix system developed at M.I.T. is a thimble-sized monitor/transmitter which uses ultraminiature components. The five

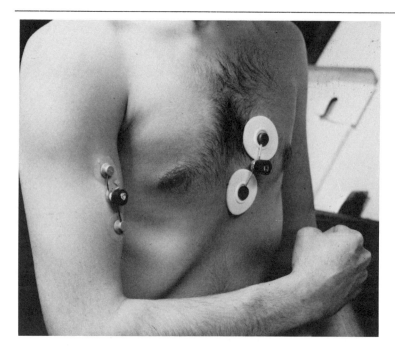

Monitronix can be attached with adhesive plates over any muscle—in this case, biceps. Second unit over chest records heartbeat. (Courtesy Midgard Electronics)

transistors that amplify and broadcast the signal are all about the size of pinheads. They are powered by a hearing-aid battery and can detect electrical signals across the entire range of body activities and transmit the signals over distances up to 130 feet. Within that range, these signals can overpower a commercial FM radio station broadcasting at or near the same frequency. Temperature, muscle activity, breathing, electrocardiogram, and brain wave activity can all be studied with this unit, giving it a potentially wide spectrum of medical application. Although the Monitronix isn't the only miniature monitor, it is the smallest and most sophisticated.

In the future

The United States Olympic Training Center in Colorado Springs is using Monitronix to study heart and muscle activity in trained athletes. Since the unit is so small and has no wires, the athlete has no activity restriction and can be monitored even at peak exercise.

Dr. Gene Hagermann, director of sports physiology at the Olympic site, has studied figure skaters, biathletes (participants in the combination cross-country skiing and rifle-shooting event) and runners with the Monitronix system. He says, "The transmitter was so small, the athletes didn't even notice it. The normal bumps and jostles of athletic activity had no effect on the signal. It remained good throughout."

Prior to this, the wires of standard monitors prohibited the study of muscle during intense activity. The Olympic Training Center plans to use the unit to monitor heart rate during stress testing, muscle strength, power and endurance, and more simple parameters such as temperature, pulse, and blood pressure during exercise. Correlating athletic excellence with patterns of heart, muscle, and physiologic activity can then be used to determine the limits of exercise, as well as to train young athletes.

David O. Pettijohn, the M.I.T. researcher who developed Monitronix, suggests that further applications of the miniature unit are limited only by the imagination: "Athletes are not the only individuals who benefit from muscle function recording. A hospital in New York is using it to aid their rehabilitation programs for stroke victims; and it can assess the tension of muscles in biofeedback training." Cardiologists may soon find such miniature units useful in following the heart rhythms of patients during stress testing, in cardiac care wards, or to follow ambulatory patients after a cardiac event. Electroencephalogram or brain wave recordings will be possible without the extensive wiring of to-

Monitronix transmitters attached to right biceps and chest of U.S. biathalon team member Ken Alligood enables physiologist Dr. Gene Ingerman (seated) to study heart and muscle activity during treadmill test at United States Training Center, Colorado Springs, Colorado. (Courtesy Midgard Electronics)

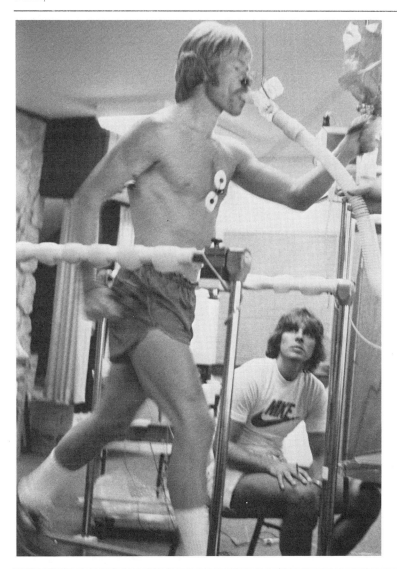

day's instruments and during a range of activities. EEG recordings currently are restricted to rest or sleep states. The Massachusetts General Hospital is also using Monitronix to observe babies at high risk for sudden infant death syndrome. It picks up the babies' breathing noises and sounds an alarm if breathing stops.

The Midgard Electronic Company in Newton, Massachusetts, is producing and further developing the Monitronix system. They feel that subsequent generations of the already miniature instrument may become even smaller, as transistor and circuit technology continues to develop.

Resources

■ The Monitronix monitor is manufactured by:

Midgard Electronics
175 California Street
Newton, Massachusetts 02158
617-964-4545

Gait
analysis

On the influence of abnormal parturition, difficult labors, premature births and asphyxia neonatorum on the mental and physical condition of the child, especially in relation to deformities.

William John Little, 1861

The childhood illness that left his foot misshapen is generally credited as the driving force behind British orthopedic surgeon William John Little's lifelong interest in deformities. In a report published in 1861, Dr. Little, the founder of the Royal Orthopaedic Hospital in London, was the first to describe a medical condition that was prevalent in his time and today affects 700,000 Americans. For years it was known as Little's disease; today it is called cerebral palsy.

Actually not just a single disease, cerebral palsy is a catch-all term given to disorders of movement that are caused by permanent brain damage encountered during birth or early infancy.

The incidence of cerebral palsy has decreased in recent years as effective prenatal and infant care has reduced the number of infants brain-damaged at birth. Prevention and treatment of Rh disease, light therapy for neonatal jaundice, and intensive care nurseries are just some of the advances that have lowered infant disease rates.

Still, cerebral palsy strikes 10,000 to 15,000 children each year. Since the disease has no cure, modern therapy is directed at recognizing the problem early, and treatment is geared to prevent further disabilities.

One major problem has always been the absence of diagnostic tools to evaluate individually each child with the condition. Definite and exacting techniques such as X rays, blood tests, and biopsies are not appropriate for cerebral palsy; the doctor instead had to depend on his clinical judgment. Now, because of a merger of the technologies of medicine, electronics, and engineering, more exact diagnostic information is available in a technique called gait analysis.

The gait laboratory was developed to provide a better understanding of the movement problems associated with cerebral palsy and other neuromuscular disorders. An outgrowth of the technology that was used to measure astronauts' movements in space, the laboratory provides an accurate and detailed assessment of each individual's condition. With this information, a clinician can rate the efficacy of a child's walk, determine which specific muscles need therapeutic exercise, and decide whether or not braces and splints are needed. Repeated gait testing at varying intervals can assess how a treatment program is progressing and what changes could or should be made. Perhaps a lighter brace would be more valuable; maybe surgery is needed to correct a shortened muscle. Whatever the choices, gait analysis enables doctors to determine the most appropriate and efficient treatment for the victims of cerebral palsy.

The gait laboratory is also being used to study the walking patterns of patients with muscular dystrophy, lower leg deficiencies, and other neuromuscular disorders. Recently, it has also aided the rehabilitation of older patients who have

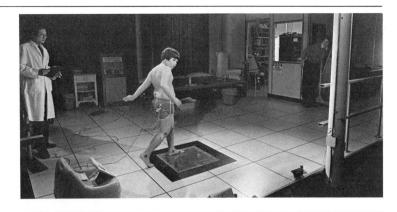

A ten-year-old cerebral palsy patient undergoes testing at gait laboratory. Force plate on floor records weight distribution; devices on knees and ankles monitor joint movement. (Courtesy Children's Hospital Medical Center, Boston)

Gait laboratory also aids rehabilitation for patients with artificial joints—here a woman with a recently implanted artificial knee. (Courtesy Brigham and Women's Hospital, Boston)

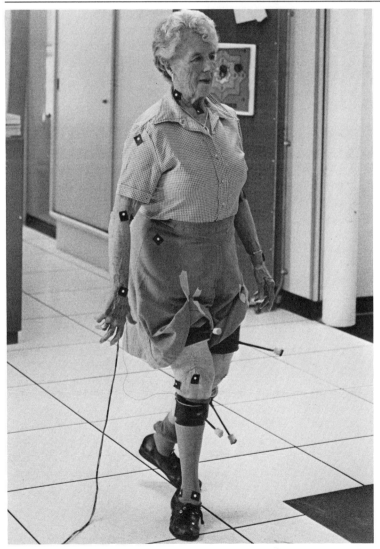

had operations to replace arthritic or injured joints with prosthetic ones.

The combined means of medicine and engineering are being used increasingly in the study of body functions. In the gait laboratory, the impact of that effort enables disabled persons to develop their full potential.

How gait analysis works

The act of walking involves more than just getting from one point to another. It is a complex relationship involving nerve impulses, muscle contraction, and bone and joint movement. In cerebral palsy the nerve impulses are disorganized and the patient does not walk in the normal coordinated way. Simple clinical observation cannot determine the nerve activity and muscle interrelationships at any given moment. The gait analysis laboratory uses electronic technology to get that information.

The gait laboratory at Boston Children's Hospital, where the procedure was developed as a joint project between Harvard University and the Massachusetts Institute of Technology, is a large, pleas-

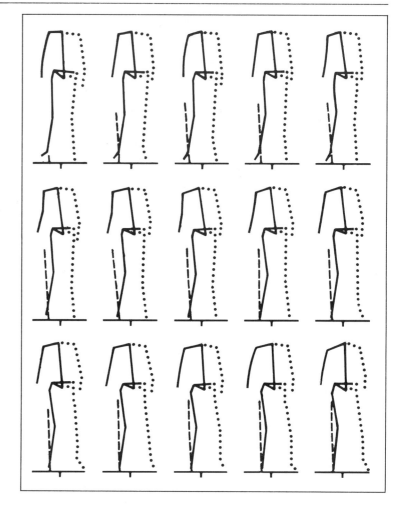

antly and brightly decorated room. The child with cerebral palsy is asked to walk across the room along a designated path. All the while, three types of information are being gathered:

■ *Electromyograph recordings of muscle activity.* Small electrodes the size of a pencil eraser are painlessly attached to the skin over large muscles such as those of the thigh and calf. The electrodes are connected by a thin wire to a recorder which measures muscle activity during the walk. As muscles contract, they generate a small electrical current which varies with the intensity of the contraction. The electrodes reveal simultaneously how hard each of the muscles works during walking.

■ *Measurements of the force of walking.* Motion occurs when

the leg muscles push against the resistance of the floor. An inconspicuous plate in the center of the floor of the gait laboratory is actually a supersensitive scale. As the child walks across the floor, the foot applies pressure on the scale, which measures the force between the foot and the floor in all directions—front to back, side to side, and twisting—giving an exact picture of the balance and how much force each part of the foot exerts while it is in contact with the floor. Dr. Sheldon Simon of the gait

laboratory at Boston Children's Hospital notes the importance of this measurement: "It may look as if a child's weight is evenly distributed between both legs, but the force plate may show that one leg is doing most of the work. The force plate also quantifies the swaying and wavering that occur when a child with cerebral palsy steadies each step."

■ *Film of the walk.* Because walking is a three-dimensional activity, motion pictures are made simultaneously from

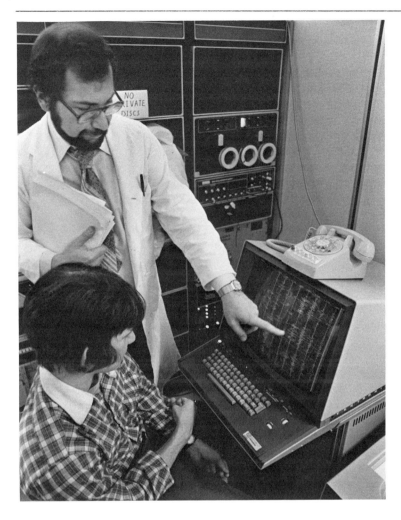

figure which provides a picture of the child's walk, showing every shift in the angles of the joints.

The computer analyzes the information from the floor force plate, electromyograph recordings, and three-dimensional films to show exactly how the limbs move, what muscles are contracting, and what force they apply to the ground at each instant during the walking cycle. Computer memory technology allows the information on each patient to be stored and recalled at any time. It also permits a permanent copy of the analysis to be placed in the patient's records.

Several walks can be filmed in five to ten minutes. Often the child is also asked to perform other movements involving arm and shoulder to assess those joints. Dr. Simon says that most children find the test fascinating and eagerly cooperate. It usually takes no more than one-half to one hour to test one child completely.

three directions: left, right, and front. Conventional cameras, however, are of little value in the gait laboratory because of the continual change that occurs during walking. Rather, high-speed cameras that operate at sixty frames per second are used. In order to observe the limb movements accurately, small pieces of tape are placed at the major joints—shoulder, elbow, wrist, hip, knee, and so forth. When the film is developed, it is projected one frame at a time over a large cross-hatched grid on a computer screen. For each frame the location of each of the pieces of tape, and therefore each of the taped joints, is recorded by tapping on the screen where the tape is seen. The act of tapping records the location of each of the joints on the computer grid. Each successive frame records a progression of movement. Noting the location of the joints on each frame enables doctors to follow the movement of each limb and joint carefully. The computer uses all these recorded points to construct and print out a cartoon-type stick

Fetal monitoring

Monitus (Latin): "to watch and to warn."

The infant mortality rate has steadily declined from almost 200 for each 1,000 births in 1930 to 16 per 1,000 births in the 1970s. Many physicians feel that increased awareness of the special problems of the fetus may reduce the prenatal death rate by another 50 percent.

In the past, the uterus and amniotic fluid which protect the fetus have also prevented direct evaluation of the unborn infant, and prenatal care has thus focused on the pregnant mother. Recently, however, modern techniques such as electronic and ultrasound technology have made it possible to monitor the unborn child's development. One process in particular, known as fetal monitoring, has resulted in major advances in the world of obstetrics.

The fetal monitor is an electronic device that records the progress of the mother and fetus during labor. Small sensors attached to the mother's abdominal wall or the fetus's scalp monitor uterine contractions and fetal heart rate and print

them simultaneously on a strip of paper for analysis.

The monitoring paradox

Modern obstetrics presents a unique paradox. After years of delivering babies while under heavy sedation—in fact, anesthesia—women now want to be awake and in control and to experience the phenomenon of childbirth. Childbirth classes prepare the mother to deal with the stress and pain of labor through the almost autohypnotic approach of breathing and relaxation exercises. Sterile, pictureless, colorless labor and delivery rooms are being replaced by birthing rooms, quasi apartments with televisions, bright colors, food, and drink where the entire family can experience the emotional interaction common to home births, while the patient remains close to the lifesaving equipment of the delivery and pediatrics units.

At the same time technology has advanced and obstetricians have learned to understand the physiologic needs and changes of the fetus during labor and delivery. The fetal heart monitor is a major evidence of this advancing technology. Now we

see wires attaching the mother and fetus to an instrument that monitors their progress during labor. Many women feel that the wires make childbirth a mechanical, dehumanized experience. Some, made more anxious by the flashing lights of the instrument and the sounds it makes with each fetal heartbeat, refuse the monitor entirely. Other mothers feel more secure with the monitor working, knowing that every flash and beat are indications that things are progressing well.

Within the obstetrical field there is also controversy on this issue. Some point to the decreasing neonatal death rates and say that technology is responsible. Others say that the relationship of technology to fetal well-being during labor is only a circumstantial one, that other factors may be at work.

CASE HISTORY

A.W. is a nineteen-year-old woman in her first pregnancy. When her membranes ruptured four days prior to her due date, she was admitted to the hospital and found to be in early labor. Her progress was slow, and fetal monitoring was begun

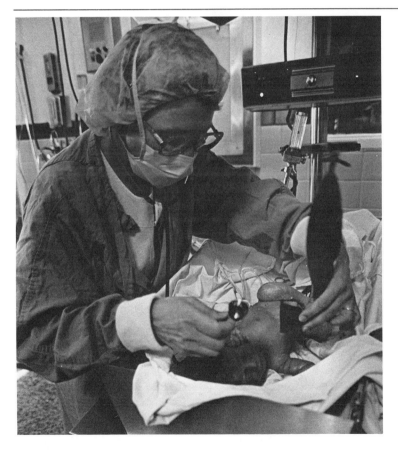

A physician checks the Apgar score of a new baby, assessing several vital functions to determine infant's overall health. (Photo by Michael J. Lutch, courtesy Beth Israel Hospital, Boston)

bed. Finally, for fear of depriving the baby of oxygen, A.W. was taken to the operating room, where a cesarean section was performed. A male infant with an Apgar score of seven was delivered. (Apgar is a system of evaluation of the new born baby based on ten observations, such as skin color and breathing. For each normal observation the baby gets one point. Scores approaching ten indicate a healthy baby; lower scores may mean distress.) After an initial two days of respiratory distress requiring close watching, the baby did well and has remained so at two-week, four-week, and six-week checkups.

How the monitor works

"The goal in treating a pregnant patient is to prevent problems from arising in the mother or fetus," writes University of Southern California obstetrics professor E. J. Quilligan.

to observe the uterine contractions and baby's heart rate. Because of interference with external leads, small electrodes were attached to the baby's scalp and an excellent tracing was obtained. At the twelfth

hour of labor, the fetus developed a slowing of the heart rate around the time of a contraction, and umbilical cord compression was suspected. The slowing persisted despite changing A.W.'s position in

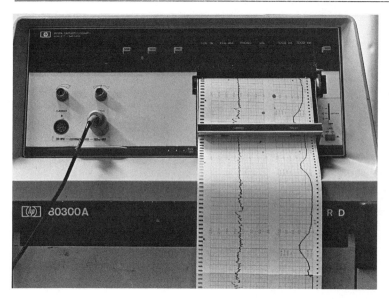

The fetal monitor records a fetus's heart rate (left) and the mother's uterine contractions (right). (Photo by Michael J. Lutch, courtesy Beth Israel Hospital)

Coordinating a symposium on fetal monitoring for the *Journal of Postgraduate Medicine* in April 1977, he emphasized that only close and careful observation of mother and fetus will realize that goal. "Communication with the fetus is mandatory, if we are to avoid potential and actual problems," Dr. Quilligan notes. However, the protective environment of the uterus makes that communication difficult.

Heart rate has been generally accepted as a good indicator of the overall health of the fetus. Throughout pregnancy, the fetal heart gradually slows and, at the time of birth, varies from 110 to 150 beats per minute. Rates of over 150 occur if the mother has a fever or if there is early decrease of oxygen delivery to the baby. Slowing of the heart rate, below 110 beats per minute, is often a sign for concern and may indicate congenital heart defect, inadequate oxygen delivery, or the effect of a maternal medication.

In response to the developing baby's nervous system activity, there is a natural variability in the fetal heart rate of from six to ten beats per minute. In fact, physicians become concerned when the natural variability stops and the heart rate becomes more regular. Dr. Quilligan points out that "infants with normal variability of their heart rate have higher Apgar scores at birth." Dr. Edward Hon, a colleague of Dr. Quilligan, comments that a fetal monitor is the only real way of appreciating the variability of the fetal heart. "A stethoscope has limited value for the early detection of fetal distress," states Dr. Hon. "With rates around 150 per minute, it is extremely difficult to appreciate variability. And the heartbeat is even more difficult to hear during uterine contractions, when the fetus may be under the most stress."

The Los Angeles physicians also point out that the fetal heart slows in response to a

uterine contraction and that three distinct patterns of slowing can be recognized. A heart rate that slows early in the contraction is probably a result of pressure on the baby's skull and is of no consequence because it is temporary. However, if the slowing begins late in the contraction or at different times during it, there is a clear association with fetal distress, probably caused by compression of the umbilical cord and subsequent poor oxygen delivery to the infant. This type of slowing is noticed frequently in monitored labors, and changing the mother's position in bed most often corrects the situation. When it doesn't, immediate Caesarean section is usually recommended. Again, a standard stethoscope cannot detect these subtle changes. Unless the rate change is prolonged (that is, remains under 110 beats per minute for at least several seconds), it cannot be picked up without a monitor. For these reasons, many obstetricians recommend that all labors be monitored. Others disagree, as we shall see.

Many hospitals monitor all labors with external electrodes, small sensors that are attached to the skin of the mother's abdominal wall with an adhesive. If interference from skin prevents an adequate signal, direct attachment to the baby's scalp is considered. Other hospitals use fetal monitoring only for so-called high-risk pregnancies, in women with poor progress in labor, toxemia, elevated blood pressure, and diabetes, or pregnancies lasting over forty-two weeks (the normal pregnancy is forty weeks). All hospitals monitor induced labors in which medications are given to speed up the process.

What are the benefits?

We have seen the potential for electrical monitoring to discover circumstances that signify fetal distress. What is the actual effect of this technology in hospitals where it is routinely used?

Most studies comparing monitored with unmonitored labors point out that fetal monitoring does lower neonatal death rates. A retrospective analysis of over 50,000 births at the Los Angeles County Women's Hospital and 15,000 births at Boston's Beth Israel Hospital showed a clear benefit of monitoring. On the other

hand, another study by Dr. Albert Haverkamp and his colleagues at the Denver General Hospital showed no difference in neonatal mortality or Apgar scores with monitored labors. There is similar controversy throughout current obstetrical literature.

Fetal monitoring does have its problems. External monitoring with electrodes attached to the mother's abdominal wall causes few or no complications, other than the obvious emotional impact of being attached to an electrical device. But when internal monitoring is necessary because of an inadequate external tracing, membranes must be ruptured. There is therefore a slight risk of infection and trauma to the baby's scalp, though obstetricians generally state that this is only a theoretical, rather than an actual, risk.

A completely randomized, scientifically valid study of the effects of fetal monitoring will probably never be done. This would require withholding the technology to groups of babies in which it has definite increased merit—that is, high-risk and premature births. Some obstetricians feel these

high-risk groups, with better prenatal evaluation, can be easily identified anyway, and will probably have Caesarean section with or without fetal monitoring.

Fetal monitoring is certainly here to stay, although the scientific community will continue to debate the actual benefit. Fetal monitoring will probably always be used in situations where complications seem likely to develop. In the end, though, monitoring may not alter what a well-trained, well-prepared obstetrician would do. Commenting on the subject in a *New England Journal of Medicine* issue, Georgetown University professor Andre Hellegers says: ''By themselves squiggles on a piece of paper do not save lives. It's what doctors do with the squiggles that matters.''

Drug therapy monitoring

The truth is, the science of nature has been already too long made only a work of brain and fancy.
It is now high time that it should return to the plainness and soundness of observations on material and obvious things.

Robert Hooke
Micrographia, 1665

Railing against the trend to solve problems by fanciful thinking more than 300 years ago, Hooke suggested that the secrets of nature could be revealed by something as mundane as closer observation. So also in medical science. While innovation and imagination have their role, the understanding of complex medical problems has always been related to the ability to observe and study those problems. The development of medical technology through the years bears testimony to scientific attempts at better observation: to wit the microscope, X rays, and nuclear medicine. Now, when the ability to examine body fluids and tissues contributes to the understanding and following of disease, the clinical laboratory

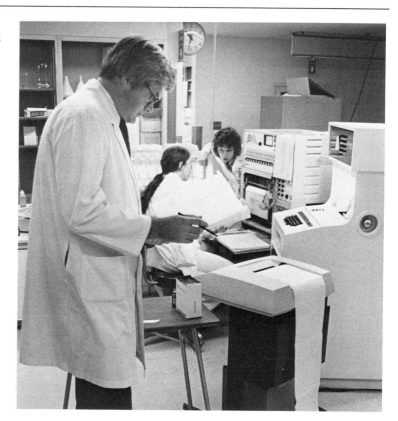

Physician checks the computer results of latest drug screening test. Computers have been important adjuncts to drug monitoring. (Courtesy Lynn Hospital, Massachusetts)

has expanded its contribution to observation with a technique called drug therapy monitoring.

Drug therapy

Drugs have been used to treat physical and emotional maladies for centuries. But drug therapy has never been an exact science because of the problem of dosage. Until recently, the physician had to depend largely on clinical judgment or trial and error to find the appropriate dose of a particular drug for a particular patient. The manufacturer's recommendation and the patient's body weight provided guidelines, but problems developed because of individual differences. With too little medication, the desired effects are not seen; with too much medication, serious complications can result. Often the range between "too little" and "too much" is very narrow.

A much more accurate way to predict a drug's effect would be to know exactly what concentration of that drug is present in body fluids. The amount of a drug that is given does not provide that information because every body absorbs, breaks down, and excretes a particular drug at a different rate. And laboratory analysis of a drug's concentration has been difficult because, by the time a particular dose has been distributed throughout the body, its concentration in any individual tissue or fluid is extremely small.

An accurate method of monitoring drug therapy finally evolved when laboratory techniques made it possible to analyze extremely small quantities of substances —often one or two parts per million. With these methods the exact amount of a drug in body fluids can be determined with great accuracy and the patient's response to the drug understood more thoroughly. In the case of epilepsy, for example, Dilantin and other medications to control seizure activity depend upon a specific blood level for their effect. If the level of anti-seizure medication is below the therapeutic range, seizures occur. If too much medication is given, the drug quickly becomes toxic to the patient. Similar situations exist with medications for cardiac and respiratory conditions and for psychoactive drugs such as Valium and lithium. Antibiotic concentrations can also be measured in the laboratory.

In addition to monitoring the specific concentration of a drug in the blood or serum, laboratory analysis can monitor a drug's effect. In the case of an anticoagulant, or "blood thinner," the effect of the drug on the blood-clotting time, rather than its concentration in the blood, can be measured. Similarly, blood counts are fol-

lowed on patients undergoing chemotherapy or radiation therapy; if the white blood count drifts too low in these patients, they may be unable to fight off an infection.

In the future

Drug therapy monitoring got its start in toxicology—the study of overdoses of medications and drugs—but its usefulness is now expanding across all of medicine. Drugs are chemicals, complicated entities that work in specific and exact ways. It is difficult to rely on formulas or clinical observations to achieve optimum drug response because those methods are not exact. With monitoring by modern laboratory methods, however, drug therapy is becoming a more exact science.

Laser surgery

One small step for man; one giant leap for mankind.

Neil Armstrong, astronaut, 1969

Armstrong's historic words were symbolic not only of the guidance and propulsion systems that took his spacecraft to the moon and back, but also of the experiments in geology, communications, and physics that were conceived on earth and were now being performed on the moon.

One such experiment begun by the Apollo 11 explorers functions to this day. Three times daily an intense, highly focused laser beam is turned on at the McDonald Observatory at the University of Texas and aimed at a mirrored reflector installed on the moon's surface by astronauts Armstrong and Buzz Aldrin. With the laser and reflector, measurements of the distance between the earth and the moon are now possible within six inches of accuracy.

The concept of a laser was developed at Columbia University by physicists Charles H. Townes and Arthur L. Schawlow and independently in the U.S.S.R. by physicists Nikolai G. Basov and Aleksandr H. Prochorov in 1958. Townes and the Soviets shared the 1964 Nobel Prize in physics for their work. The first laser, built by Theodore Maiman in 1960 at the Hughes Research Laboratory, used a ruby crystal, the major component of solid lasers even today.

At the time of Apollo 11 the laser beam was barely ten years old, and the space voyage demonstrated its value to many people for the first time. Ten years later, the laser is widely used in industry, science, and communications.

Among the many uses of the laser beam are its applications in the world of medicine. Today the laser is routinely used to remove polyps or growths on the vocal cords or the brain, to restore vision in eyes ravaged by diabetes, to remove deforming birthmarks, and to perform a variety of other operations without the complications of bleeding.

What is a laser?

A laser is a device that amplifies and focuses light. The word *laser* stands for *light amplification by stimulated emission of radiation.* Conventional light sources such as the sun, tungsten light bulbs, and fluorescent lamps are all basically hot bodies that give off spontaneous energy in the form of light in all directions. A laser differs in that the energy is stimulated rather than spontaneous, and is highly directional.

All light comes from atoms, the basic physical unit that makes up all solid, liquid, and gaseous substances. Every atom is a storehouse of energy. The amount of energy depends on the motion of electrons that orbit the atom's nucleus.

When an atom is exposed to any form of energy such as heat or light, its own energy level increases. In this state the atom is said to be excited, and the orbit of its electrons changes. When the energy reaches a critical level, the atom returns to its former state by spontaneously releasing its added energy in the form of light. This spontaneous emission produces incoherent light—light of many different frequencies and directions—because atoms release their energy irregularly.

Unlike the spontaneous

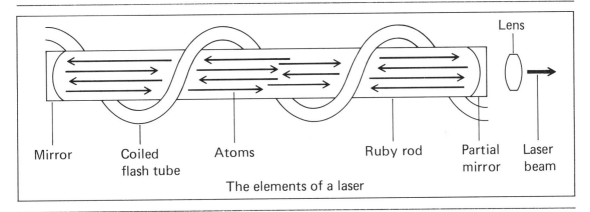

					Lens

Mirror   Coiled   Atoms   Ruby rod   Partial Laser
        flash tube   mirror beam

The elements of a laser

emission of conventional light sources, the laser uses stimulated energy emission, in which the energy released from one atom interacts with another atom that is still excited. This second atom then releases its energy, which in turn interacts with a third atom, and so on through millions of atoms. This produces coherent light; the energy released as light has the same frequency and direction as the stimulating energy.

How lasers work

Lasers can operate by stimulating the atoms in solid, liquid, or gaseous substances.

In a solid laser a crystal ruby rod is usually used. The rod is surrounded by a coiled flash tube which produces pulses of brilliant light. The powerful flash sends intense light through the ruby, exciting the chromium atoms within the ruby and changing the orbit of their electrons. Exciting atoms radiate light as the electrons drop back to their low-energy orbits. The light energy stimulates other atoms into releasing their energy. The laser light is reflected back and forth by mirrors and

continues to stimulate more and more atoms into releasing their energy. The light is then released through a small hole in the mirrors on one side and is focused intensely by a lens.

The solid laser produces a brief but intense pulse of light so strong that it can melt 1/16-inch steel in an instant. Shortly after its development it was thought wise to have a laser that was higher in power but worked continuously rather than in brief pulses. In response, Ali Javan at the Bell Laboratories developed a laser using a gas medium in 1961. Today's gas lasers use xenon, argon, or carbon dioxide as amplifying sources.

Bloodless surgery

The basis of laser surgery is the ability of the light beam to burn and evaporate biological tissues.

A laser's light beam generates intense heat. A lens can focus the beam to a point 1/10,000 inch (.0025 mm) wide. When the beam is concentrated in an area that small it can reach temperatures of 10,000 degrees Fahrenheit (5,500 degrees Celsius) and melt away any known sub-

stance, including a diamond. A laser can easily dispense with body tissues by simply evaporating them. At lower powers lasers produce heat reactions that create small burns that can seal blood vessels.

As the traditional surgeon guides his sharp scalpel through body tissues, bleeding is an inevitable complication because blood vessels surround and fill all our tissues. Much time is spent in the careful ligation (or tying off) of each bleeding point to minimize the loss of blood and prevent clot formation, which can interfere with healing and promote infection.

The surgeon using a laser beam as his scalpel has certain distinct advantages:

- The hot beam cauterizes (burns) as it cuts, and surgery can be bloodless. Much time is saved by eliminating the need to tie or cauterize individual bleeding points.

- The infection rate is lower because devitalized tissue has been evaporated, blood clots do not form, and the beam sterilizes the wound as it cuts.

- The spread of malignant cells during cancer surgery

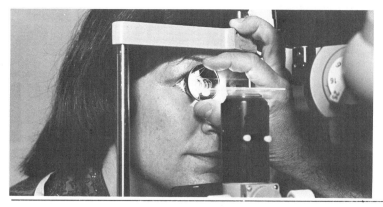

may be lessened because the blood vessels are quickly sealed.

■ Precise control and intense focus of the beam permit the involved tissue to be removed while the immediately surrounding structures are preserved.

■ Healing is rapid and thorough, without scar formation or disturbance of function.

■ Shorter, less traumatic operations reduce anesthesia risks.

■ Using flexible fiber optic devices, the beam may be delivered into any area of the body reachable through an orifice without cutting through functional tissue to get there.

■ The cost effectiveness of laser treatment may be superior to that of any other method of surgery.

Lasers and sight restoration

Perhaps the most successful and important use of the laser at the present time is in eye surgery. The light beam can pass through the clear cornea covering the eye and be directed at every tiny structure in its interior.

In the treatment of glau-

coma the laser is used to stop the overgrowth of blood vessels that eventually obstruct the normal flow of fluid within the eye and cause buildup of intraocular pressure. The laser is also commonly used in the treatment of diabetic retinopathy, one of the most insidious complication of diabetes which leads to blindness. These uses are detailed in our updates on glaucoma and diabetes (see pages 136–145 and 84–95).

Lasers and laryngeal growths

In order to reach the lungs, inhaled air must pass through the vocal cord tissue of the larynx. The area is naturally narrowed so that the cords may vibrate to produce the sounds of speech.

The vocal cords are the frequent site of cysts, tumors, and growths that may affect speech. Although most are benign, they can threaten life by obstructing the airway. If large enough, they can even interfere with feeding in the adjacent esophagus. The problem is magnified in infants where the structures are especially small and delicate.

All laryngeal growths are a

therapeutic challenge. Traditional methods of treatment have many drawbacks and often require long hospital stays. The long-term use of cortisone suppresses the adrenal gland and produces metabolic problems. Surgery is often complicated by bleeding, infection, and the risk of damaging adjacent tissue. Radiation can cause cancer of the thyroid gland many years later. Whereas some of these risks may be acceptable in treating cancerous conditions, where the treatment is lifesaving, they are certainly not acceptable for benign conditions.

The laser is a safe and effective way to deal with certain obstructions in the airway. Dr. George Simpson, an ear, nose, and throat specialist at the Boston University School of Medicine, and Dr. Gerald Healey of the Children's Hospital Medical Center in Boston have successfully treated with laser surgery over 130 cases of airway obstruction in children.

One was an eight-year-old child who had scarring of the windpipe after being bitten by a dog. Another was a ten-year-old with a neurofibroma, a benign tumor originating in

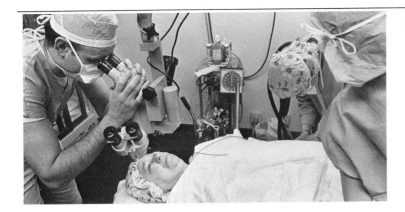

Dr. Stuart Stacy uses a microscopic laser to remove a tumor in the throat. His patients have ranged in age from eighteen months to seventy years. (Photo by Bradford F. Herzog, courtesy Boston University Medical Center)

nerve tissue. Many others were born with a narrowed airway that made it impossible to take in oxygen.

Several patients were quite young. "We are using the laser to treat airway problems in infants as young as two weeks old, an age previously thought to be too young for definitive surgery," Dr. Simpson explains.

Many of Dr. Simpson's patients would have required multiple surgical procedures, weeks in the hospital, and tracheostomy, the surgically created opening in the windpipe which, while lifesaving during laryngeal surgery, often leads to communication and learning problems.

With the laser treatment the disabilities of these patients were short. "Most patients spend less than seventy-two hours in the hospital," says Dr. Simpson. "They usually go home the morning after surgery." He further points out that the reduction in hospital stay makes laser surgery the most cost-effective of all surgical alternatives on the larynx.

Lasers and the war on cancer

One of the newest experimental approaches to cancer therapy involves photoradiation and the laser. At the Kingston Clinic of the Ontario Cancer Foundation in Canada, ten patients have been treated with the laser under the direction of Dr. James Kennedy. The technique involves the intravenous injection of material that is activated by light (photoactive material) and preferentially accumulates in tumor tissue. Within a few days the laser beam is directed at the cancerous tissue; the photoactive material becomes active and begins to destroy the cancer. The beam can be aimed directly at external tumors or, using a fiber optic endoscope (see "Breakthroughs," page 135), at an internal tumor of the bladder, esophagus, stomach, rectum, or pancreas.

Kennedy talks about his patients. "One had a skin cancer [squamous cell carcinoma] on his neck the size of an orange. We started treatment at the top and gradually worked down until the tumor was virtually gone. In another patient, the skin cancer had completely replaced and destroyed one of his eyes. All of it was eradicated with the laser."

Even though both patients eventually died of their cancer, Kennedy's group is excited about the laser's potential in cancer surgery, particularly relative to its safety. "We don't believe the laser technique will cause mutation or other cancers," he says. "A lethal effect of laser treatment does not affect DNA, the genetic stuff of life. It seems to work on the cell membranes and is probably quite safe."

Radiation biologist Thomas Dougherty, of the Roswell Park Memorial Institute in Buffalo, New York, reports that fifty patients in his institution have been treated for advanced cancer with the laser thus far. Summarizing their treatment, he notes, "The numbers are small, but the results are encouraging."

Several other cancer institutions in the United States and Europe are using the laser and photoactive techniques. All have found that the technique can be safely used in patients who have had previous multiple exposures to irradiation.

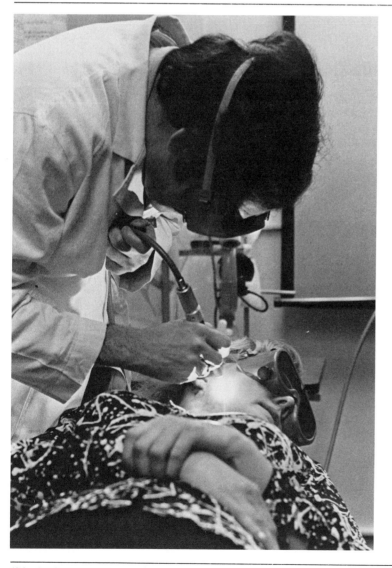

The only problem with the treatment thus far is that patients must stay out of the sun during treatment. The photoactive material reacts with any light source, particularly the sun. Since some of the material inadvertently winds up in other tissues, normal cells are then also be destroyed.

Erasing birthmarks

Almost 1 out of every 100 people is born with a "port wine stain," a flat birthmark named for its prominent reddish purple color. The "port wine stain" is actually a blood vessel overgrowth. It is three times more common in women than in men. It is not malignant, but it often affects the life-style and self-image of those who have one. Most people with port wine stains attempt to conceal them with heavy makeup and hair styles.

At Boston's Beth Israel Hospital, plastic surgeons Dr. Joel Noe and Dr. Robert Goldwyn have successfully treated port wine stains with the argon

The laser has been effective in removing large birthmarks, as seen in laser operation here. (Courtesy Beth Israel Hospital, Boston)

laser. Its blue-green beam reacts with the blood within the vessels of the birthmark to produce heat. The intense heat gradually reduces blood flow, closes blood vessels, and lightens the color. Complete treatment may take one to five visits and is done without anesthesia.

Before laser treatment became available, port wine stains were treated by surgical removal and skin grafting, tattooing, radiation, or cryotherapy, a controversial procedure in which blood vessels are frozen. Because of significant problems with scarring, most people preferred to ignore the stain despite the disfigurement.

Credit for laser birthmark therapy must go to its discoverer, Dr. Leon Goldman of the University of Cincinnati Medical School, where the technique is also used today. There are no known serious complications or side effects of such treatment.

Other uses of the laser

A handful of physicians in the country are using the laser for brain tumors. Dr. Walter Whistler, chairman of the Department of Neurosurgery at Rush-Presbyterian-St. Luke's Medical Center in Chicago, is one of them. He uses the laser primarily to remove benign tumors deep within the brain, beyond the reach of the surgeon's knife. The laser penetrates between the narrowed folds of the brain and strikes only the tiny area on which it is focused. "With the very narrow laser beam we can evaporate the tumor a few cells at a time without damage to neighboring tissue," says Dr. Whistler. "Once the benign tumor is removed, the disease is cured. We have had a high rate of success." Several of Dr. Whistler's patients had been treated unsuccessfully with conventional therapy or drugs. But with laser surgery they are doing well.

Dr. Luiz Escudero and his ear, nose, and throat specialist colleagues at the Catholic University in Campinas, Brazil, report using the laser to spot-weld or attach eardrum grafts after surgery to restore hearing. Typically, such grafts are apt to dissolve after surgery and compromise the result. "It is our opinion that the laser considerably improves graft fixation," he notes. Dr. Escudero's group in 1979 was the first to use the laser during eardrum surgery, and they have used the technique on seven patients thus far.

In dentistry, laser research has shown that the beam can rearrange and fuse the enamel surfaces of teeth and prevent tooth decay. The laser may also be used to fuse dental cements on prostheses and fix them into normal tooth structures. The laser has been experimented with as a dental drill, but it has largely been abandoned because of the potential damage to the tooth pulp from the intense heat.

Dr. Simpson comments on what may be the most important characteristic of laser surgery: "When laser treatment is appropriate, it certainly merits a trial before more extensive conventional surgery. If the laser doesn't work the first time or if the problem reappears, it can safely be used again and again. Even if it doesn't work, one still has the option of using conventional surgery later to manage the problem. No bridges have been burned."

Transplants Trans

We prayed as we started to suture the donor kidney in place—hoping that it would work. Were we amazed! The urine began to flow within ninety seconds. It came out so fast we couldn't keep the operating field dry. But it couldn't match the volume of the tears of our joy.

Joseph Murray, M.D., commenting on the first successful kidney transplant

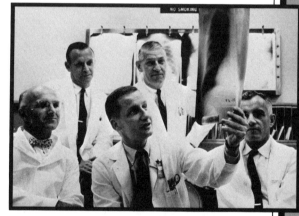

Doctors consult prior to first kidney transplant operation at Peter Bent Brigham Hospital, Boston, 1954. (Back row, left to right) Drs. J. Hartwell Harrison, Gustave Dammin. (Front row, left to right) Chief surgeon Joseph Murray, Drs. James Dealy, John Merrill. (Courtesy Peter Bent Brigham Hospital, Boston)

On December 23, 1954, a team of surgeons headed by Dr. J. Hartwell Harrison and Dr. Joseph Murray at the Peter Bent Brigham Hospital in Boston removed a kidney from twenty-three-year-old Ronald Herrick and transplanted it into his identical twin, Richard, who was suffering from kidney failure. That five-and-a-half-hour operation is considered a medical and surgical milestone because it was the first successful kidney transplantation on record. The operation had been attempted as early as 1902 but had always failed. In this case, the recipient lived for seven more years before glomerulonephritis, the inflammation that had caused his original kidney failure, also destroyed the new kidney.

Commenting shortly after the milestone operation, Dr. George Thorn, then chief of medicine at the Peter Bent Brigham Hospital, said, "It will be easier to put a man on the moon than to do what we did here." Dr. Murray himself reminisced, "I had designed an operation on laboratory dogs and knew it would work because the dogs were surviving indefinitely. The Herricks gave us the best chance to do it in humans because they were identical twins. We were delighted with our success but thought we would never get another set of identical twins with the same problem." The second

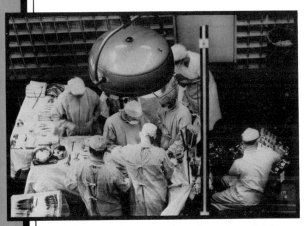

The first kidney transplant, Peter Bent Brigham Hospital, December 23, 1954. (Courtesy Peter Bent Brigham Hospital, Boston)

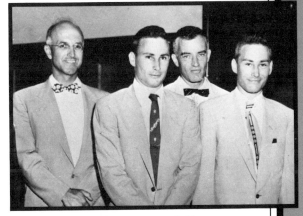

(Left to right) Chief surgeon Joseph Murray; Richard Herrick, recipient of first transplanted kidney; Dr. John Merrill; Ronald Herrick, kidney donor. Photo taken shortly after first kidney transplant operation; Richard Herrick survived for seven years after operation. (Courtesy Peter Bent Brigham Hospital, Boston)

chance came two years later, and soon other patients from all over the world began to arrive at the hospital. From this beginning, transplantation has grown into a major clinical service at most teaching hospitals.

Today, kidneys remain the most common major organs to be transplanted; thousands of kidney transplants have been successfully performed. Likewise, skin and corneal transplants and blood transfusions (though you may not realize it, this is actually a transplantation

as well) are so commonplace and successful that they might even be called routine. The advisability of heart transplants is still questioned, and routine transplantations of other major organs is still years away, but increased success has been reported. Better surgical techniques and more accurate tissue typing (comparing and matching donors and potential recipients to find the most similarities) have improved chances of survival. Although fewer than 2 percent of transplant patients die because of the operation, rejection of the transplanted organ continues to be a major problem. Many researchers feel that advances in drugs that suppress the body's response to foreign tissue will eventually eliminate rejection. In fact, tolerance to transplantation has been achieved in animal studies.

Beyond its application in life-threatening conditions, transplantation has been used as a treatment alternative in less dismal situations. Pancreas transplantation may one day provide better glucose control for the 1.5 million insulin-dependent diabetics, as we saw in the update on diabetes (see pages 84–95). Bone grafting has helped restore body contours and aided in healing where injuries or operations have resulted in bone loss. Fallopian tubes, which transfer eggs from ovary to uterus, have been transplanted to improve fertility and facilitate conception. Fingers have been moved to create a more functional hand after a severe mutilating injury; the section on microsurgery (see "Breakthroughs," pages 100–102) investigates such operations. And in a purely cosmetic sense, increasing numbers of balding men are undergoing hair transplants, in which small plugs of scalp from areas rich in hair growth are transferred to areas of the scalp with less hair.

In the next major section of the book, "Bionics," we'll look at the artificial parts of the body that can be "transplanted" to replace defective or missing joints, organs, or limbs. But in the next few pages we'll explore both the most engrossing and the most controversial transplants—those involving the kidneys, the heart, the liver, the lungs, and the skin.

Kidney transplants

The kidnew filters impurities from the blood and is vital in maintaining general health. When infection or disease restricts kidney function, impurities build up, leading to uremia, a fatal condition.

Kidney failure meant inevitable death until 1944, when Dr. Willem Kollf developed the first artificial device to filter blood—the kidney–renal dialysis machine—while working in Holland. Kolff, currently of the Institute for Biomedical Engineering of the University of Utah, later upgraded his device at the Peter Bent Brigham Hospital in Boston. Today, modern versions of Kolff's original dialysis machine are keeping thousands of patients with end-stage renal disease alive (see pages 218–220). The U.S. government estimates that by 1984, 55,000 patients in the United States will be on dialysis at a cost of $3 billion. Only one-tenth of those will ever receive a transplant. Yet if rejection problems can be solved, transplantation may someday replace dialysis treatment.

CASE HISTORY

H. C. had been feeling weak for years. She was fifty-five. "But I feel like seventy," she told her doctor. She became easily fatigued, could not sleep, and was often short of breath. She was pale and occasionally vomited dark brown material resembling coffee grounds, a material that later proved to be blood. She visited the doctor because she had difficulty walking.

H. C. was found to have chronic renal failure, a residual of a severe rheumatic infection in her earlier years. Her kidneys produced progressively less urine. What little urine there was showed scant evidence of impurities having been filtered from the blood. She was severely anemic; her blood count was less than one-half normal.

A nephrology specialist was consulted, and H. C. began dialysis with the "artificial" kidney, the dialysis machine. Three times a week she sat hooked up to the device that took the place of her own kidneys and filtered her blood. After eighteen months, a kidney donor was found whose tissues matched her own. The donor was a twenty-year-old college student who had met an untimely death in an auto accident.

The transplantation was performed successfully, and H. C. took medication to suppress rejection of the donated organ. Two years later, she returned to work as a grocery store clerk and is doing well. "I'm fifty-nine now," she commented, "but I feel fifty-nine now, not seventy."

Thirty thousand patients have had kidney transplantations in medical centers throughout the world. Each one is special, but several of Dr. Murray's stick out in his mind.

One young man needed a heart operation but had kidney failure that was so advanced he couldn't have tolerated the heart surgery. Six months after a kidney transplant, he had that heart operation and is alive today, ten years later, more active than ever.

A sixty-eight-year-old biochemist had been considered too old for a transplant at another medical center, but after his transplant surgery at Peter Bent Brigham Hospital, he finished his scientific work and presented it at a national medical meeting.

There is the special case of Doris June Huskey, age fourteen, who was involved in the first legal question of organ donations by minors. She told the Supreme Court of Massachusetts, "I cannot live with myself if I am not permitted to donate a kidney to my twin sister." She did, and the operation was a success.

Edith Helm is also special to Dr. Murary. She received a kidney from her twin sister, Wanda Foster, in 1958. After the operation she went on to bear two children. Today, she is the longest-surviving transplant patient.

Improved surgical technology and

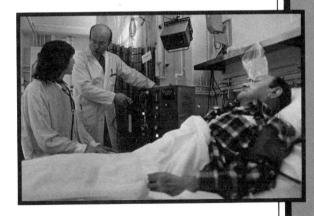

Patient awaits kidney transplant surgery on dialysis machine. (Photo by Michael J. Lutch, courtesy Beth Israel Hospital, Boston)

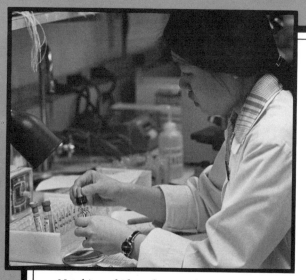

Matching a kidney donor and receiver requires painstaking laboratory testing, demonstrated by this technician comparing blood samples from potential kidney donor and recipient. (Photo by Michael J. Lutch, courtesy Beth Israel Hospital, Boston)

postoperative management have progressed so that now almost anyone with renal failure is a candidate for kidney transplantation. Years ago selection of recipients was made through a careful screening process; today, people of all ages, even those with diabetes, obesity, lung disease, and cancer, are considered for the operation.

Surgery for a kidney transplantation is standardized and, in fact, routine at most major centers. The donated kidney is placed lower than the regular site in the pelvis of the recipient, where it is surgically attached to the blood vessels in the pelvis and the bladder. In most cases the old kidney is left in place to simplify the surgical procedure, but if hypertension is present the diseased kidney may be a contributing factor and it is therefore removed.

No group of patients has been so extensively studied as renal transplantation patients, and a sharing of knowledge between transplant centers is probably responsible for the increased success rates of the operation.

Today the death rate during the first year following kidney transplant surgery is down to 5 percent for patients receiving kidneys from relatives, and 14 percent for recipients of donations from unrelated cadavers. At major centers, such as the Peter Bent Brigham Hospital, that have extensive transplant experience, those figures are 2 percent and 5 percent respectively.

There is a little controversy over whether patients with end-stage disease are better treated with transplants or dialysis, in terms of economic considerations and quality of life. According to Dr. G. Williams at Johns Hopkins University, "There is no doubt about the best treatment in the patient's mind. Virtually all the transplant patients whose grafts [transplants] failed for whatever reason chose a second operation over a life on dialysis."

Heart transplants

Dr. Christiaan Barnard, a surgeon at the Groote Schuur Hospital in Cape Town, South Africa, excited the world in 1967 when he successfully transplanted a human heart for the first time. He sutured the heart of a twenty-five-year-old woman into fifty-three-year-old Louis Washkansky, who lived another eighteen days. Across the world in twenty-two countries cardiac transplants became a virtual epidemic in the twelve months that followed, with over 100 operations being performed by sixty-four different surgical teams. Not surprisingly, doctors soon realized that there was more to cardiac transplantation than the operation itself. Infection and rejection led to dismal results, and the operation was quietly abandoned, except at one medical center. At the Stanford University Medical Center in Palo Alto, California, where the first experiments in cardiac transplantation were performed as early as 1964, research continued in the laboratory, and an active cardiac transplant program was instituted in 1968.

Dr. Norman Shumway and others at Stanford have performed more than 150 heart transplants since then. Their current success rates rival those reported for transplantation of kidneys from unrelated donors. According to Dr. Shumway's recent report in the *British Medical Journal*, 70 percent of the recipients of cardiac transplants are alive after one year, and about 5 percent die each year thereafter. Of the patients for whom a suitable donor wasn't found, 100 percent died within a year.

The Stanford group's persistence and attention to the problems of technique, rejection, and infection have shown that cardiac transplant *is* an alternative, but one that must be weighed carefully. Of the twenty or more patients referred to the Stanford center each month, only three are found to be suitable candidates. They must have advanced heart disease, usually caused by a muscle disorder leading to a failure of the pumping mechanism that can't be helped by any other form of medical or surgical treatment; and they must be stable enough emotionally to deal with the intense rehabilitation required. No patient who is over fifty-five or who has systemic medical problems that might limit survival chances (such as diabetes or circulatory problems) is accepted. "My surgeons kid me that I am always looking for what they call midwestern healthies," states Lois Christopherson, the social worker with Dr. Shumway's group.

CASE HISTORY

R. T. was a thirty-five-year-old fireman who went to his doctor because of shortness of breath. He describes his youth as normal except that "I didn't play sports. I just didn't have the stamina of some of the other guys in my class." In the previous two years he had become progressively weaker. Climbing one or two steps made him breathe deeply. He often complained of a tight, squeezing feeling across his chest.

The examination was extensive and the diagnosis disturbing: cardiomyopathy, a progressive weakening of the heart muscle. In R. T.'s case there was no known cause and no known treatment. His heart was becoming less able to pump. Blood backed up into his lungs and other body tissues. His ankles were swollen, and he gained weight from fluid buildup.

Medications stalled the progress of the condition for a while, but within a year he was virtually bedridden.

R. T. was referred to a cardiac transplantation center because there was no alternative. He was found to be a suitable candidate and took up residence near the hospital to wait for a donor. His wait was brief. Four days later, a young man died in a gunshot accident 200 miles away; his family pledged his organs, and the heart was on its way to R. T.

Within five hours the operation had begun. R. T. survived and went to the intensive care unit, where he remained for one month. Doctors checked him several times a day. He was under medi-

cation, but he found he could breathe more easily than at any time in the previous year.

After eight weeks he was discharged from the hospital. One year later, he still visits the outpatient department each month for evaluation. His physicians are planning to readmit him soon to biopsy the heart. "They want to make sure there is no rejection," he says, "I still feel as if I'm living with a time bomb in my chest, but—hey—at least I've had one good year."

Many cardiac transplant patients return to active employment. One of Dr. Shumway's patients has survived for more than ten years. Infection and rejection remain the major problems, both of which are consequences of the failure to suppress the immune system. Cardiac transplantation seems to be an alternative in a case where no other options exist, and it is expected that many medical centers will cautiously resume cardiac transplants. According to a paper on medicine in the 1980s issued recently by the American Medical Association, heart transplants "could aid an estimated 75,000 Americans annually." Many physicians disagree with that figure, saying it is dramatically high. Regardless, the National Heart, Lung and Blood Institute's director, Dr. Peter Fromer, feels that "the limiting factor for the foreseeable future in cardiac transplantation is the number of donor hearts that are available."

Dr. Fromer feels that no more than 1,000 hearts could be obtained every year from donors, so that the potential demand for transplantation will greatly exceed the number of hearts available to be transplanted. In the Stanford study about one-third of the patients who are actually selected for cardiac transplantation die before a heart is obtained for them; there is nothing like a dialysis machine, or artificial kidney, to keep heart patients alive until a donor is available.

Many centers do not perform cardiac transplants because of the enormous cost involved. The operation and hospitalization required may total $90,000 or $100,000. Some hospitals feel that such large sums of money are better distributed among their other patients. Recently the prestigious Massachusetts General Hospital decided not to embark on a cardiac transplantation program, despite the excellent results of Dr. Shumway's group. According to the hospital's director, Dr. Charles Saunders, "We were faced with the decision as to what choice would reap the greatest good for the greatest number."

Liver transplants

Since the first reported liver transplantation in 1963 by Dr. Thomas Starzl, about 300 such operations have been performed. Two centers have led the research in this area almost exclusively —the University of Colorado Medical School in Denver, where Dr. Starzl originated the procedure, and Cambridge University in England. The extraordinary challenge presented by the size of the liver and the large amount of blood and bile that the organ contains have made it technically difficult from a surgical and anesthetic standpoint. This factor and the compromised state of health of candidates for a liver transplantation have greatly restricted the number of operations even attempted.

Careful medical management offers the best hope for the most liver conditions. However, when a long-term liver problem such as cirrhosis or chronic hepatitis becomes hopeless and medical therapy has nothing to offer, liver transplantation is considered, assuming no serious disease in any other major organ. Certain cancerous conditions that originate in the liver have also been considered reason for transplantation, but cancer metastasis (spread throughout the body) has limited survival.

In the two centers currently doing liver transplantation, success rates have improved through the years. To date, only about one-quarter of the recipients survive the first year, although the figure is certain to rise as candidates for the operation are selected earlier and with more confidence that the operation will prove beneficial. Those who survive do quite well. The low incidence of rejection common to liver transplants aids chances of survival. Apparently the liver cells have fewer antigens than many other tissues and are more resistant to the body's immune systems. Some patients have lived normal lives five years or more after transplantation. One patient in the Denver group even gave birth to a healthy child and is still thriving ten years later.

Lung transplants

A visit to any hospital will demonstrate the pervasive problem of chronic pulmonary disease. Chronic bronchitis and emphysema, scarring from inhaling noxious chemical particles or vapors, lung cancer, and other conditions restrict the amount of oxygen that the lungs absorb. The patient slowly becomes thinner and weaker and gradually wastes away. A slow, horrible death with many hospitalizations is the all too frequent ending of many serious lung conditions. Despite medical advances, the inevitable outcome is only delayed. Potentially, a transplanted lung could provide new life, but the problems of lung transplantation have so far been insurmountable. Indeed, fewer than fifty have even been attempted, and no patient has survived for a year.

Donor lungs are quite rare and deteriorate very quickly when removed for transplantation. Whereas kidneys can be successfully preserved for up to seventy-two hours and still function well, lung function begins to worsen almost immediately after removal from the donor. Since the preserved and transplanted tissue must totally support the patient who receives the lung, even minimal dysfunction can be a serious problem. Furthermore, patients in need of a transplanted lung are in the worst condition imaginable, having lived with their poor lungs for years. Whereas an artificial kidney can provide excellent renal function almost indefinitely and keep the patient in good general health, no such long-term respiratory support is available.

The surgical procedure and its healing have been major factors in the poor survival rate of lung transplant patients. Lung and bronchial tube sizes vary considerably from one individual to the next. If sizes are not close, it is difficult to suture one to another. Air leakage, infection, and breakdown of the suture line result. Also, the high doses of immunosuppressive drugs (such as cortisone) interfere with wound healing.

The last problem confounding the lung transplant surgeon is recognizing when rejection of the donor lung is occurring. The X-ray evidence of early rejection approximates that of infection. Indeed, it may be impossible to distinguish between the two, making it difficult to adjust medication to overcome rejection. With this evidence, Dr. Paul Russell of Boston's Massachusetts General Hospital recently commented in a review of transplantation in the *New England Journal of Medicine*, "It is not likely that lung transplantation will become commonplace in the near future."

Skin transplants

When quizzed as to the largest organ of the body, few people would correctly answer the skin. Yet by definition skin is an organ, a body part that performs a specific function. Skin accounts for 15 percent of our total body weight and performs many roles as an organ. It covers and protects our internal cells, preventing the loss of essential fluids and chemicals and acting as an interface between the water that makes up 70 percent of our body and the dry air that is our environment. Skin is a barrier that protects our body from the assault of germs, chemicals, and physical trauma, our first line of defense. It absorbs and secretes. It helps regulate body temperature. Skin changes in size as our weight changes. With its complex of nerves, skin permits us to communicate with our world by touch.

Skin is often injured but regenerates and heals without assistance. When the injury is deep and vast, however, as in a third-degree burn where a complete thickness of the skin is destroyed, skin cannot regrow and needs to be replaced. If a large burn is left uncovered, the body's protection is gone; fluids stream out through the open surface, temperatures rise, infection sets in, and death soon follows.

Ultimately the burned area must be covered by the patient's own skin, and a skin transplant is necessary. In a skin transplant, or graft, a partial skin thickness from an uninjured body surface (such as the back of the thighs) is placed over the injury, where it grows. Since only a partial thickness of skin is removed, the donor site regenerates and heals without any problems. Such donor sites can therefore be used again and again. When the burned area covers more than 50 percent of the body surface, skin must be temporarily obtained from other sources while the patient's own donor sites regenerate. Pig skin, which resembles human skin, is sometimes used; but even with suppressive drugs the body quickly rejects pig skin, and it lasts no more than two weeks.

Donated human skin is more appropriate. Closely related living donors have the most compatible skin for grafting, but cadaver skin may also be used. In either case, the donated skin provides a temporary covering. Immunosuppressive drugs forestall rejection until the patient's own donor sites regenerate, and the related or cadaver skin is then systematically removed and replaced by grafts from the patient's donor sites. With this so-called temporary transplantation, more than half of the patients with burns covering 70 percent or more of their body surfaces can survive. Without it, severe burns are universally fatal. (However, researchers at MIT are currently experimenting with the develop-

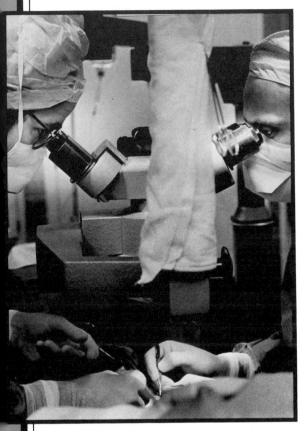

Corneal transplant operation, performed using an operating microscope. (Courtesy Massachusetts Eye and Ear Infirmary, Boston)

ment of artificial skin. See ''Bionics,'' pages 204–205).

Another form of skin transplantation, corneal transplants, have perhaps the highest success rates of any transplantation surgery. The cornea is the clear, colorless skin that covers the front of the eye. If it has an abnormal shape, becomes thickened, or is severely injured, the cornea becomes clouded and vision is impossible. The only treatment is removal of the afflicted cornea and replacement with a new one. Corneal transplants are universally obtained from cadaver donations and restore vision in 85 percent of the cases. The high success rates are achieved because the cornea is immunologically privileged. Its antigens do not stimulate the recipient's defenses, probably because small lymph vessels that carry the white blood cells that moderate the rejection reaction are destroyed in the course of the corneal transplant operation.

Preserving organs

The recent movie *Coma* depicted bodies of organ donors on artificial life support systems in suspended animation, waiting for appropriate recipients. The problems of preserving organs for transplantation are not so easily solved, however.

Low temperatures are necessary for preserving living tissues because the work of cells slows down when they are cold. They last many hours in this state without the oxygen and nutrients the blood would normally provide. Many years ago it was found that glycerol and other neutral solutes could preserve and protect living cells in a frozen state. Without such preservation ice crystals form and destroy frozen tissue, as anyone who has ever experienced frostbite knows. This method has been successful for skin and small bits of tissue. Whole organs, however, have not been successfully frozen.

Currently, when an organ is removed from a donor, it is cooled to 2 to 4 degrees centigrade and attached to a device that pumps a solution of proteins, sugar, electrolytes, and fat through its veins and arteries. This method results in less tissue damage than simple cold storage. Kidneys can be successfully preserved this way for up to seventy-two hours, making it possible to find and transport a kidney to an appropriate matching recipient miles away. In a dramatic East/West exchange, the kidney of a fourteen-year-old girl who died of a head injury in Norfolk, Virginia, was flown to Moscow and transplanted in a thirty-eight-year-old man. One month later, both kidneys of a twenty-one-year-old Moscow head-injury victim were flown to New York City and transplanted in a patient there. "The door is open in both directions with almost no advance notice," says Dr. Robert McCabe of St. Luke's Hospital in New York City, who arranged the flying kidneys.

Hearts and livers can be preserved for only six to ten hours using cold storage. Of course the technique is complex and requires paramedics for storage and support.

Improvements in organ preservation are desperately required. According to a recent article in *Surgical Clinics of North America* by Dr. Belzer and others at the University of Wisconsin, "The availability of a sufficient number of viable organs and the ability to store those organs successfully for the required times are the foundations on which the entire field of transplantation is based." Synthetic blood substitutes (see "Bionics," pages 205–207), by delivering oxygen to cells, may increase preservation time.

The problem of rejection

Upon accepting the Nobel Prize for Medicine and Physiology in 1912, American surgeon Dr. Alexis Carrel said, "From the technical point of view the problem of organ transplantation has been solved." And so it had, even in those early years. The experience of thousands of transplants has made the operation itself almost routine, at least for kidneys. The real problem in transplants is more insidious—rejection.

Everyone's tissue is made unique in cells and chemistry by the presence of substances called antigens. When foreign antigens are introduced into the body, as in the case of transplanted tissue, they are treated as invaders. Through a complicated system determined by genetic makeup and mediated by white blood cells called lymphocytes, the recipient manufactures antibodies to defend against the invading antigens. During the ensuing antigen-antibody reaction war, the antigens are destroyed. The survival of a transplant depends on the outcome of the recipient's antigen-antibody reactions.

The ideal donors and recipients for an organ transplant are identical twins. Rejection is not a problem in such cases because their tissues are identical, but rejection is a factor in all other transplants. The problem is less serious in the case of living related donors, whose tissues are similar, and more serious in the case of unrelated cadaver donors.

To minimize rejection of a donated organ the candidate for the transplantation is thoroughly studied for any complicating medical problems, then classified according to blood type and the presence of a variety of antigens that are important to transplantation. The information on each candidate is filed with the National Transplantation Registry and is available by computer recall. When a donor organ becomes available, it, too, is studied for blood and antigen groups, and the computer matches donor and recipient. In a final step, serum from the donor and serum from the recipient are combined to see if they are compatible. Tissue-typing labs work twenty-four hours a day because of the limited organ preservation time. Because the national registry enables the sharing of information between centers, organs can be sent from one transplant center to another that may be many miles away. In December 1979 a kidney was flown to Great Britain from the United States on the French supersonic transport Concorde.

The antigens important to transplantation, the HLA (human leukocyte) antigens, have been localized to the sixth chromosome in an area called the major histocompatibility complex. Within the HLA area are several series of antigens, and the accurate definition of this area has proceeded rapidly in recent years. With increased compatibility through antigen matching, the chances for graft survival are much greater. Tissue typing has succeeded to about 80 percent in living related donors, but unfortunately cadaver graft survival has not benefited to the same degree. The HLA antigen system in humans is so complex that a perfectly matched transplant from a donor is virtually impossible to obtain. Even with the best of typing to date, survival rates remain about 60 percent for the graft. Dr. Charles Carpenter of the Peter Bent Brigham Hospital in Boston, a leader in tissue typing, believes that new techniques of typing can raise the success rate to about 80 percent, however.

Because of the impossibility of a perfect match, the tranplant surgeon has to depend on drugs to suppress the rejection response, which can occur anytime from hours to months after the transplant. Most transplant patients are given azathioprine (Imuran) and cortisone preparations to minimize the rejection response and have had prolonged graft survival as a result. Fever, weakness, illness, and blood changes are signs of imminent rejection, and switching medications or changing dosage may slow or revise these responses. The suppressive medications are not ideal, as they have long-term complications. The fact that the same medications have been the mainstay of rejection treatment for the past ten years in this rapidly expanding field indicates the holding pattern that has rejection research slowed for the moment.

"Foremost among the goals of transplantation is to produce a specific and long-lasting alteration of response in the recipient that is confined to the antigens in the donor tissue," says Massachusetts General Hospital's Dr. Paul Russell. This has been achieved in some laboratories with animal studies. New excitement is being generated by an antifungal metabolyte, cyclosporin A, and irradiation directed at areas in the body that produce the white blood cells so crucial to the rejection response. Draining white blood cells off by putting a small catheter in the lymph duct, according to the researchers at the University of Colorado and Vanderbilt University, has also been effective in reducing rejection problems.

In the future

Because of the limited availability of human donor tissue, attention is increasingly being focused on synthetic devices or substances and structures from species other than our own (called xenografts), such as pig skin for burn coverings. As long as diseases continue to take their toll on body organs and systems, there will be a need for removal or replacement with more functional tissues. As advances in conquering the rejection reaction and developing more delicate surgical skills continue to be made, transplantation surgery is certain to have an increasing role in medical treatment. Other kinds of medical therapy may someday obviate the need of transplantation; that is to be hoped, since transplantation should always be regarded as a last resort form of treatment.

How to become a donor

The list of patients waiting to receive organ transplants is long; there simply aren't enough donations. Poor understanding of the donation procedure probably accounts for the limited number of donors. In this regard, here are some important points for consideration:

■ Organ donation never interferes with attempts to save a life. Organs are removed only when death occurs.

■ Donations do not interfere with funeral arrangements.

■ There are no expenses to the donor's family; the organ bank pays.

■ You can donate any one or all organs if you wish. A small sticker on the driver's license identifies a donor, but family, local physician, and hospital should be notified for their records.

All states have passed a uniform Anatomical Gift Act, which provides legal authorization to assist people in donating organs or tissues when they die. To make donation easier, most states have set up programs with state motor vehicle licensing departments which make information and donor cards available when you renew your driver's license.

Moral and religious leaders favor organ donation as the highest expression of humanitarian ideals. Not everyone can become an organ donor, though. Since organs must be removed soon after death, time is prohibitive, as is the presence of certain diseases like hepatitis and cancer that can be transmitted to the recipient.

Resources

■ The best source of information on transplantation and organ donation is the Kidney Foundation. There are several state and regional offices, usually listed in your telephone directory. The national office is:

National Kidney Foundation
2 Park Avenue
New York, New York 10016
212-889-2210

■ The following states have programs with the Department of Motor Vehicle Registration if you want to register as an organ donor at the time you renew your driver's license.

Arizona	Minnesota
Arkansas	Missouri
California	Montana
Colorado	Nevada
Connecticut	New Hampshire
District of Columbia	New Jersey
Florida	New York
Georgia	North Carolina
Hawaii	Ohio
Idaho	Oklahoma
Illinois	Oregon
Indiana	Pennsylvania
Iowa	South Carolina
Kansas	Tennessee
Kentucky	Texas
Louisiana	Virginia
Maine	Washington
Maryland	Wcst Virginia
Massachusetts	Wisconsin
Michigan	Wyoming
Mississippi	

BIONICS BIONICS

CS BIONICS BIO

ICS BIONICS B

BIONICS BIONICS BIONICS BIONICS BIONICS BIONICS

The Bionic Man may be the creation of television, but medical technology may soon make him a reality. This year alone some two to three million artificial body parts will be implanted to replace arthritis-ravaged joints and limbs destroyed by accident or abuse.

The resulting interaction between real and artificial organs creates a wondrous technological harmony that would startle even the most imaginative television writer. Today's technology produces miniature components and materials with great strength and durability that do not disrupt body tissues. The myoelectronic hand restores arm function to an amputee victim. An artificial voice box offers hope to victims of larynx cancer, while computers may someday offer mechanized "sight" to the blind and "hearing" to the deaf.

Certainly no prosthesis can replace real body parts. But today's bioengineering devices can restore function with increasing success and accuracy. The rapidly advancing bionics/prosthetics field brings to mind the old proverb, "There is a remedy for everything, if only one could find it."

Computer vision and hearing

That the eyes of the blind shall
be opened, and the ears of the deaf
shall be unstopped.

Isaiah 35: 5

When Benjamin Franklin described his
lightning experiments to the Royal
Society of London in 1751, he suggested
that the power of electricity might someday be used to restore sight to the blind and
hearing to the deaf. Today, scientists hope
to realize Franklin's dream with the development of computerized sight and hearing.
While further research is needed to perfect
such devices, current testing of electric
artificial eyes and ears has yielded positive
results, generating great enthusiasm in the
scientific community.

Eyes for the blind

The initial concept of artificial sight was
developed by Dr. William Dobelle, the
director of the Division of Artificial Organs
at Columbia University's College of Physicians and Surgeons in New York City. He
and his colleagues have successfully placed
visual implants in three blind volunteers,
enabling them to "see" simple patterns
and figures in the University's vision laboratory.

An earlier experiment inspired Dobelle's
research. In 1968 two British scientists
touched the exposed brain of a blind woman with the tips of electrified wires. With
each electrical stimulation she "saw" tiny
points of light. These brain lights, or phosphenes, similar to the visual sensations
you get when you press your eyeball, are
caused by a mechanical irritation of the
retina. Although scientists doubted that
phosphene stimulation would ever be useful to the blind, Dobelle found the concept
intriguing.

Along with computer expert Michael
Mladejovsky, Dobelle, then at the University of Utah, set to work designing a unit
that could·be implanted in the brain to
stimulate a mosaic of phosphenes, which a
computer could then organize into recog-
nizable shapes.

Dobelle's blind volunteers all have a
small Teflon plate with sixty-four platinum electrodes surgically implanted on
the surface of the visual cortex, the part of
the brain responsible for eyesight. The
visual cortex lies at the very back of the
brain in the occipital area, directly opposite the eyes, and is easily accessible to the
neurosurgeon. Tiny wires from each electrode pass out through the skull and then
are tunneled under the scalp to just behind
the ear, where they emerge through the
skin in a small black socket no larger than
a dime. The "eye" for the system, to
which the patient is hooked up, is a television camera and a room-size computer.

When the camera is aimed at a particular figure or character, the information
passes to the computer. The computer
chooses a combination of electrodes on the
Teflon plate which are stimulated to produce a pattern of phosphenes that approximate the image seen by the camera.

With this system, the patient can "see"
patterns, simple letters, and figures. Dobelle's most recent patient, a thirty-five-
year-old man named Craig, has been able
to read sentences. All the letters in the
words of the sentence, however, are in the
form of Braille dots, since the computer
can operate faster using the Braille alpha-
bet. For this man, who was blinded by a

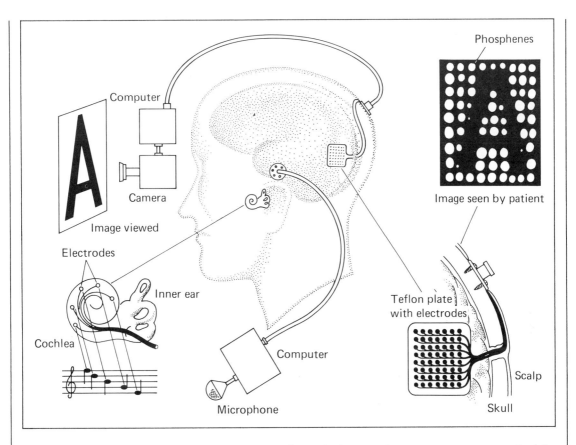

Phosphenes

Image seen by patient

Computer

Camera

Image viewed

Electrodes

Inner ear

Cochlea

Computer

Microphone

Teflon plate with electrodes

Scalp

Skull

gunshot ten years ago, the procedure yields astonishing results.

Still, this sixty-four-electrode eye requires a room full of electronics to produce vision that is hardly useful to the volunteers. But future versions of the device may be much more practical and effective.

Dobelle and his associates are now designing a microminiature TV camera that could be placed in a glass eye and attached to the eye muscles. The camera would transmit its images to a tiny computer built into the frame of a pair of eyeglasses and then through wires connected to two 256-electrode systems, one implanted in each side of the visual cortex. This system of 512 electrodes could enable a blind person to "see" people and objects in black- and-white patterns similar to the way an electronic scoreboard in a football or baseball stadium recreates images.

If this total vision system sounds like something out of "Star Trek," remember that today's microcircuits, one of the great scientific breakthroughs of the past decade, consist of chips with transistors so small that four of them could fit on the surface of a red blood cell—and 5 million red blood cells could fit onto the head of a fairly large pin.

The next stop in microcircuitry will be to reduce the size of the sight device by 100. "By the time our system has been worked out, size will not be a problem," Dobelle says. "A bigger task is to design the type and number of circuits we need and the location of electrodes on the visual cortex." Dobelle's estimates for the cost of such a system are surprisingly low. The artificial eye would cost $3,000 to $5,000, and a similar amount would be needed for surgery, hospital stay, and rehabilitation.

An ancient Greek proverb describes a blind man leaning against a wall: "This is the boundary of the world," he said. Ten thousand dollars sounds like quite a bargain for expanding the boundaries of a sightless world.

And ears for the deaf

The same sort of system might also enable deaf people to hear. The electronic signals would be diverted to electrodes implanted in the inner ear, in a structure called the cochlea. This is a snail-shell-shaped organ that houses the delicate hair cells that pick up sound waves and relay them to the auditory nerves and then to the brain. The auditory area of the brain itself is less accessible than the visual cortex, and surgery there would be very risky.

CASE HISTORY

C. G. was completely deaf for fourteen years because he had taken streptomycin years before for an infection; the drug is now known to be destructive to the cochlea and its tiny hair cells. (Many people who took streptomycin are deaf today.)

In an operation that required the continual use of the microscope, Dr. William House of the Ear Research Institute of Los Angeles removed some of the mastoid bone behind C. G.'s ear, exposed the inner ear, and placed tiny platinum electrodes along the cochlea. Wires from the electrodes were then connected to a small coil amplifier and planted under the skin. The microphone to pick up the sound was concealed in a specially designed eyeglass frame.

The surgery was successful. For the first time in fourteen years, C. G. was able to hear doorbells, birds, animals, and traffic. "This is a modern miracle to me," he wrote in his diary.

To date, three dozen patients have undergone this hearing-restoring operation. The success of the operation is limited, however, as the new "ear" cannot pick up subtle changes of human speech. The operation enables the reception only of single-pitched artificial sounds, such as horns and bells.

Dobelle's computers may solve that problem, though. His group is currently at work mapping the sound patterns within the cochlea. Once that mapping is determined, increasing the number of electrodes to record more sound patterns may make human voices intelligible. "Walter Cronkite might sound like Donald Duck, but at least he'll be understood," explains Dr. Dobelle.

The artificial ear is less complex than the artificial eye and, according to Dr. Dobelle, may hold more promise: "A little bit of hearing may be more helpful to the deaf than a little bit of vision is to the blind."

Dr. Dobelle emphasizes that his artificial senses are research instruments and are not yet alternatives for the average blind or deaf patient. Still, the next decade may very well bring hope to countless blind and deaf patients through the "eyes" and "ears" of electronic devices.

The myoelectronic hand

We can repair him. We can make him better than he was. We have the technology.

Introduction, "Bionic Man" TV series

Each year more than 1,000 people suffer accidental amputations of the hand. This dismal fact is not surprising, considering the increased role of machines in industry and society and the often violent nature of accidents in our mechanized world.

The hand is one of the most important interfaces with our environment, and victims of traumatic hand amputations face an adjustment that few of us can comprehend.

Replantation of an amputated hand by microsurgery has been achieved with only limited success. Perhaps the most famous case in recent times was that of Renee Katz, the young New York woman whose hand was severed in a subway accident. Thoughtful onlookers packed her amputated hand in ice immediately after the accident, and surgeons were able to reconnect it to her arm.

"But the frequent outcome of such surgery is a stiff, insensitive hand," explains Emory University orthopedic surgeon Dr. Lamar Fleming. "The muscles and nerves in the hand often do not regain their function after a replantation operation. The hand is there but doesn't feel and doesn't work. For these people, the replanted hand is more in the way than a help." Replantation isn't always appropriate, either. The result of many accidental injuries involving the hand is a severely mangled and crushed extremity, and the remaining tissue cannot be saved.

Most hand amputees, therefore, still must use a prosthesis, and the familiar hook is the best so far available. Working at the Woodruff Medical Center in Atlanta, Dr. Fleming's group, however, has had recent success with a prosthesis called the myoelectronic hand. Resembling a human hand and operated by a small battery, the myoelectronic hand responds to the patient's thoughts by sensing natural muscle contractions in the stump. The patient thinks "grasp" and the hand closes; "open" and the hand opens. The myoelectronic hand promises better function than traditional prostheses and certainly is more acceptable cosmetically. In the near future it may even permit sensations of touch as well.

CASE HISTORY

A. B. is a sixty-two-year-old man who lost his right arm and right leg during World War II when a kamikaze pilot aimed his bomb-laden plane directly at the navy ship on which A. B. was serving. The ensuing crash took many lives as well as A. B.'s right hand and leg. For twenty-five years A. B. wore a hook prosthesis and was able to pursue a successful career as an engineer. But there were problems. "I began to develop a neuritis in my shoulder from constant use of the prosthesis," he notes. "I was uncomfortable much of the time and in frank pain all too often."

A. B. agreed to try the myoelectronic hand in 1972. He was only the second patient to receive the device, which was attached in an operation at Emory University. He has had the prosthesis now for over eight years. He wears it sixteen hours a day, dresses himself, eats, writes, and is not limited in social or work activities. He even drives a car and flies an airplane.

The problem with hand prostheses

The major goal in prosthetic research and development has been the close approximation of normal hand function. The goal has been an elusive one because of the intricate nature of the hand. Each joint has a special function. The many muscles that operate the hand are balanced to work with and against each other, enabling subtle, delicate, and complex activities to be performed in a coordinated way. Three major nerves provide control of movement and sensation. The fingertips are among the most sensitive body tissues.

The most commonly used prosthesis for hand amputees is a hook. The unappealing nature of this prosthesis is demonstrated by its frequent appearance in literature on villainous characters, like the devious Captain Hook in *Peter Pan*. From a functional standpoint, the hook does permit limited grasp and therefore enables the amputee to perform some skilled work; but it is cumbersome to operate. The complicated system of straps, pulleys, and wires is slung over the shoulder. By lowering and raising the shoulder, the wearer opens and closes the hook. Over a period of years, hand amputees with hook prostheses complain of shoulder fatigue, pain, and neuritis.

Using the body's own signals

The myoelectronic hand has no straps or pulleys. It is, rather, a muscle-activated electronic hand that has a 12-volt rechargeable battery and motor encased within a polyvinyl chloride plastic shell and molded in the shape of a human hand with joints that open and close. The shell is covered by a rubber glove, which is tinted to match the patient's skin coloring. Without looking closely, you'd find it hard to tell the prosthetic hand from a normal one.

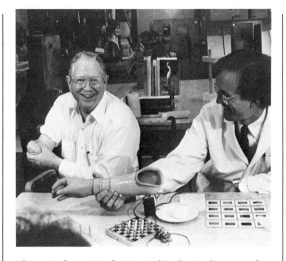

The complete myoelectronic hand unit fits over the amputee stump—and is more comfortable and easier to maneuver than a hook, which uses complicated shoulder straps. (Courtesy Emory University Medical Center, Atlanta, Georgia)

The basic concept of the myoelectronic hand is relatively simple. Biological processes within the body help to control the artificial mechanism of the prosthesis, whose motor is activated by the patient's own muscle and nerve impulses. Small electrodes are painlessly attached to the skin of the forearm stump. When the amputee thinks "open the hand" or "close the hand," the electrode detects electrochemical changes within the forearm muscles. The signal, amplified, activates the motor within the prosthesis, and the hand opens or closes. The speed of operation of the prosthesis is proportional to the degree of muscle contraction. Essentially, the harder the amputee thinks "close my hand" the harder and faster the prosthesis operates.

The myoelectronic hand permits everyday social and work activities that do not require great hand strength. Lest the reader develop visions of the Bionic Man, however, Dr. Fleming is quick to point out that the myoelectronic hand prosthesis cannot bend steel or crush rocks. In fact, "it is limited to five pounds of grip and two and a half pounds of pinch force, so it is not

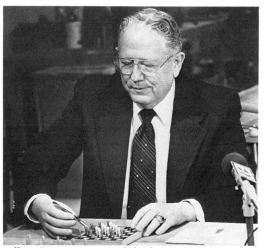

Albert Brown was one of the first patients to receive the myoelectronic hand. Now after five years, he uses the device proficiently, even to perform delicate work. (Courtesy Emory University Medical Center, Atlanta, Georgia)

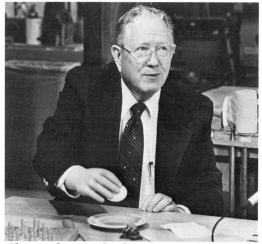

The myoelectronic hand can be controlled with such success that even a fragile egg may be safely grasped. (Courtesy Emory University Medical Center Atlanta, Georgia)

appropriate for heavy physical work." The prosthesis has a safety release which allows the index and middle fingers to break away when the load exceeds its capacity.

Seven patients have received the myoelectronic hand to date at Emory University. The first patient was a twenty-nine-year-old mechanic who had sustained third-degree burns. Now having used the prosthesis for nine years, he continues in his work as an auto mechanic. Another patient is a twenty-seven-year-old artist who also had sustained third-degree electrical burns. He continues to work as an artist, one year after getting the prosthesis. Three other patients sustained crush injuries to their hand and use the prosthesis in their jobs as minister, machinist, and freight conductor. Except for one Emory patient who has stopped wearing the hand because of painful scarring at the stump site, all the recipients use the hand fifteen to sixteen hours a day to eat, drive, write, work, and play.

The myoelectronic hand was developed in Europe, but Dr. Fleming and his group were the first to attach it to the patient's arm immediately after the amputation operation. Dr. Fleming feels this has a good deal to do with the success of the myoelectronic hand. When a suitable candidate with a crush injury is brought to the Atlanta center and evaluation determines that amputation of the crushed hand is the only alternative, the patient is introduced to the myoelectronic prosthesis and encouraged to try it before surgery to become confident that it will actually work. The prothesis is attached to the forearm skin of the normal uninjured arm, and the patient can actually practice with it. Immediately after the amputation, the prosthesis is attached to the stump.

The advantages of the immediate fit of the prosthesis are obvious. The amputee wakes up from the operation with a hand where the old one was, a tremendous psychological advantage in rehabilitation. The patient also does not establish a pattern of using only one hand because the myoelectronic hand can be used for eating and dressing as soon as the next day. Rehabilitation counseling and training using the prosthesis can begin immediately.

A myoelectronic hand costs about $4,000, not including any hospital or doctor's charges for the amputation operation. Yearly maintenance, which is usually limited to replacement of the rubber gloves that cover the unit, averages about $175 to $250.

Candidates for the myoelectronic hand

Dr. Fleming and his colleagues emphasize the importance of proper patient selection for this revolutionary prosthesis. "The patient must be in an occupation that requires cosmesis rather than heavy labor, must be intelligent and realistic enough to recognize what the prosthesis can and cannot do, and be well motivated." The patient must be willing to cooperate with occupational therapists. Therapy continues for several weeks after surgery as the patient prepares to return to home and work. Several months later, when the patient has become familiar with the use of the prosthesis and the problems in his or her own environment, he or she returns for

This woman has just received her myoelectronic hand and is learning to use the device. Later she will wear a glove colored to match her skin color. (Courtesy Emory University Medical Center, Atlanta, Georgia)

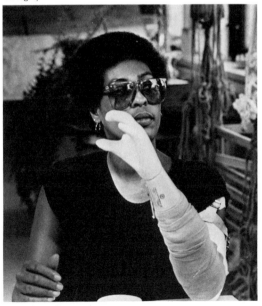

further occupational therapy, trouble shooting, and any other adjustments.

The most recent recipient of the myoelectronic hand, a thirty-year-old machinist whose hand was crushed in the rollers of a press, states, "the hardest thing to learn is to control the force of my hand's grip. I find myself crushing an egg if I try to lift it, for example." Muscles must be relaxed between movements. The amount of thought and muscle contraction that is translated into prosthesis movement must also be learned. In this regard, the faint sound of the motor seems to be a definite help, almost serving as biofeedback to control the function of the prosthesis.

In the future

The next generation of myoelectronic hands may include sensory feedback. Dr. Fleming believes this may occur within two years. Small microsensors in the tips of the glove that covers the unit will sense the characteristics of touch and be connected to individual nerve fibers in the stump to carry that information to the brain.

Similar prothesis work in responding to body signals is underway at the Liberty Mutual Research Center in Hopkinton, Massachusetts, where Dr. Allen Cudworth and his associates in conjunction with the Massachusetts Institute of Technology are refining the so-called Boston arm, a device for above-elbow amputees. The Boston arm also uses myoelectronic signals, in this case to flex and extend the prosthetic elbow joint.

Although the use of the myoelectronic hand has been limited to traumatic injuries, it may be applicable to congenital hand problems as well.

The prosthesis can never duplicate the intricacies of the human hand. Because of certain mechanical limitations, the use of prosthetics is often frustrating. But the myoelectronic hand comes the closest yet to restoring function to hand amputees.

Artificial joints

The current jogging craze may very well lead to a generation of people twenty-five years hence with the strongest lungs and hearts in our history, but with joints so worn and arthritic that they won't be able to get out of bed.

Anonymous orthopedic surgeon

Almost everyone is susceptible to some form of arthritis. The Arthritis Foundation estimates that 10 percent of the world's population, or close to 400 million people, have arthritis. Of the 50 million arthritis sufferers in the United States, some 30 million require medical attention and 5 million are disabled. Arthritis costs $5 billion per year in lost wages and medical expenses. Once joint damage occurs from arthritic inflammation, the joint never regains its normal function, despite today's advances in physical therapy and medication.

According to many doctors, the current exercise boom may bring an early onset of arthritis to thousands of eager sports enthusiasts. "Even normal activities put great strain on the body joints," says Dr. Frederick Ewald, an orthopedic surgeon at the Harvard Medical School and the Robert Breck Brigham Hospital in Boston. "The force put on knees and hip joints with normal walking can exceed three times body weight; with climbing stairs, that force exceeds four times body weight." In demanding sports such as soccer, football, and distance running, the forces on joints are dramatically increased. Each new force is cumulative, and gradually the joints simply wear away.

"It's no wonder," comments Dr. David Sonstegard of the University of Michigan Medical Center in a recent issue of *Scientific American*, "that many people go into their later years [with joints] so badly deteriorated as to be crippling."

It is now possible to replace worn and incapacitated joints throughout the body. Over the past twenty years, synthetic materials and prosthesis design have enabled more than 1 million people to receive artificial joints that promise relief of pain and restoration of normal activities. Although joint replacement is sometimes considered for traumatic injuries, the majority of candidates for artificial joints have been chronically disabled by arthritis.

CASE HISTORY

A. L., returning home after attending a convention, left the ticketing/baggage-check area of Chicago's O'Hare International Airport and walked briskly toward the departure gate. As he approached the security clearance device, the attendants noticed that he had a slight limp. As he passed through the detector, a metal alarm sounded.

A. L. was not surprised, since this scene was repeated each time he passed through a metal detector. The guard asked him to empty his pockets, but his pockets were empty. A. L. was not a security risk. He carried no knife or gun, and no keys or coins. He did, however, have a small plastic card verifying that he was "wearing" an artificial hip, a metal replacement for his own arthritis-ravaged joint that was implanted several months before. It was this metallic object that caused the security alarm to sound. He was allowed to pass through and reached his airplane in time, and was soon on his way home.

A. L. is a forty-two-year-old victim of rheumatoid arthritis, a condition he has had for about twenty years. After ten years of progressively worse pain in the hip which greatly interfered with his work as a public relations director of a major hospital, he had undergone joint replacement and was now free of pain and able to carry on his normal activities.

A. L. is one of the approximately 200,000 people who had reconstructive joint surgery in 1979. Of these, 125,000 received artificial hips, 50,000 received artificial knees, and 20,000 received artificial shoulders, elbows, or fingers. For these individuals, reconstructive joint surgery meant an end to years of pain and limitation of function. Although most do not participate in strenuous sports activities, most do lead normal lives with normal activity.

Arthritis and its destruction

Arthritis is a broad term for a group of diseases that cause pain and deformity of the joints and surrounding structures.

Although arthritis is rarely fatal, no other group of diseases causes so much suffering for so long. After heart disease, arthritis is the leading cause of activity limitation. Arthritis causes muscles to weaken, joints to become stiff and painful, and bones to become fragile and break. But most of all, arthritis causes chronic, unrelenting, and progressive pain.

Arthritis has many varieties, but osteoarthritis and rheumatoid arthritis are the major diseases. Osteoarthritis is a degenerative condition that inevitably progresses with age and the ensuing wear and tear on the joints. Rheumatoid arthritis, on the other hand, is the more disabling and actually affects soft tissue surrounding the joint itself; this disease is not specifically related to use.

In this era of advancing medical technology, doctors still cannot determine the cause of arthritis. To date, the disease has no cure. Cortisone and the newer noncortisone and anti-inflammatory drugs have done much to help arthritis victims, as have physical therapy, heat, rest, and bracing. "Notwithstanding these efforts," comments Dr. Sonstegard, "arthritis can progress to cause severe pain, limitation of activity, and disability—and it is then that surgery will be necessary."

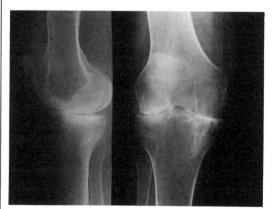

Side view (left) and back view (right) of knee joint ravaged by rheumatoid arthritis. Patient is good candidate for joint replacement. (Courtesy Frederick Ewald, M.D.)

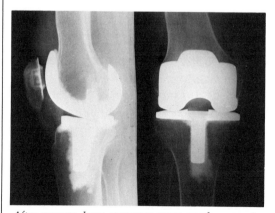

After surgery, knee structure more nearly approximates a normal joint, and pain and deformity are gone. (Courtesy Frederick Ewald, M.D.)

CASE HISTORY

M. P. is a fifty-five-year-old woman who developed rheumatoid arthritis in her mid-thirties. The disease first appeared as pain in one hip but within several years affected virtually all of the joints of her arms and legs. The pain increased so rapidly that she soon lost her desire to live. She gradually spent more and more time in bed and severely limited her activities. She had no motivation to get up. When she was referred to doctors at the Robert Breck Brigham Hospital in Boston, M. P. had been in bed completely for seven years, barely able to move her arms or legs.

Within two years the orthopedic surgeons replaced both hips, both knees and elbows, one shoulder, one ankle, and all of the knuckles of both hands. Decreased pain and increased mobility restored her motivation after the surgery. She is now totally self-sufficient and walks without support, goes up and down stairs, visits friends, shops, and does volunteer work. "M. P. holds our all-time record for joint replacement—she has eighteen artificial joints," notes her surgeon, Dr. Frederick Ewald.

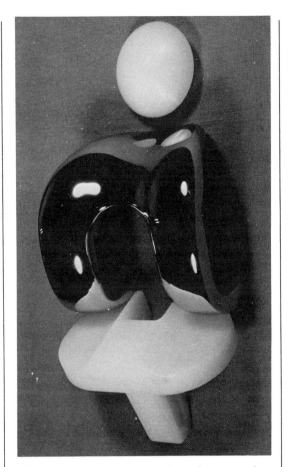

The artificial knee contains a plastic kneecap and lower leg bone. Metallic structure replaces the end of the thigh bone. As knee flexes, metal will slide through plastic joint, allowing free knee movement. (Courtesy Frederick Ewald, M.D.)

It is not unusual for orthopedic surgeons to see patients for the first time who have been in bed with fevers and immobile joints and who require expensive operations even to enable them to sit without pain. "Joint replacement should not be a salvage operation for a destroyed patient," comments Dr. Robert Poss, also of the Robert Breck Brigham Hospital. "Such surgery could more sensibly have been performed as each joint required it, and the patient could have continued walking or working in the interim rather than retreating to a wheelchair or a bed."

Early efforts

Restoration of joint function by surgery has been a challenge for many years. French surgeon Ambröise Paré in the sixteenth century gave birth to joint surgery when he removed diseased joints completely in the hope of avoiding amputation for incurable joint infections. Surgeons used modifications of his techniques for nearly 400 years. Although this operation preserved the extremity, inevitably scar tissue formed and fused the bone ends, making the "joints" stiff and unusable. It was clear that a replacement was needed for the excised joints. In the 1930s British orthopedist Smith-Peterson, used crude synthetic metals to replace the resected (removed) bone for the first time. His work has been the foundation of all subsequent efforts.

The real credit for successful joint replacement, though, belongs to British surgeon John Charnley of the Center for Hip Surgery at Wrightington Hospital in Lancashire, England. In 1958 he performed the first total hip replacement, substituting both parts of the joint, the hip bone, and the hip socket with prostheses fashioned from Teflon. Now, more than twenty years later, thousands of hip replacement operations have been performed with amazingly good results. In December 1976 Queen Elizabeth II knighted Professor Charnley for his contribution to orthopedic surgery.

Today's successes were not easily gained, however. Charnley was initially successful with his first 200 patients, but in 1965 he reported that after years of use, the Teflon had begun to disintegrate. Pieces found their way into the bloodstream and migrated into the heart and lungs of his patients.

It was clear that Teflon could not hold up to the forces of even normal activities. Attention was next directed to metal prostheses. But metal damaged adjoining bones when used to replace a section of a joint. An all-metal replacement joint creaked, groaned, and often became stuck from friction.

Today's major joint prostheses (for hips, knees, elbows, and so forth) are called metal-to-plastic joints. In a normal joint, the cartilage surfaces over the bone rub against each other; in today's modern joint prostheses, one bone end is replaced by metal, the other by plastic. The joint interface is therefore metal gliding over plastic. The metal half is a stainless-steel alloy containing cobalt, chromium, and molybdenum and is so hard that it must be cast in a wax mold. It cannot be cut or machined. The plastic part of the joint is a high-density polyethylene. Metal on polyethylene creates a very smooth-gliding surface, and the wearer is not aware of any friction.

Replacing major joints

The major indication for joint replacement is elimination of pain. Increased motion is another benefit, but most orthopedic surgeons will not perform the operation only for increase in motion. There is no age limit, as general physical and mental states are clearly more important than the patient's age in this regard.

Joint replacement is carried out under general anesthesia. During the procedure, the ends of the diseased bones that make up the joint are carefully removed, and the replacement prostheses are cemented in place to the bone ends with a cement called methyl methacrylate. Now in use for fifteen years, the glue is universally used to bond the metal and polyethylene substitute to bone. In eleven years of use in the United States and fifteen years of use in Europe, fewer than 1 percent of prostheses have loosened.

Following surgery, the patient remains in bed for five to six days, then gradually starts to use the joint. The patient is usually discharged from the hospital in about two weeks and must restrict activity for one month or more.

Many patients who undergo joint replacement surgery have had fused, fixed, immobile joints for as many as twenty-five or thirty years. As a result, the muscles of that extremity have severely weakened. After surgery those muscles must be strengthened again in order to permit proper function. Surprisingly, "weight training is never used," emphasizes Dr. Ewald. "Even though the muscles surrounding the joint have been severely weakened because of limited use, normal activity restores their function quickly."

The major complication of joint replacement is infection, which can force removal of the prosthesis and result in pulmonary embolism. Careful attention to aseptic procedures and the use of anticoagulants has reduced the possibility of this complication. Some prostheses may loosen after years of use, and the patient's pain will return. A second operation for joint replacement may then be necessary.

Is the patient "as good as new" after major joint replacement? Dr. Frank Stinchfield of the Columbia-Presbyterian Medical Center in New York City, widely regarded as the dean of American orthopedic surgeons and one of the first to do joint replacement in the United States, answers emphatically, "No artificial joint is as good as a God-made joint. Motion may be somewhat limited, but if the operation is successful, pain is gone. That was after all the major reason for doing the operation in the first place."

Most patients return to their previous occupation, even when that involves heavy manual labor. Dr. Stinchfield explains: "We do know joint replacement will last years if the patient doesn't do anything extra-strenuous. I do permit my hip replacement patients to play tennis, but encourage doubles only, and golf, but prefer they use a golf cart. I do not do joint replacement, however, just so they can play tennis or golf."

Dr. Stinchfield feels that even those restrictions may not be necessary. Years from now, he says, "many patients may ask, 'Why did you limit me? My joints have held up perfectly.'"

Dr. Stinchfield may be right. Recently, sixty-five-year-old Joe Ardito of Chicago and his partner won the Super Masters doubles tournament in the United States Handball Association National Championships; Ardito has an artificial hip. Despite the hard running, sudden stops, and pressure of handball in a tournament involving four straight days of competition, Ardito boasted; "My hip didn't even get stiff or sore." His physician, Dr. William Melcher of Skokie, Illinois, understandably wasn't happy when he heard about it, fearing the danger of a break in the prosthesis. Ardito will continue to play, though, as his wife attests: "Joe has never played an easy game of handball in his life—he doesn't know what it's like to take it easy."

Replacing finger joints

Although rheumatoid arthritis strikes each victim differently, it frequently involves the hand in a very frustrating and disabling manner.

Victims of rheumatoid arthritis in the hand often cannot hold a cup of coffee or turn a doorknob. The disease process in rheumatoid arthritis is not confined to the joint surfaces. Joint linings are inflamed, tendons and muscles are involved, pain occurs throughout the hand, and the joints become abnormally positioned and severely deformed. The usual rheumatoid hand deformity is called ulnar deviation. The fingers become angulated away from the thumb at the knuckles, and eventually the joints become dislocated and unusable.

Whereas relief of pain is the primary indication for surgery in the larger joints of the body, restoring function is the major consideration in hand surgery. As for all patients, physical therapy and medication are the first choices in treatment for rheumatoid arthritis in the hand, but surgery is considered when these options fail.

Joint replacement in the hand began in 1964 with Dr. Alfred Swanson, an orthopedic surgeon at the Blodgett Hospital Medical Center in Grand Rapids, Michigan. Prior to his work a variety of metallic implants had been tried but without success. Dr. Swanson's technique was intriguingly simple but required a sophisticated synthetic material to make it work. He replaced the finger joints with a flexible one-piece hinge made of silicone rubber, which he chose because it is accepted well by the body's tissues and is strong and flexible.

The extraordinary results of Dr. Swanson's work promise lifelong restoration of function to victims of rheumatoid arthritis. "After several design changes to im-

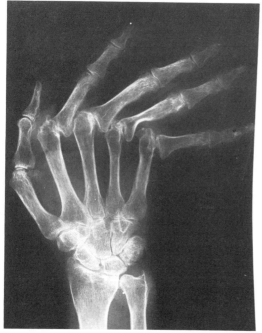

X ray of rheumatoid arthritis hand. Joints have been destroyed and bones cannot maintain normal alignment. (Courtesy Albert Swanson, M.D.)

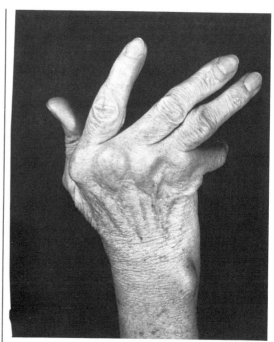

Joint destruction due to rheumatoid arthritis. (Courtesy Albert Swanson, M.D.)

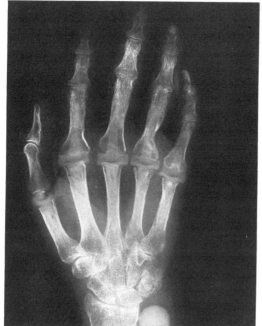

Artificial spacers, or joints, have replaced the destroyed knuckles, restoring normal finger positions. (Courtesy Albert Swanson, M.D.)

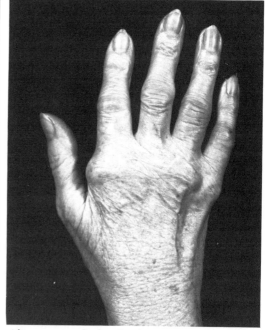

After surgery, the hand is functional once more and fingers are returned to normal positions. (Courtesy Albert Swanson, M.D.)

prove the dimensions of the implant, the latest version is a result of six years of machine testing," says Dr. Swanson. "It has been flexed from 0 to 90 degrees more than 600 million times without failure." More than 300 clinics in 83 countries have used the implant, and several hundred thousand patients now attest to its success.

In the finger joint replacement operation, which may take more than two hours, the diseased ends of the bones of the joint are surgically removed. The thin ends of the implant are then inserted into the hollow ends of the finger and hand bones. After the operation, and to keep the fingers in the proper position, the patient wears a brace continuously for three to four weeks and at night for another month. A supervised exercise and stretching program continues for three to six months thereafter, at which time the patient is able to use the hand in the normal way. During the healing process, natural body tissues accept the implant, surround it, and hold it securely in place.

Dr. Swanson comments on the difference between finger implants and larger joint prostheses: "Finger implants are not actually joints; they are spacers—that is, they hold the bone ends apart, prevent scarring, stiffness, and fusing of the joint, and permit reasonably normal function."

At a symposium on finger and hand implants in San Francisco in February 1979, several specialists from around the world compared their results and noted that the initial problems with the operation have led to much ignorance on the part of patients and practicing physicians alike about the results of today's more successful surgery. As a result, many patients with stiff hands haven't been properly counseled about this alternative to their current treatment program. "This is especially true of patients with deformities secondary to trauma or osteoarthritis," emphasizes Dr. Françoise Aiselin, a professor at the French College of Orthopedic Surgery at the University of Paris Medical School in France. "Many of them can also benefit by hand implants."

Hand implant surgery is being performed with increasing frequency at medical centers and community hospitals across the country. Surgeons also report similar success with silicone rubber implants in the wrists and the joints of the feet and toes.

In the future

Dr. Ewald, who has been responsible for the design of many of the prostheses currently in use, stresses that research is still ongoing in this field. "Materials are being improved all the time to be stronger and more resistant to the severe stresses placed on the joints." A new cement may soon be available to bond prostheses directly to the collagen fibers that make up the body's connective tissues. Still other prostheses under development may permit the body tissues to grow directly into them as they now do with replaced blood vessels.

At Boston's Beth Israel Hospital, biomedical engineer Dr. Wilson Hayes is working with orthopedic surgeons in the Department of Biomedical Engineering to design new prostheses that will take advantage of the natural tendency of bones to respond to stress by overgrowing and hardening. The result of their work may soon be a prosthesis that becomes more tightly attached with use rather than looser, as is currently the case.

Joint replacement is a major form of surgery and involves many complications. If an answer to how and why arthritis occurs in the first place finally becomes available, prevention of the deformities may obviate the need for joint replacement at all. But until then, joint replacement now promises people crippled with chronic arthritis a return to a functional life.

Restoring the voice

**And like music on the waters
Is thy sweet voice to me.**

Lord Byron
"The Prisoner of Chillon," 1816

Cancer of the larynx, or voice box, is among the more common oral cancers. Its cause is not known, but it seems to be related to cigarette smoking. Treatment for this cancer involves radiation and most often surgery. A natural outcome of surgery for cancer of the larynx is loss of the voice.

About 10,000 patients each year have their voice boxes removed for cancer. Most learn esophageal speech, a crude voice produced by swallowing air and then belching to vibrate the soft tissues of the esophagus. Others use an electronic device which is held up to the neck and produces robotlike speech.

At the First International Symposium on Surgical Restoration of the Voice held recently, Dr. James Stallings of Mercy Hospital in Des Moines, Iowa, reported a new procedure for restoring near-normal speech to people whose voice boxes have been removed. He has operated on 100 patients thus far, and the results have been more gratifying than previous options for restoration of speech.

Most patients who undergo surgical removal of the larynx speak by means of an electronic voice box, as demonstrated here. (Photo by Paul Connell, courtesy Boston Globe)

CASE HISTORY

W. L. is a prison watch commander in California whose cancerous larynx was removed in 1977. During the operation, which Dr. Stallings performed, a new voice box was created out of transplanted tendons. The very day of the operation, W. L. could talk with 75 percent of his normal speech.

"Ninety-five percent of my job is speaking. I wouldn't have consented to the surgery if I couldn't talk reasonably normally afterward," W. L. said. "I wanted no part of an electronic voice box, and by the time I learned esophageal speech I would be ready to retire." W. L. was a heavy smoker in his early years but stopped in 1951. He had been a World War II navigator and was captured and held prisoner in Poland and Germany for nine months. During that period he was severely malnourished and blames that experience for his cancer.

W. L. still has a tracheostomy, an opening into the windpipe in his neck. He covers the opening with his finger when he speaks, diverting the air upward and vibrating the tendons in his new voice box.

In W. L.'s operation, Dr. Stallings used substitute vocal cords made of pieces of transplanted tendons from a patient's arm or leg which are attached near the old voice box site. Other surgeons have had good results with variations of this technique.

Cancer of the larynx now has a 90 to 95 percent cure rate when caught in its early stages and treated by radiation and surgery. Until recently, the result of treatment was a life without speech; now, new techniques of voice box replacement surgery can give these patients hope of returning to a reasonably normal life. ˙

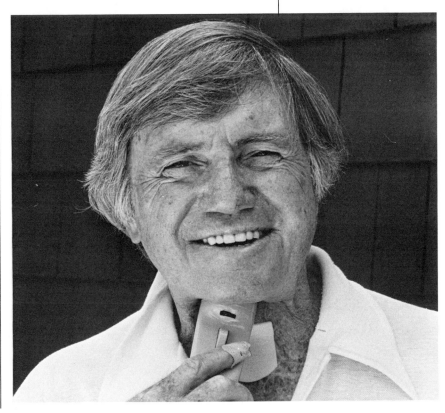

Artificial skin

Skin is the boundary between the inside and the outside, between the self and the non-self.

John A. Parrish, M.D.

A generation ago, a person with burns covering 30 percent of the body or more faced imminent death. As noted in "Update: Transplants" (see page 180), new treatments make it possible for a severely burned patient to recover today.

Researchers at the Massachusetts Institute of Technology in Cambridge, Massachusetts, and the Shriners Burn Institute in Boston may have still another advancement in burn care. Using a combination of manmade and natural materials, researchers have developed an artificial skin that promises to eliminate rejection problems and create a permanent covering for the body. The artificial skin has been used successfully in animals and may soon be used on people as well.

To treat an extensive burn successfully, new skin must be applied to replace the burned skin and restore the body's protective covering. Finding skin for this grafting can be a difficult task. Animal skin is plentiful, but the human body quickly rejects such a foreign substance. Skin from cadaver donations lasts a bit longer, but is inevitably rejected as well. Permanent skin covering must incorporate the patient's own cells; but in a large burn, the unburned areas on a burn victim that are available for skin graft donor sites may be limited.

The Boston area project uses the patient's own skin to manufacture additional skin. Professor Eugene Bell of M.I.T. and Dr. John Burke of the Shriners Burns Institute are coordinating the effort. To make their "new" skin, the Boston researchers use a mixture of collagen (a protein found in connective tissue structures), fibroblasts, connective tissue cells, and a number of other chemicals. The mixture becomes gelatinous when allowed to stand and, when poured onto a flat plate, actually forms a sheet of tissue much like the under layer of normal skin. The researchers then add a few cells from the patient's epidermis, or outer layer of skin, to the mixture. As the researchers explain, "The cells quickly arrange themselves into several layers, just the way they are in normal skin. It [the new skin] becomes quite tough; we can handle it, cut it and sew it. When we place it on the flesh of the research animal, the new skin begins to grow. Blood vessels infiltrate into it and it spreads."

The new skin has survived for over six months in laboratory tests—a figure so impressive that the investigators are now ready to try artificial skin on humans, an experiment that has just received United States Food and Drug Administration approval. Clinical trials will soon begin at Boston's Beth Israel Hospital in collaboration with plastic surgeon Dr. Robert Goldwin.

"We could grow enough skin to cover my whole body," said Professor Bell, "but it would probably take a month or so to grow that much." In burn treatment, one month is but a short time—the traditional skin graft procedure often takes years to complete. By shortening burn therapy and covering more body area, the new procedure may dramatically improve burn survival rates.

Not just for burns

The M.I.T.–Shriners project may have wide applications throughout medicine. Bell noted that the sheets of skin may be grown on cylinders, resulting in a tubular piece of tissue that could be used to replace a blood vessel and improve the success rates of vascular (blood vessel) surgery on various circulatory conditions. Another possibility involves "seeding" the connective tissue mixture with organ- or hormone-producing cells, such as the Beta cells of the pancreas. This may allow a diabetic to induce Beta cell growth, for example, and reduce or eliminate the need for insulin.

According to a recent *Boston Globe* article, the new M.I.T.–Shriners skin has been patented and will be manufactured by Flow Laboratories, Inc., a biomedical products company in McLean, Virginia.

Artificial blood

"Blood is a very special juice."

Johann Wolfgang von Goethe
Faust, Act I, Scene IV

Stories of blood shortages throughout the world are legion, since blood supplies are forever dependent on the generosity of donors. The time required to process donated blood—to match prospective donors and recipients—often create delays that compromise an individual's life. For these and other reasons, medical researchers have long sought a temporary alternative to bank blood as a lifesaving means until cross-matched blood is available and until the body's own blood-manufacturing processes can take over.

On November 11, 1979, that alternative, a synthetic blood substitute was successfully administered for the first time to a patient in Minnesota.

About blood

Blood is a vital courier that delivers oxygen and other nutrients to cells in exchange for their carbon dioxide and waste products. At their most basic level, cells need oxygen to carry out their life processes, indeed to survive. Oxygen is transported though the bloodstream by the hemoglobin molecule, a protein found in the red blood cell. Any reduction in the oxygen-carrying capacity of blood leads to poor tissue functioning and ultimately to death. It is therefore imperative that the red blood cell and hemoglobin levels in the blood be kept fairly constant and unimpeded. The typical red blood cell has a life span of 120 days. As RBCs mature and are broken down, they must be constantly replaced by newer cells more active in oxygen transport. This is the work of the bone marrow.

Sometimes, however, because of blood loss due to illness or injury, the body's blood-manufacturing capabilities cannot keep up. Then transfusion becomes necessary, and in an emergency transfusion must begin immediately.

CASE HISTORY

H. M. is a sixty-seven-year-old Jehovah's Witness with chronic anemia. Because of a nonhealing ulcer on his right leg, secondary to a progressive circulatory condition, an operation was performed to increase the blood flow. Following the surgery the patient did well, but when he was discharged from the hospital he was quite anemic, with a blood hemoglobin level of 7—about half the normal level for his age. He had refused blood transfusion because his religion prohibited it and was treated instead with iron and folic acid. At home his blood count continued to fall and his body was not making red cells fast enough. When an infection developed in the surgical wound he became gravely ill and was readmitted to the hospital. His hemoglobin level was 3.3 g, only 25 percent of his normal amount. A call was placed to the Food and Drug Administration for permission to use an experimental blood substitute, Fluosol DA. Permission was given, and 2,000 cc (2 quarts) of the artificial blood were infused intravenously. H. M. began to respond immediately. He was awake and talking within ten days. He was discharged one month later with a hemoglobin level of 8 g, and he continued to improve, although he was still anemic.

Some weeks later H. M. died of his dis-

ease, still refusing transfusion. But there was no doubt that the synthetic substitute worked at least temporarily. Dr. Robert Anderson, the surgeon at the University of Minnesota who coordinated H. M.'s care, observed: "There was electrocardiogram evidence of oxygen improvement one hour after the treatment began." Word of the successful use of synthetic blood spread quickly in the medical community.

Substitute blood

The story of artificial blood begins in 1967, when Dr. Robert Geyer of the Harvard School of Public Health began looking for chemicals that could do the work of red blood cells by transporting oxygen and carbon dioxide to and from body tissues. His investigations led to fluorocarbons, organic compounds containing fluoride that can absorb large amounts of gases such as oxygen and carbon dioxide and are not reactive or toxic to the body. (Most kitchens contain a relative of fluorocarbons—Teflon, the "magic coating" on frying pans and utensils.) Rather than binding to the gases as hemoglobin does, fluorocarbons permit the oxygen and carbon dioxide to dissolve as fluids circulate. Normal diffusion enables the oxygen to pass into the cells and the carbon dioxide to pass out. Original experiments were performed on laboratory rats, and by 1973, Dr. Geyer comments, "they could survive for ten days or more with their entire blood volume replaced by fluorocarbons. As new blood was regenerated it gradually replaced the fluorocarbons in the circulation."

With this as an impetus, Japanese investigators developed a synthetic blood that contained two fluorocarbons. The first tests on humans were performed at Germany's University of Mainz on patients who had brain death but were kept alive by respirators. Even amounts as large as 1 or 2 quarts of the artificial substance were found to sustain life safely. Further experiments in Japan included patients with rare blood types.

The current preparation, Fluosol DA, contains, in addition to the two fluorocarbons, an emulsifier that permits fluorocarbons to be dissolved in blood. It also contains sugar, electrolytes, and hydroxethyl starch, which acts as a volume expander in place of normal blood proteins. Without the volume expander, the preparation would diffuse immediately into all the body tissues.

When synthetic blood is used

The ability to transport oxygen and carbon dioxide is only part of the function of blood. Blood is a complex substance that contains white cells necessary to the body's defenses against infection and other challenges, platelets and other factors responsible for clotting, albumin, and plasma proteins. No one expects that fluorocarbons or other synthetics will replace human blood. Current thinking indicates that the use of synthetic blood may be restricted to:

■ Emergencies when properly cross-matched blood is not immediately available. The blood substitute would temporarily provide oxygen and carbon dioxide transport while the body's blood-generating capacity catches up with the need, or until appropriately matched blood is available. Rescue paramedic units and emergency departments would find great use for such a substance.

■ Surgical procedures such as heart or blood vessel replacement which ordinarily require large amounts of blood.

■ Keeping donated organs viable until they can be transplanted (see ''Update: Transplants,'' page 182).

■ Testing drugs on certain donated organs. This is important because federal regulations prohibit most drug testing on humans.

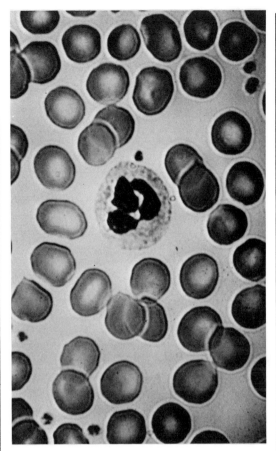

Real blood contains red and white blood cells and plasma. Artificial blood replaces the oxygen-carrying capacity of the red blood cells.

Artificial blood, similar to glucose and electrolyte intravenous solutions, does not have to be cross-matched. Because it can be given to all patients without specificity, it is very valuable and quick in an emergency. The artificial blood preparation is strictly experimental, however, and its use has thus far been restricted to life-and-death situations. Because concentrations of fluorocarbons have been found in the liver and spleen, lymph, and other tissues, some investigators question its safety, and extensive testing will no doubt shed more light on this problem. At least for now, however, we know that artificial blood, when used judiciously, can be a lifesaving substance.

Carbon tendons

In this era of surgically implanted prostheses it appears the nylon athlete has arrived.

Physician and Sports Medicine Journal, August 1978

All prostheses are made of artificial material implanted in the body to replace destroyed or nonfunctioning natural tissues. And all foreign material, no matter how apparently inert, has the potential for causing adverse reactions. The ultimate prosthesis is one that will replace a damaged or destroyed body part initially, then gradually dissolve while encouraging normal body tissues to regrow and replace the old. Such a procedure may be at hand for tendon and ligament restoration if the initial results of work on animals at the College of Medicine and Dentistry in Camden, New Jersey hold true in humans as well.

The potential of carbon tendons

One unfortunate result of vigorous activity is damage to ligaments and tendons, the strong straps of connective tissue that join muscles to bones and bones to each other. Currently, torn ligaments and tendons are treated with casts and suture repair. But such treatments require long periods of immobility for healing, and the resulting structure is weakened.

A team representing several medical and physical disciplines at the New Jersey college has developed an artificial tendon consisting of a composite of carbon fibers and polylactic acid (PLA). The PLA-carbon is a mesh that is sewn in place of damaged tissue. The tensile strength of the carbon is similar to that of the tendon. As the PLA matrix gradually changes to lactic acid in the body, the carbon is degraded completely over time. The mesh acts as a scaffold or framework for new tendon tissues to grow; while the new tissue is immature and weak, the carbon carries the load. As the tissue matures, it accepts more stress and the carbon tendons begin to degenerate.

Commenting in a recent issue of *Sports Medicine*, the New Jersey doctors feel the PLA-carbon scaffold and mesh will have wide applications in reconstructive surgery and orthopedics to replace knee, ankle, or hand tendons that have been damaged by vigorous activity.

In their work with animals, the New Jersey team, headed by Dr. Andrew Weiss, and Harold Alexander, Ph.D., found that in sixty-three days new tendon tissue has completely overgrown and enveloped the prosthetic mesh, and during that period the animal is free to move about without restrictions.

The team does not expect such quick results in humans. For example, dog tendons grow and mature more quickly; humans may have to restrict activity for a longer time. The result, however, may be a tendon as strong and functional as the original.

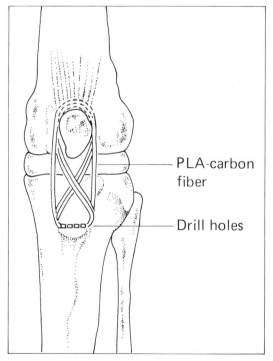

PLA-carbon fiber

Drill holes

In this drawing of a dog's leg, you can see where the coated carbon fibers have been drilled into the bone. Normal tissue grows along the fiber strands and gradually replaces them.

The artificial heart

The heart is the most noble of all the members of our body.

St. John Chrysostom
Homilies, in the *Ondes Statutes* (X),
ca. 388

From early in recorded history the heart has been recognized as the physical center of life and given philosophical significance. The word *heart* has come to represent many of our positive emotions—affection, love, courage, tenderness.

Within the medical profession research on the heart attracts the largest grants and the biggest scientific egos. Heart surgeons are considered a breed apart. Entire wards with technology costing in the millions are built for the care of cardiac victims. Cardiopulmonary rescue programs train people to intervene in acute cardiac arrest.

Such preoccupation with heart disease is not surprising. Heart and blood vessel conditions kill over 1 million people each year, amounting to one-third of all deaths in this country. Small wonder than, that of all the artificial organs, none receives as much publicity and money as the artificial heart.

While a successful artificial human heart continues to elude development, some exciting research has brought that goal closer in the past two years. In the Willem Kolff Laboratory at the University of Utah in Salt Lake City, calves have been kept alive for six months or more with arti-ficial hearts, until the young animals outgrew the devices. And in humans, partial artificial hearts called LVAD (left ventricular assist devices) have saved the lives of at least six patients. These successes have prompted many scientists to speculate that a complete artificial heart is now a real possibility.

The LVAD

The LVAD unit is mounted outside the body on the chest wall and connected to the heart by two tubes, each containing a pig's heart valve, to keep blood flowing in the right direction. One tube removes blood from the apex of the left side of the heart—the left ventricle—and directs it to a small pumping chamber. The second returns blood in the circulation to the aorta. Pumping is provided by an external air source.

The LVAD provides a temporary replacement for the main pumping chamber of the heart—the left ventricle. The pump was successfully used in calves for eight years before it was tried in humans. Now it is used only when all other alternatives

The left ventricular assist device (LVAD). Large metal area pumps blood; white tubes connect to heart and blood vessels; long transparent tube connects to air supply to operate pump. (Courtesy Boston University Medical Center)

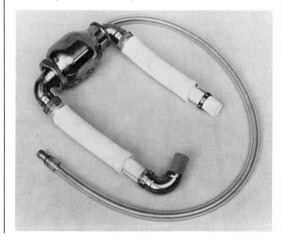

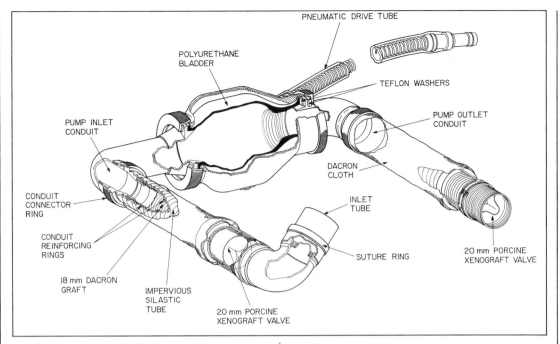

Detailed structure of LVAD. (Courtesy Boston University Medical Center)

have been exhausted and the only remaining course is to declare the patient dead. Whereas pacemakers provide an electrical stimulus to the heart's muscles, the LVAD is used in patients whose heart muscles are so deteriorated that not even a pacemaker will make it beat. The patient or his family must sign a detailed consent form pointing out the LVAD's potential hazards and benefits before the procedure is undertaken.

CASE HISTORY

R. B., a sixty-year-old painting contractor, suffered the first of three heart attacks in March 1976. Angina pectoris began to rule his life. Within two years he could not even get dressed in the morning without experiencing heaviness and pressure in his chest, a sign that his heart was not getting enough oxygen.

An X-ray study confirmed this suspicion. Three major coronary blood vessels were blocked and unable to deliver blood to the heart muscle. R. B. was scheduled for coronary bypass surgery to replace all three arteries with small vein grafts.

The graft surgery performed at University Hospital in Boston in April 1978 proceeded smoothly, but when the heart-lung bypass machine was disconnected after the operation, R.B.'s own heart would not pump blood.

When it became clear that the only alternative was to turn off the equipment and declare R. B. dead, cardiac surgeon Dr. Robert Berger implanted a partial artificial heart, or LVAD, a procedure that took about one hour. For four and a half days the LVAD functioned in place of R. B.'s heart. When it was determined that R. B.'s own heart could take over, the LVAD was disconnected. He did well and was discharged from the hospital six weeks later, in his words, "to just sit in the yard and soak up some sun." He is still alive and well.

R. B. was the first patient after twenty previous failures to be given a new lease on life by the LVAD. Subsequently, the LVAD has been used successfully on two more occasions by Dr. Berger at University Hospital in Boston, twice by Dr. William Pierce at Pennsylvania State University in Hershey, and once in Houston at the Baylor University Medical Center by Dr. John Norman.

If six successes out of more than fifty attempts seems unimpressive, Dr. John Watson, who heads the artificial heart program at the National Heart, Lung, and Blood Institute, thinks otherwise. "The program shows that the LVAD can stimulate a patient's circulation and allow the patient's own heart to recover and restore its own function by giving it a rest period," he notes. Dr. Watson should know. Since 1965 the institute has spent more than $125 million toward their goal of developing an artificial heart.

When is the LVAD used?

During cardiovascular surgery, a heart-lung bypass machine temporarily takes over the work of the heart and lungs and diverts the blood for several hours while the surgical team completes its task in a bloodless field. After the operation, the machine is disconnected and the patient's own heart begins to work again. Nearly 1,000 patients die each year on the operating table, however, because their hearts cannot take over after surgery, usually because disease has deprived their hearts of adequate blood flow for so long prior to surgery.

Thus far, the National Heart, Lung and Blood Institute has restricted the use of the LVAD to those patients who cannot be "weaned" from a heart-lung machine. But an even larger number of cardiac patients may also benefit from the LVAD.

Many thousands of people die each year from cardiogenic shock following a massive heart attack, when such a large area of

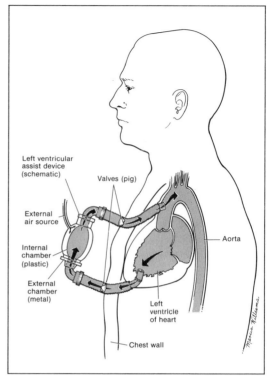

Diagram illustrates how LVAD operates. Dark arrows represent blood flow. (Drawing by Marcia Williams, courtesy Boston University Medical Center)

their heart muscle is injured that it can no longer pump blood effectively. Their blood pressure drops precipitously, and death is the frequent outcome. "By stepping in early, attaching the LVAD, and taking a load off the heart muscle, we can allow the heart to rest," comments Dr. Berger.

The NHLBI now intends to devote $2 million over three years to help finance the cost of the LVAD in up to 100 of these patients. If this effort is successful, each year many thousands of patients deemed to be in imminent cardiogenic shock may be hooked up to the LVAD.

Surgeons at Baylor University in Houston feel that the LVAD may also be important in cardiac transplantation. An article in a recent issue of the medical journal *Lancet* stated that "the biggest logistical problem is supporting the prospective recipient until a suitable donor can be found. The artificial heart can solve this problem." There are currently over 1,000 potential heart transplant patients in the United States alone. (See "Update: Transplants," pages 176–178.)

In the future

The LVAD is a temporary replacement for a poorly functioning heart. The ultimate —a permanent replacement—may be only a few years away.

Doctors at the Department of Artificial Organs at the Cleveland Clinic Foundation are developing a miniature LVAD, small enough to be attached to the heart and left inside the body for years. Dr. Yukihiko Nose explains: "An implanted battery pack will transmit power to a small pump propelled by a contact electrical motor functioning much like today's pacemakers."

Developing the artificial heart has given scientists a new appreciation for the endurance of the real heart. As one researcher says, "Very few mechanical devices can function 100,000 times per day, day after day, year after year, without rest and without failing. Yet, at seventy beats per minute, that is how often the human heart pumps blood. Our challenge is to find an artificial variety with that kind of stamina."

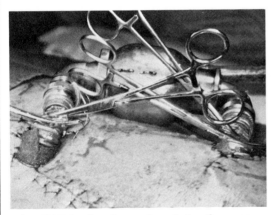

The LVAD in place in a patient during the operation. Chest wall is seen in lower part of photo; stitches hold skin together. (Courtesy Boston University Medical Center)

Medical sculpture

Art imitates nature.
Richard Franck
Northern Memoirs, 1658

Each year thousands of people are disfigured from radical cancer surgery, burns, accidental trauma, and birth defects. Whenever possible, reconstructive plastic surgery is the best solution for cosmetic and functional repair. Reconstruction, however, is expensive and sometimes painful, and it often requires many operations over months and years. There are limitations on how the plastic surgeon can use living skin, bone, and cartilage, and some types of defects simply cannot be repaired. Despite the best of attempts, the patient is often left to face life with an obvious deformity and an ugly scar.

At the University of Michigan Medical Center in Ann Arbor, Professor Denis Lee, a sculptor and medical illustrator by training, has provided another alternative for thousands of disfigured patients. His lifelike body parts, fashioned and tinted to match the patient's own, demonstrate the enormous potential of today's cosmetic prostheses to re-create a normal and socially acceptable appearance.

A new idea?

Lee began his work ten years ago with the encouragement of Dr. Reed Dingman, then chief of plastic surgery at the University of

Michigan. Dr. Dingman was struck by the crude, almost repellent character of prostheses then available. "They needed an artistic touch," he noted. Lee set out to develop that artistic quality in a home workshop. Today he is in charge of the Department of Medical Sculpture, which makes 300 prostheses per year with a skill that would make even classic sculptors envious. He also runs a training program in prosthesis sculpture. If these creations are striking and innovative, the idea for cosmetic prostheses is not new. As long as there have been artists and inventors, there have been people attempting to fashion replacement body parts. Records of their work can be found in literature and in the paintings of the great masters.

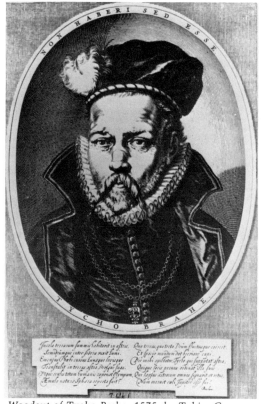

Woodcut of Tycho Brahe, 1575, by Tobias Gemperlin, showing obvious artificial nose. (Courtesy Karen Brahe's Cloister, Odemse, Denmark)

CASE HISTORY

In the Karen Brahe Cloister in Odense, Denmark, hangs on oil portrait by the German painter Tobias Gemperlin. The subject is Tycho Brahe, a sixteenth-century Danish astronomer and mathematician. He is pictured in the costume of his day with long, flowing mustache and pointed beard—and with an obvious nasal prosthesis.

Tycho Brahe lost the bridge of his nose on December 10, 1560, during a rapier duel with Danish nobleman Manderup Parsbjerg to settle an argument as to who was the better scholar. The nasal disfigurement had an enormous impact on his life. He became aloof, vengeful, and condemned the lives of his peers. He immersed himself ever more in his work.

To correct his disfigurement, Tycho replaced the missing part of his nose with wax, made a prosthesis out of copper and silver, and painted it in oil to match his skin. He always carried a small box of glue to fix the prosthesis in place.

Tycho Brahe continued his work in astronomy, which today ranks with that of Copernicus, Galileo, and Newton. When his skeleton was exhumed in 1901, his skull still bore the bright green stain of copper around the nasal defect. The legendary prosthesis however, was missing, perhaps taken by a fortune-hunting gravedigger.

Brahe is symbolic of patients with disfigurement today. Many refrain from jobs with personal contact; others withdraw from friends, family, and society, fearing that they are repulsive. Children are especially subject to ridicule from their peers.

Reconstructing a body

If the idea for cosmetic prostheses is not new, the materials with which they are constructed are new and in fact are responsible for the great success of medical sculpture today.

Most prostheses are made of silicone rubber, a soft, lifelike, textured material that is easy to work with, yet strong enough to stand up under constant use. It is also easily tinted to match the patient's own skin.

Professor Lee's medical sculpture unit at the University of Michigan creates more than 300 prostheses a year, including ears, noses, eyes, and fingers. But the most commonly requested prostheses are breasts.

Ninety thousand women have mastectomies each year. Although some accept the loss of a breast in stride, most find it traumatic and a blow to their sexual identity. Five percent have surgery to reconstruct their missing breast. Most of the others wear breast prostheses.

"Ask any woman if she is happy with her prosthesis and she'll say 'no,'" says Professor Lee, commenting on the poor quality of most commercially manufactured breast prostheses. "She'll also open a drawer to show you several that she's tried and discarded because she wasn't happy with them." Most commercial prostheses are too heavy or too light, fail to fill in defects, and feel unnatural. Most women shopping for prostheses have been subjected to salespeople with poor knowledge of their product, and to products made with little or no attention to individuality or comfort.

Lee's prostheses are being worn, however, and no wonder. They are individually fashioned in clay on a plaster cast of the patient's chest to match the remaining breast and then molded in silicone. Both skin and nipple are tinted to match the patient's own. Fluid is added to bring it up to the proper weight and to provide the positional changes in contour that are typical of normal breast tissue. The latest adhesives permit the prosthesis to be worn with confidence all day, even during sleeping, swimming, or other athletic events —and under all kinds of clothing. "It so mimics my normal breast," says one of Lee's younger patients, "that I even wear my prosthesis without a bra under a T-shirt and no one can tell."

Lee's latest development in breast prostheses is a kit that enables women to measure themselves at home. The kit's instructions explain which dimensions to measure, and it includes several templates to fit on the remaining breast for sizing and color swatches to match skin tones. The breast prostheses have also been used for patients who have lost both breasts to cancer or severe burns. In these cases, "the disfigurement is even more extreme and the prostheses therefore even more useful," notes Lee.

The ravages of cancer are not limited to

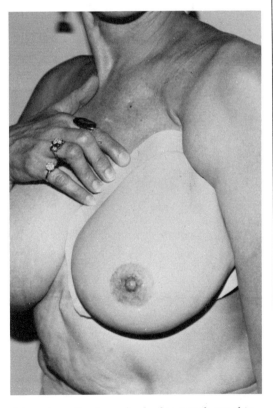

A breast prosthesis can be dyed to match any skin color. The structure can virtually duplicate a remaining breast—a far cry from store-bought prostheses. (Courtesy Prof. Denis Lee)

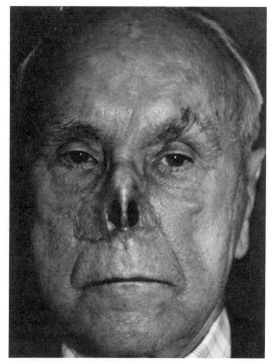

This sixty-year-old man has his nose removed in cancer surgery. He had worn gauze bandages over the deformed area for twenty years.

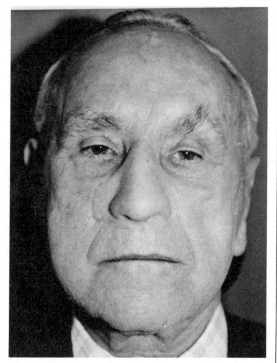

The prosthetic nose has given him a social and psychological rehabilitation. (Photos courtesy Prof. Denis Lee)

the breast. Some patients lose part or all of their nose or ears or other facial parts to radical cancer surgery. This type of deformity is particularly emotionally disruptive. One man wore gauze over the hole where his nose had been for twenty years before coming to the Michigan Medical Sculpture Department. He rarely went out and associated with few people. With his new prosthesis he has returned to an active social life. "A nose prosthesis is the most difficult to conceal," admits Lee, "but by making appropriate use of natural skin folds, makeup, and glasses, we can make it blend pretty well with surrounding tissues."

Young children may lose an eye and the surrounding tissue to a cancer called retinoblastoma. Here again, a prosthesis can be most realistic. It may even include eyelashes and eyebrow made from a patient's own hair.

Among Lee's most common problems are the congenital absences of one or both ears, a reconstruction in young children. Ear reconstruction is rarely possible by plastic surgery, but Lee feels the ear is the easiest body part to replace with a prosthesis and probably the most undetectable, particularly given today's long hair styles.

Facial areas often have varying pigmentations, so Lee's group spends hours tinting and coloring with the attention of a portrait artist. They even have a "suntan" lotion that temporarily colors the prosthesis to match the patient's skin as it tans.

Other prostheses have been used on patients who have lost part of their hands or feet in lawn mower or factory machine accidents, or on patients born with missing finger parts. Naturally, the prostheses don't move independently, but these devices at least remove the stigma of obvious deformity. Looking at the prosthesis held

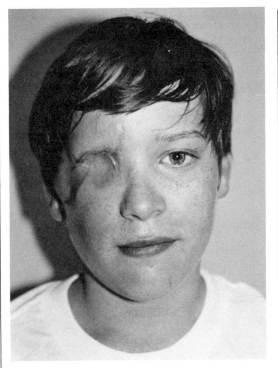

This thirteen-year-old boy lost his right eye in a gunshot accident.

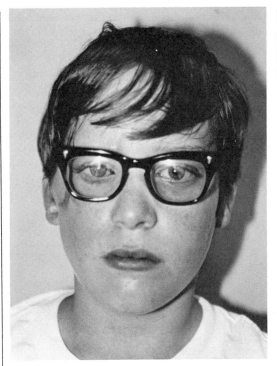

The prosthesis consists of an artificial eye and socket; the edges are hidden by eyeglass frames. (Photos courtesy Prof. Denis Lee)

in place with adhesives and with edges concealed by watches, watchbands or rings, a close observer literally cannot tell that the body part is false.

A new specialty

"A lot of people play around with cosmetic prostheses," notes Lee. "Some do fine work, others not so good. The problem is that it is hard to find consistent training or continuing education programs in this field." Along with other experts, Lee has formed an association for medical sculpture to help fund and regulate training programs for talented artists who want to enter this field. The association will also certify specialists. Certification will undoubtedly regulate consistency of quality in medical sculpture work.

Newer materials continue to result in better prostheses. Lee's current cosmetic prostheses last two years or more unless they are bleached from chlorine in pools or stained by the sun or other chemicals. Hand prostheses, for example, are often replaced every six months because of staining from food, ink, and so forth.

Cosmetic prostheses are far less expensive than reconstructive surgery and surprisingly inexpensive, given the emotional rehabilitation they provide. The average prosthesis costs several hundred dollars, including application.

For all the success of medical sculptors, many doctors still don't know of their work. Although most of the referrals to medical sculpting departments stem from private physicians, primary care doctors (such as pediatricians and internists), and plastic and general surgeons, many still don't know where or even that such work is being done at all. "We have a major education problem here, obviously," comments Lee. He goes on to say, "There are undoubtedly a lot of people out there without an ear or a nose who are afraid to go out. That isn't necessary anymore. They can be helped now."

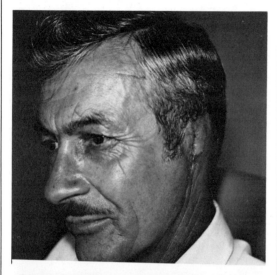

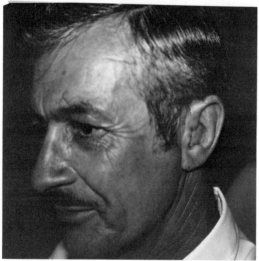

Having lost his ear from cancer surgery, this man now wears a prosthetic ear. (Photos courtesy Prof. Denis Lee)

A kidney in a suitcase

Falstaff: What says the Doctor to my water?
Page: He said, Sir, the water itself was good healthy water; but, for the party that owed it, he might have more diseases than he knows for.

William Shakespeare
Henry IV: Part II, ca. 1597–98

In the eighteenth century Parson Swift, who described urine as yellow gold, devised a system of examining the urine to permit the diagnosis of forty-one medical conditions. Today urinalysis continues to be an important part of medical diagnosis. As Shakespeare noted, the mere passage of urine is no indication of health. The kidneys are filters, and what they conserve or permit to pass out of the body has much to do with overall health.

The kidneys are as vital to the body as the heart or lungs. Should they fail, all body organs would malfunction as well. The gradual buildup of impurities in our blood leads to a condition called uremia which destroys body tissues and leads inevitably to death.

Early in the twentieth century work was begun on ways to filter impurities from the blood when the kidneys could no longer work. The first successful results were achieved during the early 1940s in Nazi-occupied Holland, where Dr. Willem Kolff, now director of the Institute for Biomedical Engineering at the University of Utah, devised the first artificial kidney using cellophane sausage casings as a blood filter. Kolff subsequently was invited to the Peter Bent Brigham Hospital in Boston, where his system was upgraded using modern plastics, metals, and electronics—and dialysis was born.

Dialysis methods

Most patients with chronic kidney failure go to a hospital-based or independent dialysis center where the long and tiring process of blood filtration is carried out three time a week for four to five hours at a sitting. During dialysis blood is routed from an artery in the patient's arm into an artificial kidney for dialysis filtration, then returned to a vein. Dialysis treatment at such a center is expensive—$25,000 per year on the average—although government funding often absorbs the entire bill.

Many dialysis patients today have an artificial kidney in their home. Home dialysis is cheaper—$15,000 per year on the average—and permits greater freedom, but such patients are still quite restricted in travel and other pursuits. They must have access to their artificial kidney devices every other day.

The chronic kidney failure patient now has prospects for greater freedom and mobility. Dr. Eli Freedman and his associates at the Downstate Medical Center in Brooklyn, New York, working with National Institutes of Health contract support, have developed a kidney in a suitcase. The portable lightweight dialysis device uses the latest computerized systems and needs only running water and an electrical outlet to make it work. Many of Dr. Freedman's patients have traveled throughout the United States and abroad, using their "suitcase kidney" in recreational vehicles, motels, and hotel rooms with good results.

Other treatment developments

With NIH sponsorship, three investigators

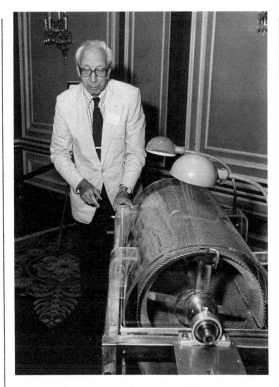

In December 1979, on the twenty-fifth anniversary of the first kidney transplant operation, Dr. Willem Kollf demonstrates the first artificial kidney, developed in 1948. The original device used sausage casings as filters. (Photo by Daniel Bernstein, courtesy Brigham and Women's Hospital, Boston)

are continuing the development of an intriguing technique which uses the lining of the patient's abdominal cavity as a replacement kidney. Dr. Jack Moncrief and Dr. Robert Popovich at the University of Texas in Austin and Dr. Kenneth Nolph of the University of Missouri Medical Center are studying continuous ambulatory peritoneal dialysis (CAPD), a simple and relatively inexpensive form of home dialysis that frees the patient from machine hardware.

A patient on CAPD therapy attaches a plastic bag filled with 2 liters (approximately 2 quarts) of a solution similar in composition to that of body fluids to a small tube that has been surgically implanted in the abdominal cavity. The patient hangs up the bag and lets gravity drain the solution into the belly. When the bag is empty, the patient rolls it up and tucks it away under a belt and returns to normal activity. After four to five hours the patient places the empty bag on the floor and lets gravity drain the fluid, which is now filled with blood impurities, back into the bag. Then the patient disconnects the old bag, hooks up a new one, and repeats the procedure.

Patients on CAPD go through this process early each morning, just before bed, and twice more in between for a total of four times per day. Unlike dialysis with an artificial kidney machine, CAPD treatment must be undertaken every day, but the patient does have much greater mobility. CAPD patients have an extra 2 liters of fluid in their body at all times, but this doesn't appear to cause problems.

CAPD is a direct outgrowth of peritoneal dialysis, which has been used on hospitalized patients for many years. Dr. Moncrief explains: ''Unlike machine dialysis, we don't use a cellophane bag as a filter in peritoneal dialysis. Instead, we use the peritoneal membrane, the fine tissue sheet which surrounds the bowel. The peritoneal membrane has a rich blood supply. Water impurities pass from the blood through the peritoneal tissue and into the dialysis solution.''

CAPD does have one major drawback: a high potential for peritonitis, an infection of the lining of the abdominal cavity. Careful treatment has made this an infrequent occurrence, however. CAPD is now being used successfully in many medical centers and on several hundred patients around the country.

CAPD costs about $8,000 per year. If it gains wide acceptance, the device might save hundreds of millions of dollars from the government's annual dialysis bill.

Any form of artificial device is still an imperfect solution to the problem of chronic kidney failure. Besides filtering impurities, the kidney has other important func-

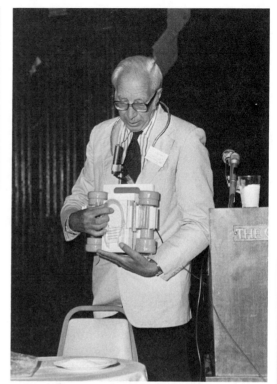

Dr. Kollf shows the latest artificial kidney—small and portable enough to be carried in a suitcase. (Photo by Daniel Bernstein, courtesy Brigham and Woman's Hospital, Boston)

tions such as the production of hormones that are important in blood pressure. Kidney transplantation is still considered the ultimate solution to this serious medical problem. But for those who are awaiting transplantation, or for those who are not candidates for it because of medical reasons, the new methods of dialysis and artificial kidneys are providing better treatment and are certainly boosting morale.

Harvey—the bionic patient

PROBLEM: How to expose medical students and doctors in training to patients with rare or unusual problems when there are few of those patients to be found.

ANSWER: Harvey.

PROBLEM: How to permit medical students and doctors in training to practice and sharpen their examination skills without overtiring or embarrassing a patient.

ANSWER: Harvey.

PROBLEM: How to prevent large numbers of students and instructors from examining the same patient for teaching purposes.

ANSWER: Harvey.

Harvey is a synthetic patient, a revolutionary teaching device that simulates the symptoms and physical findings of several common and unusual cardiovascular medical conditions.

Dr. Michael Gordon, a Miami cardiologist, originated the idea of the mannequin in 1967. Along with a consulting group of physicians, Dr. Gordon is responsible for its continued development, which to date has cost $7 million. The program is sponsored by a combination of federal and private funds. Dr. Gordon compares Harvey's role to that of a flight simulator for teaching pilots: "Harvey is not intended to be a substitute for a living patient any more than a flight simulator is for actually flying a 747, but it is an adjunct, an aid to make medical teaching more effective.

Harvey is a mannequin covered by a polyvinyl chloride skin which closely resembles human skin. Harvey's "brain" is a computer that controls a series of levers, pumps, cams, and speakers within the mannequin.

Harvey boasts veins and arteries which can be felt to measure pulses. The thrust of Harvey's heart can be felt by placing a hand over the left chest wall, and it can be heard with a stethoscope. Harvey's lung function can be watched by noting the abdominal skin rise and fall in simulated respiration. The computer can alter any of these to correspond to the state of Harvey's "health."

The intent of the teaching mannequin is to sharpen the students' bedside skills. It is appropriate, then, that Harvey should have been named after Dr. W. Proctor Harvey, a cardiologist at Georgetown University renowned for his attention to physical examination and bedside skills.

Dr. Joel Felner, a teaching scholar of the American Heart Association and an associate professor of medicine at Emory University in Atlanta, is one of the doctors overseeing Harvey's development. "Each heart condition has its own examination findings—sight and sounds, if you will —which are peculiar to it. Harvey can realistically simulate over twenty of these conditions, such as angina pectoris, hypertension, and a number of valvular problems. The student examines the mannequin as he would any patient."

By adding a small cassette tape, the student can select a particular disease, listen to and compare the sounds with other similar conditions, and begin to appreciate the nuances of findings that could one day mean life or death to a real patient.

Each disease cassette is accompanied by a "workup" prepared by the development group. The workup explains the patient's history and symptoms, electrocardiogram

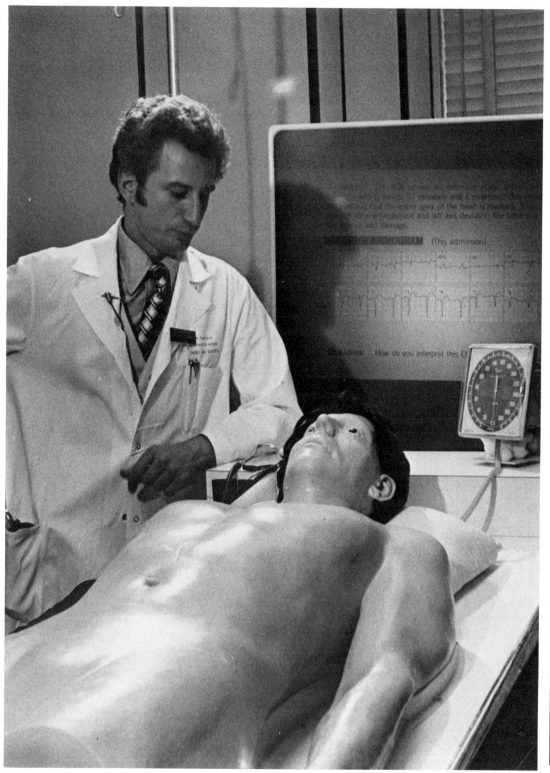

results, blood and other tests, and stress or echo cardiogram studies, and displays the results on a screen. In case the condition requires surgery, films of an actual operation of that type are available.

The advantage of the synthetic patient is obvious. Students can become familiar with rare or unusual cardiovascular conditions that they might otherwise never encounter during their training period. Students can learn at their own rate any time of the day that they choose. Harvey is always available and is never tired. In fact, the "down time" for the computer system in Harvey averages less than one hour per day.

The National Heart and Blood Vessel Institute is currently evaluating the usefulness of Harvey and comparing the performance of students who have been exposed to the mannequin with that of others who have not.

Harvey mimics only cardiovascular disease, but Dr. Felner feels the mannequin is the forerunner to a series of simulated patients that will have other medical conditions. The Bascolmb-Palmer Institute in Miami currently is working on a mannequin to simulate ophthalmic problems. Its eyes would dilate as drops are placed in them; they would react to light, get bloodshot, age, and even become tense and bulging, as with glaucoma.

Five Harveys, costing over $100,000 apiece, can now be found at the medical centers of Emory University in Georgia and Duke University in North Carolina, and the Universities of Miami, Nebraska, and Arizona. But Harvey is so innovative and well received that there is a long waiting list with many orders. Eventually the mannequins could be programmed for interns, residents in training, nursing stu-

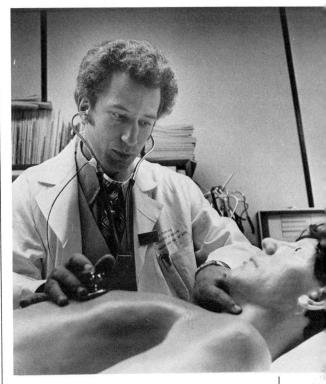

Dr. Joel Fellner examines Harvey—a synthetic patient that can simulate the physical symptoms of numerous cardiac conditions. (Courtesy Emory University Medical Center, Atlanta, Georgia)

dents, and a variety of other health care professionals. Everyone associated with Harvey today feels that in the years to come synthetic patients of this type will be found in every major teaching center around the country.

PROBLEM: How to create the ultimate hypochondriac.
ANSWER: Harvey!

Harvey comes complete with a programmed instruction course (seen on slide tape in background). Cardiologists such as Dr. Joel Fellner are continuously upgrading the material. (Courtesy Emory University Medical Center, Georgia)

Genetics Genetics

Would it be too bold to imagine that all warm-blooded animals have arisen from one living filament which the Great First Cause endued with animality . . . and thus [possess] the faculty of continuing to improve by [their] own inherent activity, and of delivering down those improvements by generation to its posterity, world without end!

Erasmus Darwin
Zoönomia, 1794

The unique nature of each living species and the relationships between species have long fascinated scientists. For centuries, most men of science believed each species fixed since the time of Creation, a point of view shared by theologians. So when early theories of evolution were introduced, they were rebutted by scientists and theologians alike. How ironic, then, that modern genetics should have its beginnings in a monastery garden. With his well-planned crossings of pea plants and the study of their characteristics, Gregor Mendel, an Austrian monk, demonstrated in 1865 that small packets of information, called genes, determine the particular traits of a living thing, and that these genes are inherited. Around the same time Charles Darwin was ad-

vancing his grandfather's theory that plants and animals, including man, evolve and survive according to their ability to deal with their environment.

From these obscure beginnings, only later recognized as cornerstones of biology, the science of genetics today has literally exploded with information.

Public awareness of genetics is in many cases limited to the knowledge that obvious individual traits such as eye and hair color and afflictions such as Tay-Sachs disease and sickle cell anemia are passed from one generation to the next. Many also know that some conditions, such as diabetes and heart disease, tend to recur in the same family. Until recently, however, the specifics of these family tendencies have been clouded.

All this is changing dramatically. It is now apparent, for example, that a specific gene or genes may make a person susceptible to certain medical conditions. The electron microscope, biochemical studies, radioassays, and other technological advances make it possible to identify such genes, or markers of them—proof that the genes exist. One marker might be a particular chemical found in the blood or urine. The gene or marker is not always a guarantee that the disease or condition will develop, only that the individual is susceptible to the disorder. As Cornell University

Genetics Genetics Genetic

scientist Dr. Zsolt Harsanyi described in a recent article in the *New York Times*, "The genetic defect may be the gun, but an environmental factor pulls the trigger."

Slowly, then, the old environment-versus-heredity issue, debated through so many generations, is becoming irrelevant. It is fairly universally agreed that both heredity and environment are important in the final determination of health and illness. Genes direct the basic shape of your body—stocky, lean and lank, or muscular. Your nutrition and exercise habits, together with your overall state of health and environmental factors, mold that shape into the final body sculpture. Similarly, heredity may predispose someone to diabetes, for example, but the disease will not manifest itself unless and until something in the environment—just what is not yet known—triggers it.

Genetic markers have been found for emphysema, diabetes, some types of arthritis and cancer, and several other conditions. Many more are on the horizon. We will discuss some of these diseases and their genetic markers in the next few pages.

It is entirely possible that in the near future, medical screening tests may take on new importance. Rather than ordering such basics as blood chemistry or

sugar determinations, Pap smears, and stool tests for blood, all of which detect a condition that already exists, a physician may be able to order a blood or urine test for genetic markers—that is, for susceptibility to certain diseases. Each patient would then be able to obtain an inventory, a laundry list, of his or her genetic markers, the diseases they represent, and any environmental factors and risks that might precipitate the appearance of the diseases.

Today's concept of public health and preventive medicine maintains that all individuals are in equal danger of disease and should therefore seek or avoid those environmental factors known to affect their health. Although well meaning, such generalizations have been largely ineffective—witness the number of cigarette smokers, despite the well-known relationship of cigarette smoke to lung disease. Genetic markers make possible preventive medicine at a more basic level—prediction—and emphasize that each individual is different and must live accordingly.

Genes

Genes determine every characteristic that makes us unique as individuals—from something as obvious as body height and shape to the intricate chemi-

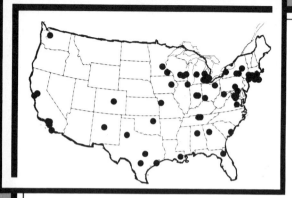

Locations of birth defect registry resource centers around the U.S.

cal structures that make up our cells. These bits of information constitute the blueprint of our bodies, and each cell in the body contains a complete set of those plans. Humans possess at least 100,000 genes, which together oversee the production of the proteins that form all body tissues.

Thanks to the work of American zoologist Thomas Hunt Morgan in the 1920s, we know that genes are located within the nucleus of the cell, strung out in an orderly way like beads along threadlike structures called chromosomes. There are twenty-three pairs of chromosomes, forty-six in all. One member of each pair originated in each of our parents, so each parent contributes one-half of the plan that makes us complete. Genes are composed of the chemical DNA, a molecule so long and so thin that if stretched out it would be the length of a football field. But in its double-helix coiled state, it can fit easily on the point of a pin. DNA gives the code of life to our individual bodies.

Each gene has a specific location on a particular chromosome and, except for abnormal translocations, that location is constant. The gene that determines blood Rh factor, for example, is located near the short arm of chromosome one. Work is under way to map all chromosomes for the genes they carry; so far about 250 of the estimated 100,000 genes have been identified and located.

Genetic counseling

Long before the word *genetic* was invented, grandparents boasted about the family characteristics that could be expected in their prospective grandchildren. They were genetic counselors of sorts to their children.

Today genetic counselors are medical specialists who use a highly organized network of information to advise the blind and deaf, patients with birth defects and their families, and others with known hereditary conditions about the relative risks they face from those conditions and the chances that their offspring will inherit them.

CASE HISTORY

When their first child died shortly after two years of age, the young couple consulted their pediatrician, who was also the director of medical genetics at the local medical school. The child had seemed normal at birth but soon afterward began to stare inattentively. At six months he was weak and could not sit. By one year he could neither crawl nor lift his head and could not hold objects. Soon he was entirely blind. The diagnosis was Tay-Sachs disease, a universally fatal condition occurring almost exclusively in Jewish families. The couple wanted to know if another child would have the disease.

The pediatrician turned to a computer terminal and punched out the code for

Tay-Sachs. The console printed out several pages of information about the diagnosis, complications, and inheritance patterns of this tragic genetic problem. Armed with this information, the pediatrician counseled the parents about the relative risks of a second pregnancy. Each parent carried the gene for Tay-Sachs; there was one chance in four that a second child would have the condition, a three-out-of-four chance that the child would carry the gene. They decided against having another baby.

The National Foundation—March of Dimes notes that 250,000 infants are born each year with birth defects, the single most serious child-health problem in the United States. New attention is focusing on birth defects throughout the world. To keep track of the new information, the Foundation is establishing a computer registry of birth defects. To date the registry has stored all the available data on 1,005 types of birth

Technician checks computer terminal at birth defect registry center to gain access to vast amount of material on birth defects stored throughout the network. (Photo by Michael J. Lutch)

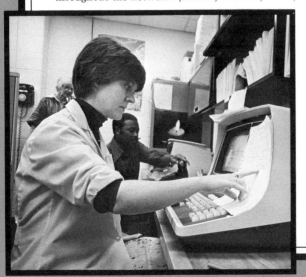

defects, from Aarskog syndrome to xeroderma pigmentosum, for instant retrieval. Eighteen genetic-counseling services across the country are connected to the system, which is based at the Center for Birth Defects Information Services, a division of the Tufts–New England Medical Center in Boston. "Without the system," notes Dr. Marylou Buysee, medical director of the center, "information about some of the more rare birth defects would take hours of painstaking searching through the medical literature."

The computer is being programmed to give diagnoses as well. Dr. Arthur Bloom, professor of human genetics and pediatrics at Columbia University in New York, reported at the recent press conference held to unveil the computer system that he expects to punch in signs and symptoms and get back probable diagnoses. He further notes that the computer may sort out new syndromes, as yet unknown. "It is by no means a replacement for the physician's judgment," he emphasized, but "it is a vast storehouse of information obtainable frequently and rapidly."

Amniocentesis

Collecting information about a patient is the first step along the road to successful diagnosis and treatment. In this regard the fetus has emerged as an important patient. Until recent years, the protective environment of the uterus prohibited diagnosis and treatment in the prenatal period, that is to say, in utero. Now the technique of amniocentesis makes it possible to learn much about the general and genetic health of the fetus. Because it is often used to gain information on which to base a decision to terminate a pregnancy (as in the case of a fetus with Tay-Sachs disease, which has no treatment and is universally fatal within the first years of life), amniocentesis has sensitized and polarized many ethical and religious groups. However, the major purpose of the technique is to reassure families when no abnormality is found. And, as seen in the unusual case history that follows, amniocentesis can be used to gather information that can save a developing baby's life.

CASE HISTORY

Three months after the New England couple had their first child, the enthusiasm of parenthood turned to tragedy as the child inexplicably weakened and

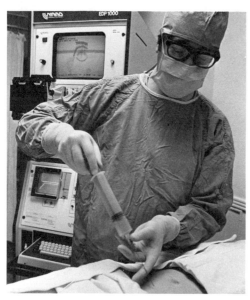

During amniocentesis, doctor inserts needle into uterus of pregnant woman and withdraws sample of amniotic fluid. Ultrasound device in background guides needle so doctor will avoid baby. (Photo by Michael J. Lutch, courtesy Beth Israel Hospital, Boston)

died. Subsequent study showed that the child died of methylmalonic aciduria, a rare condition in which the body is unable to break down protein; the victim becomes mentally retarded or dies. Because it is a recessive inherited disease, it occurs only when two carriers of the gene conceive a child; such a child has a 25 percent chance of developing the disease. When the woman became pregnant again, amniocentesis was recommended to see if that baby also had methylmalonic aciduria. To the couple's frustration, the second child was similarly afflicted. However, Dr. Mary Ampola, a specialist in genetics at the Tufts–New England Medical Center, thought it might be possible to treat the child while still in utero. Massive doses of vitamin B-12 were given to the mother in the hope that some of it would pass through to the fetus and counteract the protein defect. The treatment was continued for the last six weeks of the pregnancy and was completely successful. The healthy daughter had normal protein and vitamin B-12 levels. She still has the defect, of course, and that means a lifelong abstention from protein, except in small amounts. But the growing girl, now eight years old, is doing just fine. Subsequently a third child free of methylmalonic aciduria was born to the family.

The case marked the first time in medical history that a child was treated for a genetic defect while still in the womb. Early diagnosis by amniocentesis made it possible.

An obstetrician performs amniocentesis during the sixteenth to seventeenth weeks of pregnancy. Ultrasound studies are used to locate the baby's position. Then, after administering a local anesthetic, the physician inserts a needle through the abdominal wall and into the uterus, withdraws an ounce or two of amniotic fluid, and removes the needle. A small Band-Aid covers the procedure site.

The amniotic fluid, which completely surrounds the fetus as it develops, contains many proteins and other chemicals that provide clues about the health of the child. An elevated level of alpha-fetoprotein in the amniotic fluid, for example, is a good indication that spina bifida or another congenital spinal cord defect is present. The fetus also sheds a few skin cells into the fluid, and since each cell contains all of an individual's chromosomes, they can be studied for chromosome defects such as Down's syndrome. Cell study can also tell the sex of the fetus, but that alone, according to most obstetricians, is not enough to justify amniocentesis.

Even though amniocentesis can detect eighty or more hereditary or developmental defects, most obstetricians see its major benefit as confirming a normal pregnancy. For a family at risk for conceiving a child with a congenital defect, amniocentesis can be very reassuring when it determines that the child has been spared of the problem. Over 99 percent of all amnioceteses reveal normal development.

The most common indication for amniocentesis is the age of the mother. Though statistics vary from study to study, analyses of births show that the risk of chromosome abnormalities increases as the mother's age when she conceives increases. For Down's syndrome, an abnormality at the twenty-

first chromosome, the risks are 1 in 1,900 births at age twenty, 1 in 1,200 births at age twenty-five, 1 in 900 births at age thirty, 1 in 350 births at age thirty-five, 1 in 100 births at age forty, and 1 in 30 births at age forty-five.

Other indications for the procedure include a family history of a genetic defect, or a previous delivery of a child with a problem known to be genetic in origin.

A recently published study of over 3,000 consecutive amnioceteses at the University of California Medical School concluded that "prenatal diagnosis [by amniocentesis] is safe, highly reliable and extremely accurate." The risk of spontaneous miscarriage following amniocentesis is minimal when the procedure is performed in a hospital where it is common and routine. Hospitals strictly monitor a physician's results and techniques, and supportive equipment is generally available to increase the safety of the procedure. Ultrasound equipment, for example, which can locate the position of the placenta and fetus, reduces the risk of amniocentesis considerably. Occasionally the needle must be inserted more than once to obtain enough fluid for study, which also increases the risk of miscarriage. The California report, however, indicates that proper pretest evaluation makes multiple needle insertions unnecessary in most cases.

Amniocentesis costs between $250 and $300 and the results are available in three to six weeks, depending on the processing laboratory. Because many samples are sent to laboratories some distance away, they can deteriorate or become contaminated, resulting in the need to repeat the amniocentesis. In

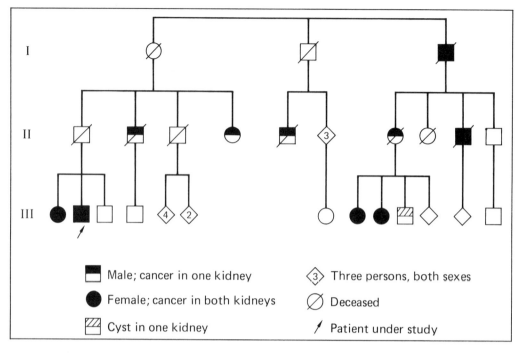

Male; cancer in one kidney

Female; cancer in both kidneys

Cyst in one kidney

Three persons, both sexes

Deceased

Patient under study

Pedigree of family with hereditary cancer of the kidney, showing patient under study and two previous generations. (Courtesy Beth Israel Hospital, Boston)

most respected genetic centers, failure to process a specimen correctly occurs less than 1 percent of the time.

Anyone contemplating amniocentesis should request serious and extensive discussion with a genetic counselor. The procedure and all its risks should be carefully explained. Each family's circumstances are unique, and genetic counseling can help put it in perspective.

Chromosomes and cancer

CASE HISTORY

When the thirty-seven-year-old man was told by his physician that he had cancer in his kidney, he wasn't surprised. Several other members of his family were known to have had the same condition. This unusual circumstance prompted Dr. Robert Brown and colleagues at Boston's Beth Israel Hospital to begin a thorough study of the patient's family by examining living relatives, hospital records, autopsy reports, and death certificates of deceased members. Their findings, reported in 1979, made medical history—a specific type of cancer was traced to an abnormal chromosome pattern inherited in a family.

Abnormal chromosome patterns had previously been associated with cancer. Wilms' tumor, a kidney cancer affecting children, is associated with an abnormal eleventh chromosome. Retinoblastoma, an eye cancer, occurs in people with an abnormal thirteenth chromosome. But neither of these conditions is familial. Of the many types of cancers that do "run in families," no specific chromosome pattern had been found prior to Dr. Brown's work.

In-depth study of the family tree of Dr. Brown's patient revealed that six of his relatives had kidney cancer and five had already died of the disease. Testing of all apparently healthy family members revealed a previously unknown kidney cancer in three others. In all, ten people over three generations of the family had cancer of the kidney, and the average age at diagnosis was forty-five. Typically, people who develop cancer of the kidney do so when they are well into their sixties.

Electron microscope photo showing chromosomes of woman with cancer of the kidney. "Chromosome translocation" has caused cancer in this instance; arrows show piece of third chromosome is attached to eighth chromosome. (Courtesy Beth Israel Hospital, Boston)

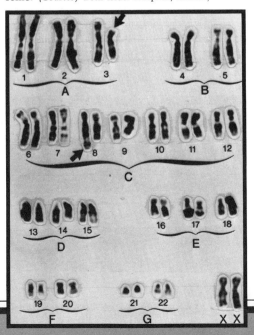

Chromosome studies revealed that each of the family members with renal cancer had a chromosome translocation—in every case, part of the third chromosome was attached to the eighth chromosome. Family members without kidney cancer had normal chromosomes. Commenting on the findings of Dr. Brown and his associates, the *New England Journal of Medicine* stated, "In other familial cancers there have been no methods for identifying individuals at high risk, but in this instance the individuals can be identified at any age." Indeed, they can even be identified as a fetus. A carrier of the genetic abnormality in this family has an 85 percent chance of developing cancer of the kidney by age sixty. By contrast, in the rest of the population kidney cancer occurs in 1 out of 1,000 people at that age. The implication is obvious. Genetic screening of members of such a family permits early diagnosis, and early diagnosis leading to early treatment is the key to survival in cancer.

HLA markers

On the sixth chromosome, an area called HLA has recently been localized. The genes within this site have the ability to direct the formation of proteins called antigens on the surfaces of cells; the proteins are called HLA (for human leukocyte) antigens. Several genes can exist at the HLA site. Since each gene determines a specific antigen, several different antigens are also possible. The known antigens have been grouped into five categories, and several antigens are known to exist in each group. A total of sixty-nine antigens of HLA type are known; they were first discovered during organ transplantation research and were found to be important components of the rejection response (see "Update: Transplantation," pages 172–185). Recently, though, it has been determined that the presence of one or a combination of these antigens is associated with different illnesses.

Immunologist Dr. Frank Lilly, at the Sloan-Kettering Institute for Cancer Research in New York City, discovered in 1964 that the counterpart of human HLA genes and antigens in mice determines their tendency to develop a virus-caused form of leukemia. His landmark research demonstrated that the antigens were genetic markers of the susceptibility to leukemia in these animals. When the antigens were present, the virus could cause leukemia; when they were absent, leukemia did not occur. The first break in associating HLA antigens with disease in humans was made in 1973, when two research groups independently reported the association of the gene that determines antigen B27 with ankylosing spondylitis.

A form of arthritis of the spine known since at least 1000 B.C., ankylosing spondylitis (AS) is called Marie-Strümpell's disease after the two doctors who first described it, and "poker spine" because patients with the condition have a stiff, poker-like back that won't bend. Now virtually all people with AS are known to have the gene for the antigen B27. It is, in fact, one of the highest associations of genetic markers with disease. People without the gene for B27 simply don't get AS, or at least they get it very rarely. Although almost no black people carry B27, it is present in 7 percent of white Americans and up to 50 percent in some Indian tribes. As

expected, blacks almost never have AS, but whites get the disorder frequently and American Indians still more frequently.

Not everyone with the gene for B27 develops ankylosing spondylitis; in fact, only one of six with the marker actually develops the disease. One does not, therefore, inherit AS; one inherits the *tendency* to it. Some other unknown factor takes advantage of that susceptibility and "causes" the disease to appear. The unknown factor in AS is presumed to be an infectious agent, probably a virus.

Ankylosing spondylitis is much more common than previously thought. Its major early symptom—low back pain—is so common that many patients and physicians tend to ignore it or treat it as muscle strain. A common medical teaching premise warns, "You never find what you don't look for." Now that doctors are looking for AS, they encounter the disease with increasing frequency.

The implications of a genetic marker for AS are far-reaching. Some large industrial firms have begun screening for the disease. If the symptoms are caught early enough, proper anti-inflammatory drugs (rather than the muscle relaxants so commonly used for low back pain) and an exercise regimen can prevent deformity and preserve reasonably normal activity. Children of individuals with B27 markers can be taught early in their lives what activities and occupations they would be best suited for. And, if the presumed virus is ever isolated, a vaccine may even be possible to immunize B27 carriers against AS.

The gene for B27 also occurs in 90 percent of people with Reiter's syndrome, an arthritic condition accompanied by skin rash, eye inflammation, and discharge from the penis (urethritis). Its cause is also unknown, but Reiter's syndrome frequently follows a gastrointestinal infection.

In a bit of medical investigation that would have made Sherlock Holmes proud, Stanford University immunologist Dr. James F. Fries and Dr. Andrei Calin, and his wife, Dr. Jane Calin, proved the association of *Shigella* bacterial dysentery and Reiter's syndrome with the B27 antigen marker in 1970. Earlier, in 1962, two days after the departure of the U.S. Navy cruiser *Little Rock* from its port in Trieste, Italy, 1,300 of the 2,000 crew members came down with bacterial dysentery due to the *Shigella* organism. Reporting four years later in the *Journal of the American Medical Association* about the epidemic, the ship's doctor noted that ten of the affected sailors also developed Reiter's syndrome two weeks after their bout with the intestinal problem. None of the 700 sailors who escaped the original dysentery developed the Reiter's symptoms. Thirteen years later, Drs. Fries and Calin and their colleagues attempted to track down the ten sailors who had both dysentery and Reiter's —no small task since their names were never published in the original article, all had subsequently left the navy, and the massive military bureaucracy was anything but helpful. After a tedious search that took the better part of a year, six of the ten sailors were located. All had the B27 antigen, and all had symptoms of ankylosing spondylitis as well.

Researchers have made other interesting HLA-disease associations in recent years. Rheumatoid arthritis has been associated with three markers, HLA genes D4, D7, and D10. People with HLA type B8 are ten times more likely to develop celiac disease, an intestinal disturbance characterized by intolerance to the gluten in wheat; four times more susceptible to hepatitis; and four times more susceptible to myasthenia gravis, an often fatal condition marked by muscle weakness and fatigue. Eighty-five percent of patients with multiple sclerosis have HLA genes A3 and A7. HLA typing has also helped to distinguish early insulin-dependent diabetes. In children who develop diabetes before age ten, genes for B8, B15, and DW3 are inevitably present; these genetic markers apparently predispose the child to develop the disease early in life. HLA typing of other children in families in which one child has insulin-dependent diabetes can pinpoint fairly accurately their risk of developing the disease.

Several more projects are under way across the country to establish other ties between HLA types and certain diseases. It is interesting to note that many of the relationships so far suggested are with diseases long suspected to be caused by viruses. It may just be that the HLA site on chromosome six determines how and why certain viruses express their disease states.

Anemia markers

Red blood cells and their oxygen-carrying hemoglobin molecules live about 120 days in circulation before they are replaced by newer, more capable cells. Hemolytic anemia is a hereditary disease that decreases the life span of the red blood cells. Most often seen in African blacks, Mediterraneans, and their

Ancestry and genetic vulnerability

African black: Albinism, anemias (sickle cell, thalassemia, glucose-6-phosphate dehygrogenase G-6PD, milk intolerance (enzyme lactase deficient)

African white: Porphyria (abnormal breakdown and excretion of hemoglobin pigment leading to abdominal pain and skin rashes)

American Indian: Arthritic conditions, milk intolerance

Arabian: Anemias (sickle cell, thalassemia)

Armenian: Familial Mediterranean fever (recurrent fever with abdominal and chest inflammation, arthritis—unknown cause)

Askenazi Jewish: Plasma lipid abnormalities, Bloom's syndrome (sun skin sensitivity and leukemia), clotting problems (factor XI deficient), dystonia musculorum (a degenerative nervous system disease), Riley-Day Syndrome (a nervous disease with sweating, pain, and taste, temperature, and blood pressure abnormalities), Gaucher's Disease, Niemann-Pick Disease, Tay-Sachs Disease (abnormal lipid diseases with nervous system problems), abnormal sugar accumulations in the urine (pentosuria, fructosuria)

Asian: Anemias (sickle cell, thalassemia), G-6PD

British Isles/Ireland: Paget's Disease (abnormal bone resorption), skin cancer, various enzyme deficiencies leading to mineral problems

Chinese: Anemias (thalassemia, G-6PD)

Eskimo: Adrenogenital syndrome (female masculinization), myasthenia gravis (muscle weakness due to nerve impulse transmission)

Finnish: Congenital nephrosis (a kidney malfunction)

French Canadian: Amino acid and protein problems

Japanese: Amino acid problems, milk lactose intolerance, sulfur metabolism problems leading to bone, cardiovascular, and nervous system disease

Lebannese: Elevated blood cholesterol and abnormal sugar metabolism

Mediterranean (Italian, Greek, Sephardic Jewish): Anemia from G-6PD, Mediterranean fever, liver problems due to abnormal storage of starch

Northern European: Amino acid problems, cystic fibrosis, lipid diseases

Scandinavian: Alpha 1 antitrypsin deficiency (abnormal protein breakdown leading to early emphysema and liver problems)

Explanation

Persons of various ethnic origins often have increased chance of specific diseases because of certain genes. Consanguinity (intermarriage) may lead to the clinical presentation of genes that otherwise are recessive. The best known example of such genetic pooling is hemophilia, the "bleeder's disease" that showed up in European royal families after centuries of inbreeding between cousins, nieces, half-brothers and -sisters. They thought their blood to be noble and wanted it pure, unmingled with inferior commoner blood.

descendants, the different forms of hemolytic anemia affect millions of people throughout the world. Red blood cells literally explode, and the hemoglobin molecule is unable to carry out its work of oxygen delivery. Although hemolytic anemia has many causes, one of the most common is the lack of glucose-6-phosphate dehydrogenase (G-6PD), an enzyme important in producing energy within the red cell.

CASE HISTORY

M. N. is a thirty-six-year-old black woman whose parents were born in Sri Lanka. Although basically healthy, she had frequent minor illnesses. Flu, colds, and other illnesses seemed to last longer and affect her more severely than most. She often stayed home from work on that account. In fact, in the previous two years, she had lost two jobs because of frequent absenteeism due to minor illness. For years she was told that she was anemic. Except that she was extremely tired, her two successful pregnancies were normal. Recently she visited her physician because of painful urination and fever and was found to have a urinary tract infection. Shortly after starting therapy with a commonly used sulfa medication, she became very weak, passed blood in her urine, and required hospitalization. She was severely anemic with a hemoglobin count of 6 g (normal is 12 g) and required blood transfusion. Her diagnostic workup revealed hemolytic anemia due to G-6PD deficiency. The sulfa was discontinued and another antibiotic started in its place and M. N. has done well ever since.

When G-6PD is absent from a person's red blood cells, they become fragile and weak, and are easily damaged. The life span of the cells is shortened, and the person becomes anemic as the bone marrow lags behind in red cell production. When such an individual is exposed to anything that by itself is also a threat to red blood cell survival, anemia develops quickly as red cells explode. Patients so affected may pass blood in the urine, develop heart failure, and even die. In M. N.'s case, a medication took advantage of the G-6PD deficiency. Typically the sulfa and antimalarial drugs, phenacetin (found in many over-the-counter pain relievers), vitamin K, and the antibiotic chloramphenicol all pose a threat. Often a viral or bacterial infection can as well.

Medical sleuths uncovered another G-6PD deficiency trigger several years ago on the island of Sardinia. For generations some people on the Mediterranean island were observed to become weak and listless during a two- to three-month period each spring. While studying this phenomenon, medical researchers found that the affected people had hemolytic anemia due to G-6PD deficiency. After traveling down many blind research alleys, they came up with an explanation for the worsening of their anemia each February. The fava bean flowers at that time. Exposure to its pollen or eating the bean itself took advantage of the G-6PD deficiency, and the residents became anemic. Screening of the island population revealed that 35 percent were so affected. Now that they know to avoid the fava bean, Sardinians no longer experience the February blahs, now known as favism.

History can teach us many lessons if

we care to learn. All too often we pay no attention because we don't understand. The Greek philosopher Pythagoras knew about the perils of the fava bean as early as 500 B.C. and admonished his followers to avoid any contact with the bean or its plant. Now, some 2,500 years later, we know why.

Lung disease markers

The familial nature of emphysema has been known for many years. Since cigarette smoking is the most clearly associated cause of emphysema, it may be that air pollution generated by smokers within a family is responsible. However, a genetic factor is now also tied to emphysema. Alpha-1-antitrypsin (AAT) is a protein important to the structure and strength of lung tissue. AAT is also a genetic marker. Its presence in the bloodstream signifies that the M gene is present. Most of the population has two M genes (genotype MM), which direct proper levels of AAT to be made. Individuals who have two Z or two S genes (genotypes ZZ or SS) instead of two M's have a greater tendency to develop emphysema. It is common for ZZ or SS people to develop cough, congestion, difficulty in breathing, and other symptoms of chronic obstructive lung disease by their twenties or thirties. Fully 75 percent of them eventually develop emphysema; but individuals who smoke cigarettes or who work in chemical plants or other areas where they inhale noxious fumes develop it ten to fifteen years earlier than the average.

People who have one normal M and one Z or S genes (genotypes MS or MZ) have some AAT in their bloodstreams, but less than the MM individuals. There is controversy over whether they have an increased tendency to emphysema. Most respiratory specialists advise their patients with this genetic type to avoid respiratory irritations just in case. Dr. Hugh Evans, a Brooklyn specialist in AAT disorders, commented recently in the *New York Times:* "While I would never deny anyone with one Z or S gene a job, I would definitely advise that person to avoid a profession where he or she would come in any contact with respiratory irritants. Personally, if I had a single Z or S gene, I wouldn't work as a copper smelter or in a cotton mill. I'd learn other skills until the verdict was handed down." The eventual verdict is of great importance, given that 10 percent or more of our population has one Z or S gene.

Less complete information is available about another protein found to be a cause of lung disease. Aryl hydrocarbon hydroxylase (AHH) is an enzyme found in white blood cells. Increased concentrations of AHH, which is also genetically determined, have been associated with cancer of the lung.

Given the pervasive and restrictive nature of lung disease, any marker permitting early diagnosis or indicating susceptibility is of great interest. Lung pollution is something that can be avoided. Perhaps the presence of a marker indicating high risk of lung disease would be just the factor to motivate a person who "just can't seem to quit smoking."

DNA research: tampering with nature?

DNA is the molecule of heredity. Each gene consists of DNA, a double-stranded chain of nucleic acids; the particular arrangement of acids within the DNA chain determines the function of that gene. The American biochemist Linus Pauling has said, ''The discovery of the double helix of DNA and the developments that resulted from the discovery constitute the greatest advance in biological science and understanding of life that has taken place in the last 100 years.'' Since the Nobel Prize–winning efforts of England's James Watson and Francis Crick in identifying the structure of DNA in 1952, much work has been done to determine the sequence of acids in individual chains. This is no easy task, since a given strand of DNA contains several thousand nucleic acids in a specific sequence. In 1977 the Laboratory of Molecular Biology at Cambridge University identified and published the full sequence of 5,375 nucleic acids in the DNA of the virus Phi-X-174. The DNA information in a human cell is about one million times that size.

DNA sequencing study is accomplished by using enzymes to break down strands of DNA into fragments of varying length. Each fragment can then be catalogued and studied. According to Dr. Walter Gilbert, a molecular biology professor at Harvard University, ''The techniques are now available to work out in detail the structure of any gene.'' Dr. Gilbert's group recently did work out the structure of the hepatitis B virus and that of the gene in the *Escherichia coli* bacteria which controls the protein that breaks down lactose.

Once the structure of DNA in a particular gene is determined, it can be used to manufacture the protein for which that gene is responsible. The technique, called the recombinant DNA technique, involves moving fragments of DNA from one living source to another. Bacteria are used as the host media because they have a simple structure and are quite well understood. Furthermore, whereas the DNA of higher animals is contained in chromosomes and complex genes, the DNA of bacteria is contained within small structures called plasmids. The plasmids freely pass through bacterial cell walls and can easily go from one bacteria to another. Bacteria thus transfer DNA between themselves.

Researchers using recombinant DNA techniques splice a section of DNA (for example, the sequence that determines insulin production) into a plasmid that has been isolated from a bacterium. The plasmid is then placed back within the bacterium, which incorporates the new DNA as its own. When the bacterium multiplies, the new DNA is reproduced millions of times. If bacteria are given the DNA codes to produce insulin, bacterial multiplication results in greater insulin production. Researchers at the Joslin Diabetes Foundation in Boston and at the University of California have recently succeeded in doing just that.

Bacterial factories will undoubtedly be used in the future to produce many human proteins in large quantities. Besides insulin, other candidates for bacterial production include cortisone, antihemophilia factors (currently available only through large numbers of blood and serum donors), growth hormone used to treat dwarfism (now available only from cadavers, and fifty cadavers are required to obtain the amount needed to treat one child for a year), and interferon, the potent antiviral, anticancer protein. In a recent issue of the *Journal of Current*

Prescribing, Dr. Wallace Rowe, chief of the Laboratory of Viral Diseases at the National Institute of Allergy and Infectious Diseases, comments, "The list of diseases that recombinant DNA techniques can potentially alleviate, either through increased understanding of the basic clinical disturbances or through production of therapeutic and preventive substances, is staggering."

As recombinant DNA research unravels the mysteries of genetic structure, many possibilities unfold. Individuals with sickle cell anemia, Tay-Sachs disease, and other genetic conditions may someday undergo "gene therapy," in which the abnormal gene is repaired or "turned off" and a normal one substituted.

Information contained in DNA directs all of a cell's activities. Many researchers feel that changes in DNA can alter the signals regulating cell division and growth and can therefore be responsible for cancer. Exactly how a normal cell changes into a continuously dividing, cancerous one is still a fundamental question in cancer research. DNA research is likely to play an important role in answering that question.

Critics of DNA research say that "tampering with nature" is sure to bring consequences, some of which may be lethal. They feel that altering the genetic structure of laboratory bacteria is essentially creating new life forms, some of which may be stronger than their ancestors—indeed, resistant to current antibiotics. They warn that even the finest of safeguards cannot prevent a leak, which would release a potentially dangerous bacterium into the environment with an "Andromeda Strain" type of epidemic as a result.

DNA researchers counter that the strain of bacterium *E. coli* used in laboratory research has, in the course of passing through several thousands of generations, become completely dependent on the laboratory environment to survive. It cannot, they say, even exist in the human body any longer, much less cause disease. The few scattered reported infections involving laboratory research around the world in the past twenty-five years seem to verify their point. In any event, the government has established rigid DNA research guidelines. Whether for or against the methodology of DNA research, one has to agree that the technology is a major scientific advance.

Through the years, many researchers and critics of research have based their objections to the study of genetics on moral grounds, perhaps fearing consequences typified by the following prediction, allegedly made by the French physiologist Claude Bernard in the mid-nineteenth century and ascribed to him by biographer Edmond de Goncourt: "Claude Bernard . . . was reported to have announced that after a hundred years of physiological science, one would be able to make laws for organisms and carry out human creation in competition with the Creator himself." Also concerned about such a consequence, the biographer added his own opinion to Bernard's prediction: "We made no objection, but we do believe that when science has reached that point, the good Lord with white beard will arrive on earth with his key chain and tell mankind, just as they do in the Art Show at five o'clock: 'Gentlemen, it is closing time.' "

Resources

■ Referrals to genetics counseling centers are available from:

Your doctor, your state medical society, or the *International Directory of Genetics Services*, published by:

National Foundation/March of Dimes
1275 Mamaroneck Avenue
White Plains, New York 10605
914-428-7100

■ The following medical centers are among those tied into the National Foundation's computerized birth defects information service:

Northeast United States

New Haven, Connecticut
Yale University Medical Center
203-436-8208

Boston, Massachusetts
Tufts–New England Medical Center
617-956-7400

New York, New York
Columbia-Presbyterian Medical Center
212-694-3998

Valhalla, New York
Westchester Medical Center
914-347-7627

Hershey, Pennsylvania
Hershey Medical Center 717-534-8412

Philadelphia, Pennsylvania
Jefferson Medical Center
215-928-6958

Midwest United States

Indianapolis, Indiana
University of Indiana Medical Center
317-264-2542

Lexington, Kentucky
University of Kentucky Medical Center
606-233-6296

Ann Arbor, Michigan
University of Michigan Medical Center
616-774-7803

Kansas City, Missouri
Children's Mercy Hospital
816-471-0626

Cincinnati, Ohio
University of Cincinnati Medical
Center 513-559-4760

Western United States

Los Angeles, California
Harbor General Hospital 213-533-3667

Honolulu, Hawaii
University of Hawaii Medical Center
808-948-6843

Albuquerque, New Mexico
University of New Mexico Medical
Center 505-277-5551

Seattle, Washington
Children's Orthopedic Hospital
206-634-5088

Southern United States

Birmingham, Alabama
University of Alabama Medical Center
205-934-4968

New Orleans, Louisiana
Louisiana State University Medical
School 504-568-6221

Richmond, Virginia
Medical College of Virginia
804-768-9632

■ Another source is the National Genetics Foundation, which also supplies genetic literature and information.

The National Genetics Foundation
9 West 57th Steet
New York, New York 10019
212-759-4432

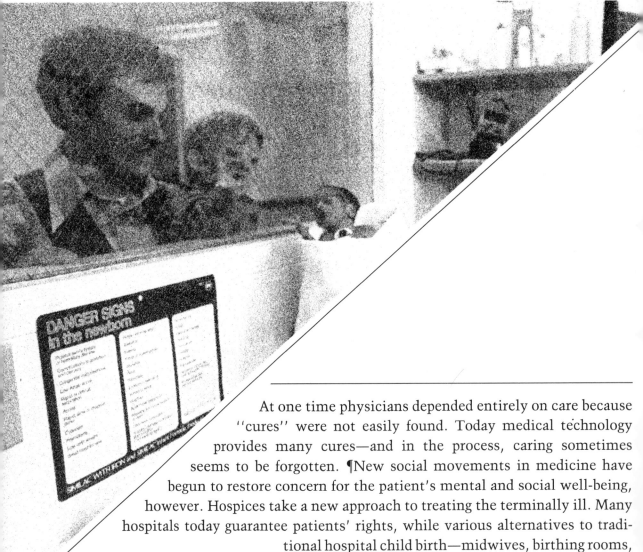

At one time physicians depended entirely on care because "cures" were not easily found. Today medical technology provides many cures—and in the process, caring sometimes seems to be forgotten. ¶New social movements in medicine have begun to restore concern for the patient's mental and social well-being, however. Hospices take a new approach to treating the terminally ill. Many hospitals today guarantee patients' rights, while various alternatives to traditional hospital child birth—midwives, birthing rooms,

C T I V E S

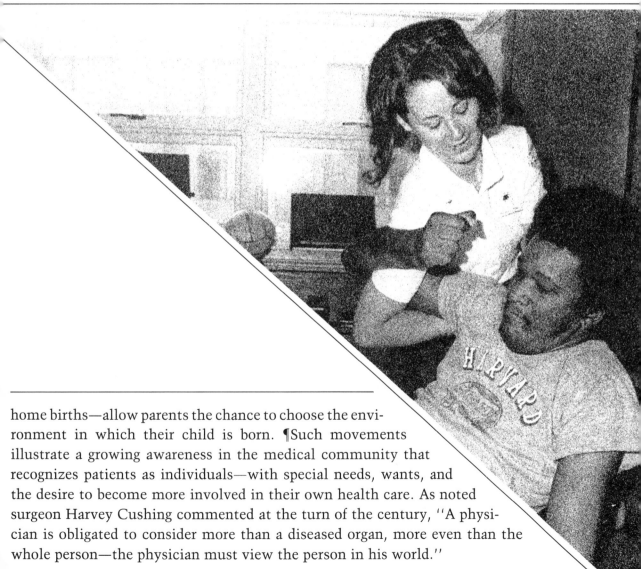

home births—allow parents the chance to choose the environment in which their child is born. ¶Such movements illustrate a growing awareness in the medical community that recognizes patients as individuals—with special needs, wants, and the desire to become more involved in their own health care. As noted surgeon Harvey Cushing commented at the turn of the century, ''A physician is obligated to consider more than a diseased organ, more even than the whole person—the physician must view the person in his world.''

Patients' rights

We have talked long enough in this country about equal rights. We have talked for one hundred years or more. It is time now to write the next chapter—and to write in the books of law.

Lyndon Baines Johnson, first address to Congress as president, November 27, 1963

In 1972 Boston's Beth Israel Hospital became the first in the nation to adopt a patients' bill of rights. The bill, which spelled out a hospital's responsibilities to its patients, was a landmark idea, one that hospitals throughout the country have since adopted in various forms.

Many Beth Israel staff members initially feared that the document, which was prominently displayed and available to every patient, would lead to a barrage of complaints and unrealistic expectations that would disrupt the smooth flow of medical care and interfere with the doctor-patient relationship. Others thought it might even lead to more malpractice suits.

These fears have not been realized, as Beth Israel Hos-

pital director Dr. Mitchell Rabkin noted in a recent interview: "Once in a while a patient would use the document to complain and the complaint was usually justified. But our incidence of malpractice action has declined, and the ratio of praise to blame has improved considerably."

If a written bill of rights for patients seemed revolutionary in 1972, the items in the document certainly were not. They merely confirmed a standard of conduct that hospitals had been or should have been striving toward for years.

Despite acceptance by the American Hospital Association and the American Medical Association, not all physicians and hospitals have accepted the patients' rights movement. Some have moved only after repeated nudges from patient advocates and patients' rights activists. Other, less progressive institutions resist the movement altogether and wait for laws to force their action.

Nevertheless, the patients' rights movement is gaining momentum. Largely gone is the passive patient, an unknowing and sometimes unwilling spectator and subject of

medical care. In greater evidence is the active patient who wants to know all the alternatives and participates along with the medical staff in the decision-making process.

Legislation is appearing in all states to extend the rights of patients and the responsibilities of medical providers. Insurance companies are using financial clout to encourage and even require second opinions before major or complicated medical and surgical procedures. Boards of medical discipline are being given greater authority to enforce quality care standards.

The ultimate result, it is hoped, will be to improve the quality of health care and to help control escalating medical costs as well.

Your rights as a patient

The commitment to provide quality medical care gives health care providers certain responsibilities. They must respect your individuality, your dignity, your right to know about your illness and to participate in decisions that affect your well-being.

Accordingly, you have

certain rights as a patient. Following is the Beth Israel Hospital patients' bill of rights.

- To receive the best medical care possible, without regard to your sex, age, race, religion, national origin, or ability to pay.

- To be treated respectfully and fairly and to be addressed by your proper name without undue familiarity.

- To expect that your individuality and your cultural and religious background will be respected.

- To know the name of the doctor who is coordinating your care and the names and roles of all others involved in that care; and to have anyone unrelated to your care leave at your request.

- To ask for and receive complete and current information to help you understand your diagnosis, your medical outlook, and all diagnostic and therapeutic procedures prescribed for you. If your doctor feels that it is not medically advisable for you to receive this information, it will be given to an appropriate person on your behalf.

- To refuse any or all diagnostic and treatment procedures; nevertheless to receive the best help your doctor can give you under the circumstances.

- To leave the hospital against your doctor's advice, unless you have a contagious condition that may endanger others or are unable to maintain your own safety as defined by law. If you decide to leave against advice, you will be asked to sign a form releasing the hospital and doctor from any harm that your discharge may cause you.

- To have every consideration for your privacy, and to have any discussion with doctor, nurse, health worker, or administrative officer conducted discreetly and confidentially.

- To receive second or other opinions on your medical condition, as you desire.

- To have a full explanation of any research or training program before you agree to participate, as well as the right to refuse to participate.

- To seek and receive adequate instruction in self-care, to enable you to prevent dis-

ability and maintain your health as much as is possible under the circumstances.

- To examine your medical record. (As a general rule it is recommended that you not examine your record in the middle of your hospital stay. It is usually incomplete until your care is completed and serves more as a worksheet for doctors and nurses than as a clear-cut listing of the pertinent medical facts of your case. It is much more helpful to ask questions of your doctors or nurses.)

- To examine a full and itemized hospital bill and receive an explanation of any and all charges.

- To inquire about possible financial aid to help pay your bill and to receive prompt and courteous assistance in obtaining any aid for which you may be eligible.

Your responsibilities as a patient

If medical care is to become a more cooperative effort, patients must understand their responsibilities as well. The following describes your role in the doctor-patient relationship:

- To respect and be considerate of other patients and, when hospitalized, to see that your visitors are considerate as well, particularly with regard to noise and smoking, which can be annoying to others nearby.
- To give the health care team all the information they need in order to provide appropriate care. This involves a thorough and honest disclosure of all medications and drugs you are taking, social and work habits, and past personal and family medical history.
- To be as cooperative as possible with necessary diagnostic and therapeutic procedures.
- To ask for clarification when in doubt. Failure to ask obvious questions often leads to confusion and needless worry.

Getting a second opinion

In 1978 the Subcommittee on Oversight and Investigation of the United States House of Representatives released a report that challenged surgical practice in this country. The report found wide discrepancies between medical communities and even between hospitals and doctors in the same community in the indications for performing many operations. The results of the surgery also varied, in terms of success, mortality, and complications. Quality controls were inconsistent, and steps to control unnecessary surgery and discipline incompetent physicians were often ineffective, according to the report. The subcommittee further estimated that 10 percent of the 20 million operations performed each year were not necessary, at a potential cost of 10,000 lives and $4 billion.

The American Medical Association and various specialty societies strongly objected to the report. While admitting that there are incompetent physicians and that some "inappropriate" surgery is performed, the organizations stressed that these were isolated instances nowhere approaching the volume the subcommittee estimated. The AMA pointed with pride to the many efforts of the medical profession to assure quality medicine and to police itself. Hospitals hold daily medical conferences within specialty groups where physicians discuss interesting and difficult cases. Medical and surgical review panels review individual cases to assure consistent and quality care that is in line with national and community standards. State Boards of Medical Discipline investigate and deal with incompetence and unethical behavior.

Although the debate has never been resolved, it has provided a spark for the already growing consumer movement toward second opinions.

Today, Medicare and Medicaid agencies and most insurance companies strongly suggest second opinions for serious, complicated, and controversial problems and will pay for most, if not all, of the cost of getting those opinions. Other plans insist on second opinions before they pay for complicated treatments at all.

Voicing the concern of many physicians about mandatory second opinions, one specialist says: "There may be many correct ways to treat a given problem; a second opinion, though different from mine, is not necessarily any better. At the very least, the patient may become confused, because he or she does not have the background knowledge to choose between alternatives. At the worst, the patient may opt for no treatment at all, or lose confidence in my abilities."

Most physicians accept second opinions and willingly discuss the options with their patients. Second opinions tend to deepen patients' knowledge and get them more involved in their care.

When should you get a second opinion?

- If you are told that you have a rare or unusual condition, one that is not seen frequently in your community or by your doctor.

- If you are told that you have a condition that is inevitably fatal. In either situation, ask your doctor to refer you to a specialist whose area of interest covers the problem.

- If you have gone directly to a surgeon and have not consulted a generalist or internist. Although there are exceptions, an internist often does a more complete history and physical examination and can find complicating medical conditions that might interfere with the surgery. The internist might also point out a medical treatment that might be tried first.

- If you have any doubts about a physician's competence or judgment, particularly if the physician's personality is not reassuring to you.

- If the physician has not made a persuasive case that this is the most efficient way of dealing with the problem.

- If the physician does not discuss all the options.

- If the physician thinks that a second opinion is desirable.

Getting a second opinion is your opportunity to satisfy yourself that you are getting the best and most current therapy available. You should be sure that you have the answers to several questions:

- Is this therapy necessary at all?

- Is there another way of accomplishing the same thing?

- Are there any complications, and how can they be minimized?

- Exactly what is the treatment, how does it work, and who will perform it?

- How will the treatment affect my life? Will I have to change my life-style?

How can you get a second opinion?

- Ask your doctor. Many people are afraid to do this, but a good doctor should not be offended. Responsible physicians are confident in their judgment and want you to be confident as well. If your doctor objects, ask why. If you don't get a satisfactory answer, get another opinion. Remember that no one is perfect.

- Insurance carriers often have second opinion referral services.

- Medicare patients should call their Medicare or Social Security office.

- Medicaid patients should call their local welfare office.

- State medical societies can provide the names of several appropriate specialists.

- The administration offices of local hospitals can give the names of doctors within particular specialties who have privileges to practice in their institutions.

■ The federal government has a toll-free second opinion hotline: (800) 325-6400. This program, set up and managed by the Department of Health and Human Services, coordinates over 150 referral agencies throughout the country. You will be given the name of an agency or a physician to contact.

A two-way street

The New Physician, a medical journal for medical students and physicians in training, recently described American medicine as "a system that makes young people sacrifice and suffer to enter its highest rank, at each step become more convinced that if they make it to the top, they sure as hell will be gods. It is a system wherein hundreds of thousands of concerned, intelligent Americans allow information about their health, their lives and their bodies to be kept from them or dispensed only in little bits at the discretion of their doctors."

This "medical mystique," which regards the doctor's advice as infallible and not to be questioned, is the target of the movement for patients' rights. Physician attitudes may have fostered this mystique, but they are clearly are not solely responsible for it; patients have contributed to it as well.

Patients often do not wish to "bother" their physician with a question they feel may be stupid; and they don't want to appear ungrateful or challenging, or to take up the physician's time. Such patients remain unsatisfied, and their doctors seem all the more detached.

The ultimate goal of the patients' rights movement is better health care. Reaching that goal requires two-way travel: mutual communication between doctor and patient and sensitivity to each other's roles and needs.

It is a goal that can be reached only by voluntary effort, not by legislation. Laws can change actions, but not attitudes, and the patients' rights issue is more attitude than action. Cardiologist and medical author Dr. Michael Halberstam, the editor of *Modern Medicine*, states it this way: "Legislating good health produces neither good legislation nor good health."

Resources

Most hospital administration offices can advise you about your rights as a patient. For further information, contact:

■ American Hospital Association
840 North Lake Shore Drive
Chicago, Illinois 60611
312-286-6000

(State hospital associations are listed in your telephone directory.)

■ American Medical Association
535 North Dearborn
Chicago, Illinois 60610
312-751-6000

■ United States Department of Health and Human Services tollfree second opinion Hotline
800-325-6400 (in Missouri, 800-342-6000)

Alternative childbirth

I believe that birth is too important an event to be left to the obstetrician, that a newborn and his mother need a loving artist's attention, not the impersonal manipulation of a highly trained engineer.

Dr. Frederick Leboyer
New York Times Magazine,
1974

F rench obstetrician Dr. Frederick Leboyer became an international celebrity when he challenged established methods of childbirth. "We must think of the child," he argued, contending that a brightly lit, cold, and glistening labor room frightens the infant and lessens the bond between mother and child.

But Dr. Leboyer's voice was only one of many calling for alternatives to traditional birth practices. Reacting against the sedatives, anesthetics, forceps, and monitors that have become fixtures in hospital labor and delivery suites, an ever increasing number of women have begun to demand less technology, more naturalism, and more personal and family involvement in the important event of birth.

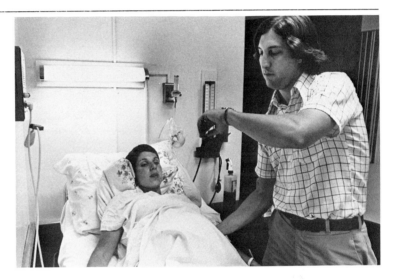

Alternative birth practices are designed to involve husband and wife as a team in the birth process. Here a husband times his wife's contractions. (Photo by Janet Knott, courtesy Beth Israel Hospital, Boston)

While considered reactionary at first, alternative birthing methods today are common practice. Progressive hospitals now routinely offer homelike birthing rooms, natural or prepared childbirth classes, and midwife-assisted deliveries. The birth of a baby is no longer treated as a pathological event. Alternative methods make childbirth more normal and dispense with any interference except what is required for safety and comfort.

Leboyer births

Before entering private practice, Dr. Frederick Leboyer was a scholar and teacher on the Faculty of Medicine at the University of Paris. After delivering several thousand babies in the traditional manner, Dr. Leboyer developed a revolutionary concept about childbirth that emphasized that birth is the most traumatic of human experiences. "Babies are small people," he said, "with feelings, aware-

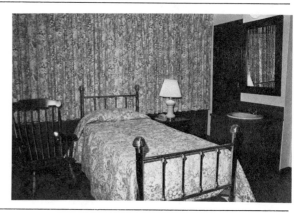

Birthing rooms such as this one at Lynn Hospital in Massachusetts often resemble well-decorated apartments more than labor and delivery rooms, but are only a short distance from traditional delivery units. (Courtesy Lynn Hospital, Massachusetts)

ness, and sensitivity.'' His method of childbirth eases the baby's entrance into the world by creating an environment that does not frighten or upset the infant. Leboyer babies arrive in softly lit delivery rooms where physicians and nurses speak in hushed voices. After birth, the baby is immediately placed on the mother's abdomen, where it can retain the curved prebirth shape of its spine, while mother, husband, and doctor gently massage it until the umbilical cord stops pulsating and can be severed. The baby is then bathed in a basin of warm water—"a comfortable return to the environment from which it has just emerged.'' During pregnancy and after delivery, Leboyer treats his patients in standard ways.

If Leboyer's ideas are revolutionary, they are also controversial. Critics regard his method as amusing, foolish, and even dangerous. "Safety must take precedence over psychology,'' one doctor states, maintaining that a well-lit delivery room is essential to check the baby for proper breathing and to watch for problems in the birth process

such as bleeding or tears in the birth canal.

On the other hand, followers of Leboyer feel his methods lead to emotionally healthier children with closer bonds to their mother. They also argue that maternal and child safety is not compromised. Dr. Odile Herdner, an anesthesiologist who has assisted Leboyer during many deliveries, emphasizes that "before the baby is presented, everything is done in the normal way with the latest equipment . . . if problems arise we switch on the lights and act as any team would in an emergency.'' Hospitals that use the Leboyer method exclusively support its safety with statistics. At the Maternity Hospital of Pithviers in Loiret, France, infant mortality actually dropped from 20 per 10,000 births to 12 per 10,000 births after instituting Leboyer's methods, even for forceps, breech, and cesarean births, which are traditionally high-risk and complicated deliveries.

Can the birth environment influence the psychological state of the infant? Many obstetricians and obstetrical

nurses comment that Leboyer babies are more alert, sleep less, and are more interested in their surroundings. This can encourage more cuddling, holding, and eye contact between mother and infant and a potentially stronger bond between them. Psychologist Dr. Danielle Rapaport of the Sorbonne feels that the brief "nonviolent'' birth which Leboyer advocates can have long-range effects on the infant as well. She followed 100 Leboyer babies up to four years of age and found that they ate and slept better, and were more precocious and interested in the world and people, when compared with infants delivered in a conventional way. She also felt that they were more positive and social, based on their performances in the widely used Gesell test, which measures social adjustments among young children.

Although not generally accepted as routine, many of Leboyer's techniques have been adopted by teaching and community hospitals alike. The warm water baths are often eliminated, however, because it is thought that immersion in warm water may

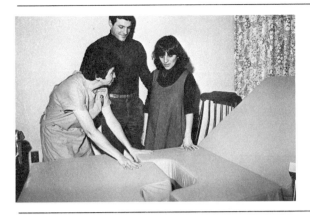
Labor and delivery nurse shows the features of a birthing room bed to an expectant couple. (Courtesy Lynn Hospital, Massachusetts)

lead to heat loss by evaporation or breathing problems.

Home births

Few physicians still do home deliveries, but feeling that home births can be an extraordinarily rich experience for families, a few physicians join their ranks each year. In contrast to hospital deliveries, which can easily cost $2,000 or more, doctor-attended home births cost only about $500. There is evidence to suggest that babies born in medically supported home deliveries that are carefully screened and provided with adequate support do very well compared with hospital-born babies. But the same cannot be said for home deliveries that are not medically supported.

The increasing number of home deliveries in this country is of great concern to those individuals involved in the medical aspects of the birth process. According to the American College of Obstetrics and Gynecology, 40 percent of home births in 1977 were attended by people with no medical or paramedical license. In eleven states that accumulate data linking fetal

and newborn deaths with place of birth, the risk of dying is two to five times higher in home-born babies; the stillborn rate is also particularly high. "Home births are the earliest and most profound form of child abuse," states one obstetrician, typifying the lack of support of most of the medical community for this type of birth. Although up to 90 percent of all deliveries are uneventful and might occur safely at home, obstetricians emphasize that it is difficult to predict which births will have problems, despite screening.

According to Dr. Sheila Gottshalk and her associates at the Louisiana State University Medical Center, up to 16 percent of all pregnancies identified as low risk on admission to the delivery unit become high risk during labor because of cord or placental problems requiring immediate medicine or surgery that would not have been available at home. Dr. Kenneth Edelin, chief of the Department of Obstetrics and Gynecology at Boston City Hospital, has put into words what many obstetricians think: "If you're in this profession long enough, you develop

a healthy respect for childbirth. The potential is there for every woman who goes through pregnancy, labor, and delivery to develop complications—even to die."

The birthing room

The heightened risks during home births have led to the evolution of an alternative —the birthing room. Even though they are located in hospital delivery units, birthing rooms are a far cry from typical labor rooms. They are designed to simulate a home environment and are comfortably furnished. Cheery wallpaper, carpeting, color-coordinated bedspreads, drapes, and pictures replace hospital blues, greens, and whites. Flowers, televisions, and brass beds are often in evidence. Families are encouraged to be present.

Labor and delivery take place in the same room, avoiding the anxiety of moving the woman to the delivery room at exactly the right time. Surgical tables and instruments are brought into the birthing room immediately prior to the delivery. The patient may give birth with her feet on the bed rather than in the traditional

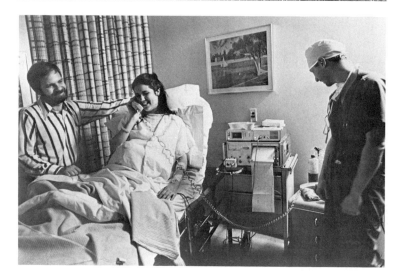

Fetal monitors are not standard in birthing rooms, but can be brought in if a need arises. (Courtesy Beth Israel Hospital, Boston)

stirrups. Fathers have assisted at the delivery and, under supervision, in many cases have eased out the baby's head and even cut the umbilical cord. In some cases mother and infant stay in the same room until discharge. Celebrations are encouraged, and in some hospitals champagne and wine are even made available. Yet the birthing rooms, for all their comfort and homelike atmosphere, are only a matter of feet from all the technology and equipment of the operating and traditional delivery rooms should unforeseen problems or emergencies arise.

Birthing rooms are intended for low-risk deliveries. Every attempt is made to screen women carefully to avoid complications. There are some considerations that may prevent women from using birthing rooms, including:

■ Age—women younger than sixteen and older than thirty-five are considered higher risks.

■ A history of obstetrical complications, such as previous miscarriages, cesarean births, postpartum hemorrhage, and difficult labor.

■ A history of major medical disorders such as heart disease or diabetes.

■ Known addiction to heroin or other mood-altering drugs.

■ Complications, including the fetus being in a difficult position, or multiple births.

Routine fetal monitoring of all patients is not performed in birthing rooms. However, monitoring equipment can be brought into the birthing rooms should the need arise.

Birthing rooms in and of themselves do not guarantee the sharing emotion of a home birth. It takes more than a few pictures on the wall or printed bed sheets to create a positive experience. Obstetrical staffs must be supportive and sincere in their attitudes toward families that prefer this childbirth alternative.

Birth centers

Still controversial, but appearing with greater frequency, are out-of-hospital alternative birth centers. These are specially designed facilities for labor and delivery which may be on hospital grounds or at some distance from the hos-

A midwife shows an expectant woman's son how to read his mother's blood pressure. (Photo by Don Robinson)

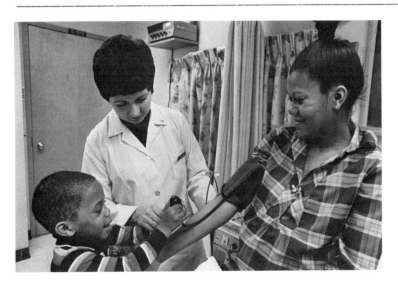

pital but are not within the hospital building per se. Out-of-hospital birthing centers generally offer extensive education programs during pregnancy, covering topics from body control during labor to infant care and nutrition. These classes are usually included in the birthing center fee. There is also an extensive screening program to rule out high-risk deliveries, because birthing centers are usually not prepared to handle emergencies such as transfusions and cesarean births. The cost of out-of-hospital birthing cen-

ters is about half to two-thirds the cost of the hospital birth. Some obstetricians insist that out-of-hospital birthing centers guarantee the best safety for the patient only when operated as a unit of a hospital. Critics feel that hospitals should offer such a choice, but a connection with a hospital would almost invariably signal a rise in costs.

Midwives

Midwifery is as old as recorded history. In the fifth century B.C. Hippocrates began a school for midwives, and

throughout the ages thereafter, midwives have attended women all during childbirth. Today, midwives deliver 80 percent of the world's children. Most of the fifteen countries with a lower infant mortality rate than the United States' use the skill of the midwife.

Midwives in this country, on the other hand, have always had the aura of the unskilled and untrained "backwoods granny." But today midwives are making a comeback, assisting at and performing deliveries and attending to pre- and postnatal care.

A modern midwife is a registered nurse with special training at one of twenty midwife schools. Advanced training in obstetrics, newborn care, and family planning is required for certification in the Amcrican College of Nurse Midwives. Midwives most often work under the supervision of physicians and are trained to recognize immediately any complications that would require an obstetrician's expertise. Some do home deliveries. Most, however, work in hospitals as part of a health care team. Midwives follow patients in prenatal clinics, manage labor, perform uncomplicated deliveries, and see patients during the postpartum period. They do not perform cesarean births and are less likely to perform episiotomies (the surgical cutting of the perineum to allow more room for the infant's head). Part of midwife training is to learn to ease the infant's head gently through the birth canal to avoid the tearing that often accompanies the birth process.

"Midwives are easier to talk to," comments one patient. "They are not rushed and give me straight answers to all my questions." One nurse midwife explains: "We talk more about feeling and help the patient with her reaction to the pregnancy." Prenatal care for the midwife is more than blood pressures and uterine measurements; it is assisting in the whole experience of pregnancy and childbirth.

Although some obstetricians resent the intrusion of the midwife into their professional domain, most feel that the professional midwife enhances good obstetrical care and is a vital member of the health care team. Many experts go further, claiming that the professional midwife gives a greater chance for a good birth experience.

The benefits

In an attempt to meet the psychological and emotional needs of patients while providing a medically safe environment, alternatives to the traditional hospital delivery are now in greater evidence. The Leboyer technique, birthing rooms, birthing centers, and midwives have all resulted in closer contact between mother and infant sooner after birth. Many specialists feel that this increased contact will have long-term positive benefits. Cleveland pediatricians Dr. Marshall Klaus and Dr. John Kennell published the results of a carefully controlled study in the *New England Journal of Medicine* and in a subsequent book. They noted that mothers who spend more time with their infants in the first hours and days after birth show more fondling and eye contact during feeding throughout the first year. Even up to five years later these mothers are generally more concerned; they ask more questions during physical examination and are reluctant to leave their children in the temporary care of others. While it has long been known that animals experience an immediate bonding with their young after birth, until recently this had not been demonstrated between mother and child.

Today there are many alternatives for the pregnant woman about to deliver. Alternative birthing methods are encouraging the warm, caring experience that the birth of a new child can be, but they must be kept in perspective. Alternative birthing methods are not for everyone. The modern technology that characterizes the progressive hospital's labor and delivery suite is essential. Many lives of infants and mothers alike would have been lost had it not been for the medical and surgical intervention of technology. It is fair to say, though, that technology is necessary in only the minority of cases. Childbirth is a natural experience that mother and family should share and experience to the fullest.

Resources

■ The National Association of Parents and Professionals for Safe Alternatives in Childbirth (NAPSAC) has names and addresses of physicians and midwives in home-birth practice, birth rooms, and training programs. NAPSAC also holds conferences on the issues.

NAPSAC
P.O. Box 1307
Chapel Hill, NC 27514

■ The International Childbirth Education Association (ICEA) has a similar role.

ICEA
P.O. Box 1284
Mission, Kansas 66202

■ Alternatives in your area can be determined by discussion with your obstetrician or family physician, local hospital or its maternity unit, or state medical society. Or contact:

American College of Obstetricians and Gynecologists
Suite 2700
1 East Wacker Drive
Chicago, Illinois 60601
312-222-1600

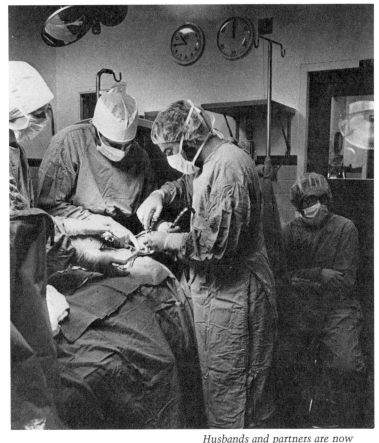

Husbands and partners are now allowed in labor and delivery rooms, and can even be present during a cesarean section. The expectant father sitting on the stool awaits the imminent birth. (Photo by Janet Knott, courtesy Beth Israel Hospital, Boston)

New approaches to pain

But pain is a thing that is glad to be forgotten.

Robinson Jeffers
"Post-Mortem," 1926

The scene is repeated day and night in doctor's offices, emergency rooms, and clinics throughout the world. A pale elderly woman sits in the corner and stares, gently stroking her gnarled fingers. A young overweight man winces as he shifts from foot to foot, unwilling or unable to sit. A young woman moans, clutching her stomach and rocking back and forth in her chair. These desperate people of all ages, from all walks of life, from every background, have one thing in common: chronic pain. No hour of their life is spared from agony. Some cannot sleep; most cannot work; none can rest or be comfortable.

Chronic pain is America's third largest health problem. It can originate with medical illness, surgery, or an accident, and it can last for six months or several years.

The average victim of chronic pain has had three operations, has spent $50,000

to $100,000 in doctors' bills, and is a habitual user of pain medication. For back pain alone, 200,000 operations are performed, 5 million people are disabled for at least two weeks, and $1½ billion is spent on hospital and doctors' bills each year. The National Institute of Arthritis, Metabolism and Digestive Disorders estimates that the 6 million people in pain and disabled by arthritis spend over $10 billion annually. Another $1 billion is spent for over-the-counter pain relievers and $300,000 for habit-forming prescription drugs such as codeine and propoxyphene (Darvon, Dolene, and other drugs). If the figures are staggering, they are also frustrating. Most of the money spent on surgery and drugs for pain is spent in vain. The treatments do not work, and the patients' pain continues.

To the physician faced with managing chronic pain it is one of the most frustrating problems of medical practice. The doctor feels impotent; the patient feels frustrated.

Finally, however, the situation is beginning to change. Medical technology has produced biofeedback instruments

to develop concentration and control muscular tension, and nerve stimulators to block the brain's perception of pain. The 100-year search for painkilling drugs that are not addictive is at last showing promise. And most importantly, the medical profession has begun, finally, to distinguish chronic pain from the medical condition that causes it and to help the patient deal with pain in specialized treatment centers.

Pain units—therapeutic communities

A pain unit is a therapeutic community, a live-in center (often within a hospital) where people spend day and night for several weeks learning to understand and cope with their pain. Chronic pain inevitably brings isolation to the sufferers because they can't concentrate on anything else; a pain unit provides the opportunity to overcome the isolation of pain and to share experiences with others who have pain. Psychiatrist Dr. Gerald Aranoff, director of the Boston Pain Unit at Massachusetts Rehabilitation Hospital, one of fifty such live-in units in the country, comments that there is no morbid pooling of misery in pain units. "Even though all our patients have chronic and debilitating pain, there is a sense of optimism. The patients understand each other. They share something in common—their pain. Their understanding encourages each other and gives each other support."

CASE HISTORY

H. L. is an eighty-year-old woman in her fourth week in the pain unit. She cracked a vertebra twenty years ago and has been in pain since. In the past two years she has spent twenty-two hours a day in bed. Two operations and two spinal nerve blocks have not helped her pain. "What a shock this place is. They won't let me baby myself. I've had to be on my feet all the time." H. L. explained her depression when she entered the unit: "I was isolated because of my injury. Here there are people to talk to. At home I did nothing." When she entered the pain unit, H. L. was stiff because of her inactivity. Now, with great fervor she eased out of bed and demonstrated her loose walk and straight stance. She swiv-

eled her hips, first one way and then the other.

Chronic pain may be the result of migraine headaches, muscle strain or spasm, slipped discs, abdominal surgery, or other causes. By the time such patients reach a pain unit, however, their original problem has been treated with everything imaginable and is now secondary; the pain has become their disease. Pain units review the patient's medical record and may order a few basic medical studies or specialty consultations where appropriate. Usually, though, the patients have already had thorough workups, so studies that have already been done elsewhere are not repeated. The diagnosis of a patient in chronic pain is almost never in question, rather why the patient has failed to respond to therapy.

Patients with chronic pain are often at the end of their rope. Many doctors have already told them to forget it, that it's all in their head, or that it will go away. Dr. Nelson Hender, a psychiatrist at Johns Hopkins Pain Treat-

ment Center and the author of a book on chronic pain, states: "I have rarely, if ever, seen imagined pain. If you feel pain then you have pain." Dr. Aranoff agrees, but elaborates: "When people have chronic illness it affects them psychologically and physically. To say that pain is psychosomatic may be true, but then again all illness is psychosomatic to some degree." Pain is therefore accepted as real in pain units, and the purpose of therapy is to enable the patient to deal with it.

Physicians refer patients to a pain unit when standard approaches to therapy have failed. At first glance a pain unit resembles a hospital ward; there are individual rooms, a nursing station, activity and social areas, and examination and treatment rooms. There the similarity ends.

Since all the patients have the same problem, a team approach is used. A physician, usually a psychiatrist or neurologist, is in charge. Nurses, psychologists, physical and occupational therapists, social workers, and rehabilitation specialists all play an important role. The patients also participate in each other's care. Frequent group discussions are held so that individuals can benefit by the experiences and support of others who have the same problem. During the daily medical rounds, the medical director discusses each patient's record, program, and progress in front of the group. This helps to expose those patients who are not cooperating and strengthens the unity of the community.

There are about fifty live-in pain units in the United States, but there are more than 300 pain services or clinics. According to Dr. Aranoff, it is important to distinguish between the two. A pain unit is an inpatient multidimensional center incorporating physical, medical, psychiatric, and recreational treatment. Though nerve stimulation and biofeedback technology are in evidence, the focus is clearly on attitudes and adjustment rather than equipment. The multidimensional approach creates a system of checks and balances, and the patient benefits. Pain clinics, on the other hand, are outpatient services that offer a specific treatment such as physical therapy or nerve blocks.

Some pain clinics offer little more than faith healing. Often pain clinics are simply one physician with a new gimmick. There is, for example, a neurosurgeon in the Midwest who calls his office a pain clinic, but he merely operates on everyone who comes in the door. That type of pain clinic obviously has the potential for doing more harm than good. When searching for a pain unit, a private physician can help with a referral, but the key is to look for one that evaluates the social and environmental influences as well as the physical causes of pain and offers many approaches to therapy.

Most people with chronic pain take a lot of medication, much of it narcotics. "It seems to add credibility to their pain," says Dr. Aranoff. One of his patients agrees. "If you take a lot of medication, it helps the doctor to understand how bad your pain really is." Realistically, though, doctors also contribute to the overuse of drugs by these patients. Many find it easier to prescribe painkillers than to try to understand or help the patient cope.

One of the major steps in a pain unit is to wean the patients off drugs, a process called deceleration. It is not necessarily the first step, however. The staff may decide to wait for the patient to become more familiar with the unit and gain awareness of the alternatives for dealing with pain before beginning deceleration. Ultimately, however, drugs must be reduced to zero. Doctors generally agree that although narcotics and pain relievers may be effective in treating acute pain, patients with chronic pain may benefit very little from them. Medications destroy the stabilizing support of constructive goals, interfere with rehabilitation, and alter social interaction— all attitudes that pain units stress. Nearly every patient is completely off medication upon discharge from a pain unit.

Do patients resist? "Not as much as you'd expect," answers Dr. Aranoff. "It's handled in a gradual way." Goals are set for each week. If a person takes six to eight codeine and ten Darvon per day, it is unreasonable to eliminate all of these medications at once. Rather, the dosage might be reduced by a third each week. Dr. Aranoff goes on to say that "oddly enough, once the medication is reduced, the patients don't notice much increase in pain." One reason might be that pain units stress alternatives to medication. Patients are taught to relax muscles to increase blood flow to painful areas, which can reduce pain. Physical therapy also helps, as do activity programs. Patients in pain units have little time to dwell on pain. Their days are filled with social interactions and physical activities.

The concept of a pain unit is one of patient participation. They don't lie in bed all day. Rather, they take responsibility for their life and their body. They learn about their body and about their own attitudes; their getting well depends on it. The patient with chronic pain must of necessity play the most important role in his or her treatment.

Chronic pain affects more than the individual, though. Because pain becomes a part of life-style, patients with chronic pain may become manipulative to get the attention of family, friends, and co-workers, and to satisfy their needs. Family interactions can often lead to frustration, helplessness, anger, and in some cases a worsening of pain. Although well meaning, family and friends may provide the wrong emotional support at home. Pain units therefore encourage families to attend regular sessions at the unit to meet other families and to share their experiences.

Two-thirds of patients who leave after the four- to six-week stay that is common in pain units benefit from the program. "Those who don't respond," says Dr. Aranoff, "are generally less motivated and have less family support and community resources. Sometimes these patients are so accustomed to getting emotional rewards like sympathy that they choose to stay helpless, pain-ridden people." The patients who do benefit are taught to continue the attitudes and techniques they learned in the unit at home. Gaining complete control over pain takes longer than six weeks, but with work many patients are eventually able to eliminate all pain.

Do physicians accept pain units? "Yes," says Dr. Aranoff. "Years ago the medical community thought pain units were radical. That's curious because they didn't see surgery or medications as radical. Now, though, the pain unit is seen as another viable treatment option." Dr. Aranoff sees a possible expansion of the pain unit concept out of the hospital into a sort of halfway house. With the Boston Pain Unit he has purchased a house near the Massachusetts shore where he plans to establish a live-in facility for a pilot group of his patients, particularly those who have no strong family or community to return to. Such individuals would be required to work, go to school, or volunteer. Dr. Aranoff wants to demonstrate that "if you treat people who are down and out with respect, you can get them back to a productive life."

CASE HISTORY

M. R. tore a cartilage in her knee when she was seventeen.

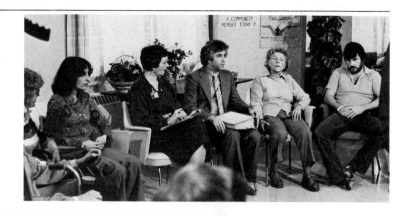

Dr. Gerald Aranoff conducts ward rounds in the Boston Pain Unit. The unit is a community where patients participate in each other's care. (Courtesy Massachusetts Rehabilitation Hospital, Boston)

Now, at twenty-one, she has had four years of pain. "The pain unit is my last step," she commented. She is wary of the medical profession. "Some of the treatment I received caused more pain than I already had. You follow these doctors, you do what they ask, you want to be strong and independent, but when you challenge them or ask questions they say, 'OK, you're only hurting yourself.'" M. R. used to take several prescription medications, including up to thirty Darvon per day. Now she throws her hands up. "I don't want any more doctors or any more medication. I just want to get better." In the pain unit she takes no drugs at all.

In 1846 Dr. W. T. G. Morton discovered how to use the chemical anesthetic ether successfully for pain. Dr. John Charles Warren operated on the first anesthetized patient and promptly announced, "This is no humbug," perhaps recognizing that the era of scientific pain relief had finally arrived.

In the years that followed,

and even today, medical research has concentrated on understanding the mechanisms of the body that lead to the pain response. The unpleasant and disturbing sensations of pain consist of two elements: (1) the input of painful stimuli, which travel from the injured area to the brain; and (2) the reaction in the brain and central nervous system to those stimuli. As an example, if an individual falls and scrapes a knee, the injury stimulates the nerve fibers, which send electrical impulses up the spinal cord and to the brain. In the brain these electrical impulses cause various biochemical reactions that result in the perception of pain. All of this—the tissue damage, the electrical impulses, and the brain chemistry—constitute the pain experience we all have known. But even that is not the whole story behind the mystery of pain. Each of us feels a different intensity of the same painful stimulus. Psychological factors can magnify pain, and they can also soothe it. It would be hard to comprehend how the hugs and comforting words that stop an injured

child from crying, the fervor of religious martyrs who allowed themselves to be burned alive, or the distracting effect of stress that makes many people unaware of serious injury have anything to do with electrical pain impulses or brain chemical perception. Clearly, an emotional or psychological response is at work.

Current excitement in the pharmacology of pain relief focuses on drugs that interfere with the brain and tissue chemicals that are involved in—in fact, mediate—the pain response rather than affect the emotional response to pain. Such drugs would have the advantage of being nonaddicting. In this regard, the Fort Washington, Pennsylvania, pharmaceutical firm McNeil Laboratories (the manufacturer of Tylenol) is eagerly anticipating Food and Drug Administration approval for a new pain reliever named Zomax (chemical name zomepirac sodium). At a recent symposium on pain relievers, Georgetown pharmacology professor William T. Beaver called Zomax "one of the most impressive compounds for pain developed so far." Zomax

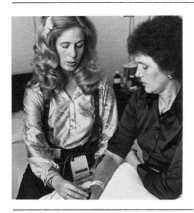

Transcutaneous nerve stimulators short circuit the pathways of pain to the brain. Electrodes are attached to the skin with an adhesive, and the unit is controlled by a small box worn around the waist. (Courtesy Massachusetts Rehabilitation Hospital, Boston)

interferes with the body's synthesis of prostaglandins, a group of fatty chemicals produced at the site of injury and recently found to be important in the transmission of the pain sensation to the brain. Its characteristics give it distinct potential advantages over pain relievers in use thus far. It is taken by mouth, and its dosage can be tailored to a broad spectrum of pain intensity. It can substitute for the relatively minor pain relief of "two aspirin" to the potent activity of 12 to 16 mg of morphine (the standard dose). In fact, in its trials with cancer patients with severe pain, it was as effective as morphine in relieving pain. All this is with minimal side effects and no potential for addiction. Zomax is similar in its chemistry to the nonsteroidal antiinflammatory drugs so important today in the treatment of bursitis, arthritis, and other similar conditions.

Nerve stimulators

Most of the technological interest in pain relief is directed at nerve stimulators. They were developed in the 1960s as an outgrowth of cardiac pace-

maker technology and are in widespread use today. Transcutaneous nerve stimulators (TNS) transmit an electronic signal through the skin to an underlying nerve to prevent the message of pain from reaching the brain. Another theory states that TNS may stimulate the brain to produce a group of morphinelike substances called endorphins that are the body's natural defense against pain. Transcutaneous nerve stimulators are portable and battery powered, and can give at least some relief for up to 70 percent of persons with chronic pain. However, they are inefficient and somewhat cumbersome and the attached wires give only temporary relief. Pain units use them to make patients feel more comfortable during periods of severe pain and as a diagnostic tool to help determine the best pain control approach.

The goal of research in nerve stimulation is an implantable unit, much like the cardiac pacemaker. Battery power is the major problem. Nerve stimulators use a lot of power, so frequent operations to replace the batteries might be necessary with im-

plantable stimulators. Some companies are working on long-life lithium batteries. The Johns Hopkins Applied Physics Laboratory is developing a miniaturized stimulator that could be completely implanted under the skin of the abdominal wall and uses space-age technology to be recharged, programmed, and monitored from outside the body. A cigarette pack–size box contains a rechargeable battery, a radio receiver, and a small computer. Wires run to the spinal cord or brain for direct stimulation and pain relief. Compared to the TNS, which costs $500, the implantable stimulator may cost $10,000 when it is finally developed and available. Even at those prices, it may be a bargain for a patient with chronic pain who may already have spent ten times that much seeking relief of symptoms. The Johns Hopkins group feels that there may be a market for these units of 1.2 million patients.

Even though the implantable stimulators may be available within the next year or two, many pain specialists disagree with the concept of a permanent nerve stimulator

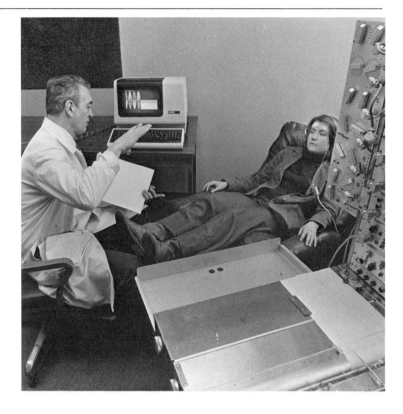

Biofeedback instruments instruct patients to recognize muscle tension and spasm and aid in relaxation efforts. (Courtesy Boston University Medical Center)

because of the possibility that the patient will become dependent on the electronic technology rather than dealing with the problem emotionally. As Dr. Aranoff says, ''The last thing these patients need is another operation, even if it is to put in a pain reliever.''

Biofeedback

Biofeedback programming uses electrical technology to teach mind and body awareness. Electrodes from the instrument are painlessly attached to a patient's skin. When the individual contracts a muscle in the area of the electrode, the monitor shows the amount of muscle tension. If the muscle is tense, the machine beeps loudly or registers a high reading on the dial. Armed with that information, the patient works at relaxing the muscle until the sound is reduced or the dial reading is lowered. Patients learn to remember the feeling of a relaxed muscle. The purpose of biofeedback programming is to teach the individual how consciously to regulate the movement and tension in certain muscles by using visual and auditory information. ''The patient can hear, see, and feel muscle tension,'' explains a biofeedback therapist. ''Often a patient has significantly tense muscles without realizing it.'' Biofeedback programs teach concentrated muscle relaxing and offer much pain relief. After practice with the biofeedback instrument, the patient develops a skill that can be used at home without instrumentation.

The future for pain relief

As the understanding of the workings of the brain and nervous system deepen, many more electrical systems and drugs for treating pain will undoubtedly reach the market. Many people feel, however, that all these devices—electrical or chemical—are mis-directed. They emphasize that individuals would do better to learn to deal with pain than to cover it up. The good doctor Oliver Wendell Holmes said, ''I firmly believe that if the whole materia medica as now used could be sunk to the bottom of the sea it would be all the better for mankind—and all the worse for the fishes.''

Austrian historian/philosopher Ivan Illich in his book *The Medical Nemesis* notes that our society is one that values anesthesia and that physicians are contributing to dehumanizing the human race by shielding human experience with drugs—in effect, performing chemical lobotomies. Illich comments: ''Such individuals still perceive pain but lose the capacity to suffer from it; the

Home medical testing

experience of pain is reduced to a discomfort with a clinical name." Illich worries about the ability of medication users to react to life's challenges in an intelligent way. "They are just at the level of domestic invalids or household pets," he warns. "Pain killing turns people into unfeeling spectators of their own decaying selves."

The medical acceptance of pain units demonstrates that the health professions are coming around to adopting this attitude as well. Pain relievers will continue to be appropriate for terminal medical problems and acute self-limiting events, but the problem of chronic pain requires a multidisciplinary approach. All of the body and mind is involved in the problem of chronic pain, and all of the body and mind must be considered in the therapy.

Most people will never experience the debilitating, dehumanizing isolation of chronic pain, but those who do can be comforted in knowing that strides are being made at last in pain control.

A private little revolution any woman can easily buy at the drug store.

Nationally distributed advertisement for e.p.t., a home pregnancy-testing kit

Americans have been treating themselves at home for years. Sales are consistently high for hundreds of over-the-counter products for ailments ranging, from constipation to the common cold. A recent survey found no fewer than fifteen medications in the average home medicine chest.

Today, home medical care is going beyond decongestants and laxatives. Over-the-counter products now intrude into a world that only recently belonged to the doctor or clinic alone—the world of medical testing.

Home kits to check pulse, blood pressure, pregnancy, diabetes, and intestinal bleeding are currently available, and others for anemia, hepatitis, cholesterol, and kidney and heart disease are under development.

Most physicians agree that patients should be more involved in their own care. A re-

cent issue of the *American Journal of Public Health* remarked that "not everyone needs carpenters to hammer in their nails."

Many physicians are critical, however, feeling that the people who tend to rely on home testing may be just the ones who need professional diagnosis and guidance. As a case in point, it is worth examining the pregnancy test, the first major and most popular home screening test.

Home test for pregnancy

Until recently a woman wondering whether she was pregnant had two choices. She could wait for the obvious physical signs, or bring a urine or blood sample to a doctor's office or laboratory for analysis. In 1976 it became possible for a woman to test for pregnancy in the privacy of her home with an over-the-counter test kit.

Home pregnancy tests are simple to perform. The woman simply adds a few drops of the morning's first urine to the contents of the prepackaged vial and waits two hours. A brown ring visible in the tube indicates pregnancy. The test measures the presence of human chorionic gonadotropin (HCG), a hormone present only during the development of a fetus. Home pregnancy tests can be used as early as nine days after a missed period, but levels of HCG begin to rise just at that time, so the test may be more reliable many days later.

The advantages of home pregnancy testing are obvious. A woman has the right to know if she is pregnant, and home testing enables her to do so privately. Unfortunately, there are disadvantages as well. Although the test is 97 percent accurate when it is positive, 20 percent of women whose tests are negative may be pregnant, although their hormone levels have not yet become high enough to indicate it. Drugs can also affect test results. Aspirin, antidepressants, or marijuana if taken within three days, and any food or drink taken within twelve hours, affect results—yet the packages do not contain this warning.

Many women use the test as a substitute for an early visit to the doctor. This practice can have serious risks, as the following case demonstrates.

CASE HISTORY

T. Y. is a twenty-two-year-old factory worker who has been in good health all her life with normal, regular menstrual periods. Fifteen days after she missed her menstrual period she purchased and performed a home pregnancy test according to the instructions on the package. The test was negative. Following the package instructions, she was waiting ten days to repeat the test. But on the twenty-second day after her missed period, she developed sudden lower abdominal pain which became very severe. She was quite weak and was sweating profusely. Her physician met her in the hospital emergency department and diagnosed an ectopic pregnancy. T. Y. underwent emergency surgery and has done well since.

T. Y. recovered, but a tubal pregnancy can be life threatening. Admittedly T. Y.'s case is unusual, but it demonstrates that home testing is no substitute for medical care. If T. Y. had had a physician perform the examination, her condition probably would have been detected.

Pharmaceutical companies agree. "Patients have a right to know," commented a representative of a company that manufactures a home pregnancy test, "but with that knowledge comes responsibility."

Other home tests

Early diagnosis remains the key to many medical problems. Simple screening tests can often provide that early diagnosis, and increased numbers of physicians and medical organizations are encouraging patients to perform regular screening tests in addition to their regular program of health care. The results have been encouraging. The recommended tests are:

- Breast self-examination. Monthly breasts checks have prompted many women to see their physician before their regular visit to check a small lump that later turns out to be cancer. Early diagnosis has saved many lives.

■ Physicians encourage their diabetic patients to check their urine for sugar daily, as a measure of insulin control. Waiting three to six months between examinations can leave a diabetic vulnerable to the ravages of uncontrolled sugar.

■ The American Cancer Society in many of its regional offices has available a kit for testing the stool for blood, an early sign of cancer. "We have a lot of stool gazers out there," commented Dr. Timothy Talbott of the renowned Ferguson Clinic for Lower GI Disorders in Grand Rapids, Michigan. Dr. Talbott feels that the preoccupation of many older people with their bowels could be put to good use by having them test their stools for occult blood and thereby pick up cancers much earlier.

Several pharmaceutical companies are at work developing home tests that will screen for anemia, hepatitis, cholesterol, and kidney disease. All are reluctant, however, to discuss the status of their current work because of its competitive nature.

As patients become increasingly involved in their own care, industry will undoubtedly capitalize on that interest by making home tests available to them.

Resources

The following companies are actively developing and producing home medical testing kits:

■ Bio-Dynamics Home Health Care, Inc.
6405 Castleway Ct.
Indianapolis, Indiana 46750
317-849-1110
(Daisy home pregnancy kit, anemia and cholesterol tests)

■ Diagnostic Testing, Inc.
767 5th Avenue
New York, New York 10022
212-758-4218
(Answer home pregnancy kit)

■ Marshall Electronics
7440 Long
Skokie, Illinois 60076
312-583-6060
(Emergency and midwifery kits)

■ Miles Laboratories
Post Office Box 340
Elkhart, Indiana 46515
219-264-8111
(Variety of home testing kits)

■ Warner-Lambert Company
201 Tabor Road
Morris Plains, New Jersey
07950
201-540-2000
(E.P.T. home pregnancy kit)

■ J. B. Williams Co.
767 5th Avenue
New York, New York 10022
212-752-5700
(Acu-test home pregnancy kit)

■ Whitehall Laboratories
685 3rd Avenue
New York, New York 10017
212-986-1000
(Predictor home pregnancy kit)

Breast feeding

The Cinderella substance of the decade—the longer one looks at it, the more elegant it appears.

Medical World News report on breast milk, February 5, 1979

Scientists are taking longer and harder looks at human breast milk, and they like what they see. In 1750 babies either were breast fed or they died. But as the eighteenth century Industrial Revolution took women out of their homes and into the work place, artificial feeding replaced breast feeding. Prior to 1900, many of these "bottle babies" died. Since then, however, proper refrigeration techniques and more sophisticated formulas that all but duplicate mother's milk in composition have given the bottle-fed baby a safe, nutritious, and convenient alternative to the breast.

The 1970s, however, saw a growing return to the breast for feeding. An estimated 35 percent of women now nurse their babies, twice the percentage of just ten years earlier. There are many reasons for this new interest. Breast feeding must begin very soon after birth and mothers are less sedated for childbirth now and are given their babies much sooner thereafter. Less attention is being paid to strict every-four-hour time schedules. Comparisons with bottle-fed babies have shown breast-fed children to have fewer infections and allergies, and there is new interest in "natural" feeding.

The Committee on Nutrition of the American Academy of Pediatrics picked 1979, the United Nations International Year of the Child, to encourage all mothers to consider breast feeding. Doctors who treat very early premature infants and severely ill children are so impressed with the benefits of breast milk that they have established breast milk banks to provide milk to infants whose mothers cannot nurse them. Here are the results of several recent studies that have begun to change previous attitudes toward breast feeding among physicians.

Immunology

This important field of study deals with the body's defenses against disease. Several recent studies show that breast-fed infants develop infections of the respiratory and gastrointestinal systems less frequently than infants on formulas. Many researchers feel that this immunity may be a result of certain proteins and cells which the mother transfers to the infant's body in breast milk.

Breast milk contains many white blood cells similar to those circulating in the blood. Ninety percent of the cells in breast milk are so-called monocytes, large white blood cells that have the ability to pick up and destroy foreign material, a process called phagocytosis. This phagocytosis is the way the body rids itself of infection and harmful foreign substances. Monocytes are formed in the bone marrow and migrate to various organs, usually the liver, lung, and spleen, where they change and acquire characteristics important to that site. In the lactating mother, however, 25 percent of the monocytes are pumped into breast milk. Once in the milk they undergo a transformation into cells that are larger and more phagocytic—that is, they pick up and destroy more foreign sub-

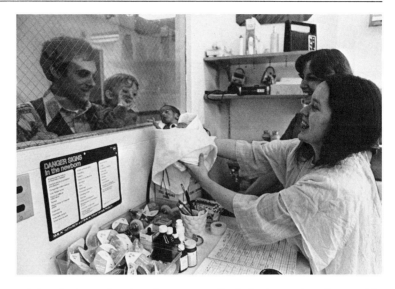

stances. In this state they are called macrophages. A chemical factor found in the liquid part of the breast milk, monophage transformation factor (MTF), is probably responsible for the change.

In the laboratory, these large macrophages, or "big macs," easily dispose of bacteria and other foreign debris by trapping them in small compartments. The "big macs" are known to produce other proteins that are components of the so-called complement system, another important factor in the body's defense and immunity system. "Big mac" cells produced by the mother are transfused into the infant through breast milk. In addition to their direct effects on the infant's disease immunity, the macrophages and MTF may also stimulate the infant's own monocyte/macrophage system to mature. So the breast milk has a double effect: it provides direct immunity from infection and stimulates the infant to develop its own immunity.

The newborn infant, particularly the premature infant, is at risk to develop severe intestinal infections. In mature adults the intestine is subjected to a variety of foreign substances, food and food products, bacteria, and a variety of chemicals. In order to protect itself from these foreign substances, so-called plasma cells in the intestinal lining produce antibodies which coat the intestine and mechanically grab onto and bind bacteria, viruses, and proteins and food. Because premature infants cannot produce all the antibodies they need, they are thus at risk for severe infection. One such infection, necrotizing enterocolitis (NEC), is seen often in premature infants on intravenous feedings in intensive care nurseries. The infection can be fatal. However, when small premature infants are fed with breast milk instead of intravenous solution, the risk of NEC disappears. One reason may be that they are receiving protection against the infection in the breast milk from their mothers. Almost unbelievably, the infant can actu-

ally help determine the specific types of antibodies that it receives from the mother. An infant with an infection transmits a small bit of the bacteria that caused the infection (or else a small amount of a chemical produced by the bacteria) to the mother by absorption through her breast skin. The mother actually contracts a mild case of the infection, and her defense system produces the right type of antibody against bacteria and chemical antigens and transmits these antibodies back to the child.

So the nursing mother and infant work together to provide immunity. The mother's much more mature defense system produces antibodies for the infant influenced by information that the infant communicates to her and her "big macs," and MTFs transmitted in the breast milk pick up and destroy foreign material in the infant's gut and stimulate the baby's monocytes to learn to do the same.

The implication of these recent findings is enormous. We know that allergies develop when a person is exposed to antigens and produces antibodies against them. This antigen-antibody reaction produces the chemical histamine, which is responsible for the symptoms. When the antibodies are transmitted in breast milk, however, uptake of the antigen and the resulting sensitization can be prevented. Some investigators believe that most symptoms of gastrointestinal upset (diarrhea, vomiting, and so forth) in the first two years of life are actually manifestations of allergy to cow's milk. Breast feeding can prevent these symptoms of allergy.

Nutrition

Until recently, breast milk was thought to be incomplete as a nutritive food. Now we realize this is incorrect. Analysis of human milk shows it may be complete as a nutritional source for up to a year. In fact, mothers in several societies throughout the world breast feed their infants for two to three years and more, and the children do not seem to be lacking in size, strength, or health as they grow. The practical composition of breast milk may just be more appropriate than any of our well-intentioned substitutes.

Fat is a case in point. Concern about fat and its relationship to arteriosclerosis and blood vessel and heart disease in later years led many pediatricians to attempt to reduce infants' cholesterol intake. It was in vogue for several years to put a child on low-fat milk, but cholesterol is important enough to the growing infant that this practice may be harmful in the long run. Infants and small children grow quickly. Their rapidly growing nerves and membranes need the cholesterol. Further, the "big macs" that are so important to defending the intestines from bacteria and viral onslaughts also need cholesterol to do their important work. Some researchers also feel that cholesterol and fat in an infant's diet prepares it to meet the challenges of dietary fat encountered as adults. Dr. Isabelle Valadian of the Harvard School of Public Health is overseeing a study that has followed blood levels of fat and cholesterol in people for more than forty years. Adults who

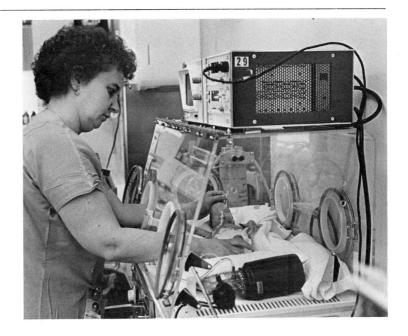

Intensive care nurseries often separate mother from child for extended periods. Breast milk banks can provide the needed milk during this time. (Photo by Michael J. Lutch, courtesy Beth Israel Hospital, Boston)

were breast fed as infants have lower cholesterol levels, regardless of the fat in their diet. Their childhood feeding experiences seem to prepare them to handle dietary fat more efficiently.

Maybe this old adage "A fat baby is a healthy baby" should be restated as "A fat baby is a fat adult." Pleasant as it is to pinch baby fat and to watch roly-poly, apparently well-nourished infants in their crib, increasing evidence shows that infants overfed in the first year of life may just be fighting obesity all their lives. A popular theory relates appetite to the number of fat cells a person has. During the first year of life overfeeding can increase the number of fat cells permanently. At most other times, overfeeding just increases the size of the fat cells, and this change is reversible.

Most bottle-fed babies tend to gain more weight than breast-fed babies. There is less of a tendency to overfeed when breast feeding. The babies take only what they need, drink more slowly, and get fewer calories. Human milk has less mineral content. There is less fluid retention, and it contains

less protein so that organs that break down proteins don't have to work quite as hard. Furthermore, the building block composition of the proteins—amino acids—differ. Those in human milk are clearly less allergenic.

Breast milk banks

Breast milk is the standard of nutrition for babies born at normal-term pregnancy and premature infants who may have special needs. Breast milk, though not perfect, tends to come the closest to their needs, acccording to most neonatologists (physicians who specialize in premature and young infants). Many infants, however, cannot get breast milk directly from their mother, as in the following situations:

■ In some cases the child is separated from the mother in a special medical care center.

■ Because of the stress of illness in the mother, breast milk may not be available in needed quantities.

■ Some premature babies weighing only three pounds or less have little or no strength to nurse from the mother.

■ In older children, a problem requiring breast milk is discovered long after the mother's milk has dried up.

For all these situations and more, donors can provide the breast milk. Breast milk banks have therefore been set up in several locations across the country. Any nursing mother in good health whose baby is thriving can become a breast milk donor. The milk is collected at home, frozen, then brought to a regional collection center, where it is stored for future needs. Often it is shipped to hospitals far away. Each breast milk donor can provide between 1 and 8 ounces a day. As evidence of the need, some older children on breast milk therapy may require 50 ounces a day or more.

Breast milk centers are becoming more widely recognized by nursing mothers. In the nursery of the Hahnemann Hospital in Worcester, Massachusetts, one of fourteen regional breast milk banks in the United States, 150 women donate approximately 20,000 ounces of breast milk each year. But the need at this center and the others is much greater. Babies all over the country need breast milk.

Resources

Women who are pregnant or nursing owe it to themselves to become acquainted with the rapidly changing field of infant nutrition. Your best sources are your obstetrician, pediatrician, and the La Leche League, an organization whose goal is the dissemination of information on breast feeding. The La Leche League has offices in most major cities.

Breast feeding will continue to increase in the United States and throughout the world as women recognize the valuable source of information of nutrition their bodies can provide to their babies.

■ The most reputable and reliable information on breast feeding and breast milk banks is available from the La Leche League International, which has offices in virtually every large city in the country. Many pediatricians and hospitals also offer reference material and courses. The headquarters of the LaLeche League is:

LaLeche League International
9616 Minneapolis Avenue
Franklin Park, Illinois
312-455-7730

Other reputable sources of information include:

■ American Academy of Pediatrics
1801 Hinman Avenue
Evanston, Illinois 60204
312-869-4255

■ Office of Maternal and Child Health
Program Services Branch
Bureau of Community Health Services
Health Services Administration

Room 7A20, Parklawn Building
5600 Fishers Lane
Rockville, Maryland 20857
301-443-4273

Reliable sources of nutrition information include:

■ United States Department of Agriculture
Human Nutrition Center
Room 421A
Washington, D.C. 20250
202-447-7854

■ Nutrition Foundation
Suite 300
888 Seventeenth Street, N.W.
Washington, D.C. 20006
202-872-0776

■ National Nutrition Education Clearinghouse
Suite 1110
2140 Shattuck Avenue
Berkeley, California 94704
415-548-1363

Rehabilitating patients with spinal cord injuries

God may forgive you your sins, but your nervous system won't.

Alfred Korzybski, 1879–1950

Many body tissues regenerate after injury, restoring normal function. Not so the nervous system; it is is rarely forgiving, and injuries to it are usually permanent.

Five hundred years ago, Leonardo da Vinci recognized the importance of the spinal cord to life. In his experiments he found that "the frog dies instantly when the spinal cord is pierced; yet it can live without heart, without head or any bowels, or intestine or skin; and here, therefore, it would seem, lie the foundations of movement and life."

The spinal cord is vital . . . and vulnerable. It is surrounded by the vertebral bones, thirty-three in all, stacked one on top of the other like building blocks. The arrangement permits flexibility, bending, twisting, turning . . . and injury. Violent movement can shear the bones apart and disrupt the normal alignment. The neck or back can be easily fractured, pinching and sometimes tearing the delicate spinal cord within it.

The spinal cord contains many tracts of nerve fibers lying close together. The fibers are extensions of nerve cell bodies in the brain and ganglia (groups of nerve cells) throughout the body. The nerve fibers may be very long, carrying messages as they must from the head to the fingers and toes. If the tracts are damaged, the fibers must regenerate along many feet—an impossible task.

A spinal cord injury is permanent. Once lost, function cannot be reclaimed. The injured patient has no feeling or movement below the point of injury.

It remains for the determined patient and innovative rehabilitation specialists to use the areas of the body that still function. Therein lies the goal of rehabilitation for spinal cord injuries: preserve what function is left—and use it to replace what is irretrievably lost.

The primary cause of spinal cord injury is automobile and motorcycle accidents (40 percent), then falling or being struck by a falling object (21 percent), then sports injuries (15 percent). Most sports injuries are from diving, when the person hits another person or object in the water and the head is violently flexed on the neck.

Quadriplegics, paralyzed in all four limbs, have died from their injuries until recently. (Paraplegics are paralyzed in the legs only.) Modern technology now helps them to survive. Coupled with a sensitive partnership of specialists in many medical disciplines, technology is also helping them to do what also had been impossible—to control their surroundings and lead independent lives.

CASE HISTORY

It was a preseason game with the Oakland Raiders, a warmup to the bruising National Football League season. When the quarterback called his number, New England Patriots wide receiver Daryl Stingley went over the play in his mind: "Run down field, cut toward the center, accelerate, catch the ball at full stride, and head for the goalposts." It was a play he had run many times; he was

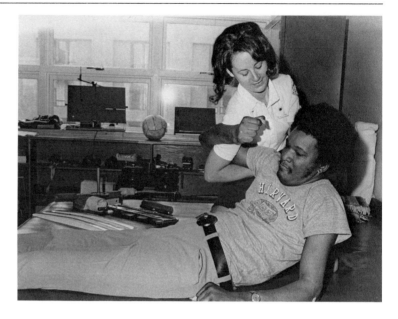

one of the best in his business.

This particular play was going to end differently. No touchdown, no long gain. It was going to be the last football play ever for the talented player.

Daryl Stingley was hit with a bone-crushing tackle. His body fell limp to the ground. Trainers and doctors rushed to his side. Their initial fears were later confirmed—spinal cord injury.

After several operations and a year in rehabilitation, Daryl Stingley returned to the field of his former glory. The fans cheered as they had so many times before, but this time not for a man in a red-and-white uniform. This time the cheers were for a man in a wheelchair. Daryl Stingley would never walk again. He is paralyzed in all four limbs.

Facilities for care

The facilities of an average hospital cannot cope with spinal cord injuries. Today patients are treated at regional centers, where the latest techniques and the most competent specialists are marshaled.

There are fourteen Regional Spinal Cord Injury Centers in the United States. In the past three years, the New England Regional Spinal Cord Injury Center at University Hospital in Boston has seen 180 patients, a little more than one per week.

Dr. Murray Freed, director of the center, comments that what the spinal cord injury problem lacks in frequency, it more than makes up in severity. "The individual paralyzed in all four limbs and trunk is returned to infancy both physically and emotionally. He must be fed, bathed, and clothed and have all his body excretions taken care of. Nothing is private." The hospital stay of a patient with a spinal cord injury averages four to six months.

The New England Spinal Cord Injury Center was the first nonmilitary center in the country to rally specialists from many fields to care for patients with spinal cord injuries; it has served as a model for the other centers. "It takes the efforts of many individuals; one can't do it alone," comments Dr. Freed, whose staff in the twenty-four-bed unit includes neurosurgeons, orthopedists, plastic and general surgeons, internists, psychiatrists and psychologists, bioengineers, social workers, and physical and occupational therapists.

Patients with spinal cord injuries can have a myriad of problems and yet have few symptoms because the spinal cord, which usually carries messages to the brain, no longer functions. The task is therefore complex: to find problems in patients who aren't even aware that a problem is present.

Operations may be necessary to relieve pressure on the cord structure. Breathing problems are frequent. Bowel and bladder functions need to be regulated. Poor urine control can lead to infection and incontinence. This, as it turns out, is a major problem in readjustment to life outside the medical facility. "You can be socially acceptable if you can't walk, but not if you can't control your bladder," notes Dr. Freed.

Even though patients with spinal cord injuries have lost all sensation, they do feel discomfort. The phenomenon is called "phantom pain"; it is also seen in patients who have had amputations. The phantom sensation diminishes in time but may be severe and lead patients to rely on narcotics. Many such patients become addicts.

The directors of all fourteen regional centers meet twice a year to share what they have learned from their patients. The information is pooled at a data research center in Phoenix, Arizona. These data show that the regional program has had a major effect in reducing the length of hospital stay. For those admitted to a regional center within four days of injury, quadriplegics stay 128 days, and paraplegics stay 110 days. For those admitted to the center after three weeks, quadriplegics stay 189 days, paraplegics 152 days. If a patient is never admitted to a regional center, the rehabilitation may take twice as long.

Technology

Regaining independence is a key to recovery and rehabilitation for a patient with a spinal cord injury. Motivating patients who cannot feel or move is difficult. "Their lives are so different, the future seems so murky, they aren't ready to ask what will happen next," Dr. Freed notes.

The technology for patients with spinal cord injuries is designed to assist what function remains naturally and replace what has been permanently lost. The latest effort by bioengineers is called an environmental control unit (ECU).

The ECU is about the size of a small radio and has twelve sockets for plugging in electrical appliances. An electrical display of lights (one for each socket in the ECU) is positioned so that the patient can see it. Each light is labeled accordingly for each socket.

If the patient wants to turn on a radio, he sucks an air hose connected to the device while the scanner proceeds from one light to another. A distinctive click sounds when each successive light comes on. When the display switch labeled "radio" comes on, the patient stops sucking, and the scanner stops. Puffing on the air hose slightly turns the radio on.

If the patient wants to turn on a light, he sucks again on the air hose until the scanner reaches the switch labeled "light" and repeats the process. "Anything that can be attached to the equipment can be operated by the environmental control center," Dr. Freed explains. "The unit helps patients to do much for themselves, an important factor in motivation and rehabilitation." The device can also be activated by a small rocking lever that can be controlled by chin or hand pressure.

The ECU system has also been adapted to wheelchairs. Appropriate combinations of puffs and sucks can control forward, backward, and turn locomotion.

Physical therapist Nancy Dutton, who teaches patients

Dr. Mary Joan Willard trains Crystal the monkey to assist paralyzed victims. Here Crystal feeds Dr. Willard, who portrays the patient. (Photo by Daniel Bernstein)

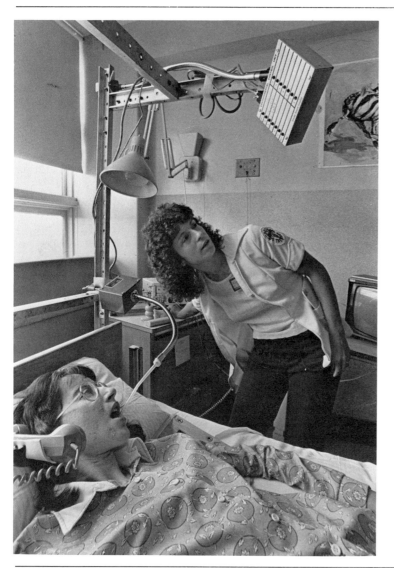

the use of the ECU at the New England regional center, says, "Patients can learn to control the ECU in five or ten minutes. They become familiar with it here at the hospital so they can use it later to control their environment at home. The unit could be on a small table in their home. Using an electric wheelchair operated by the air hose, the quadriplegic could wheel right up to the unit, take the unit's air hose, and control all the electrical appliances in the room."

Elsewhere at the Tufts–New England Medical Center, rehabilitation specialists are using *living* environmental control units on several patients with spinal cord injuries. Researchers have trained monkeys to turn lights on and off, open doors, retrieve objects, or play the radio or TV, all at the verbal command of the patient. The monkeys re-

Rehabilitation specialist demonstrates environmental control unit to a quadriplegic patient. Unit on frame controls various electronic appliances; patient selects appliance by blowing or sucking on tube. (Photo by Bradford F. Herzog, courtesy Boston University Medical Center)

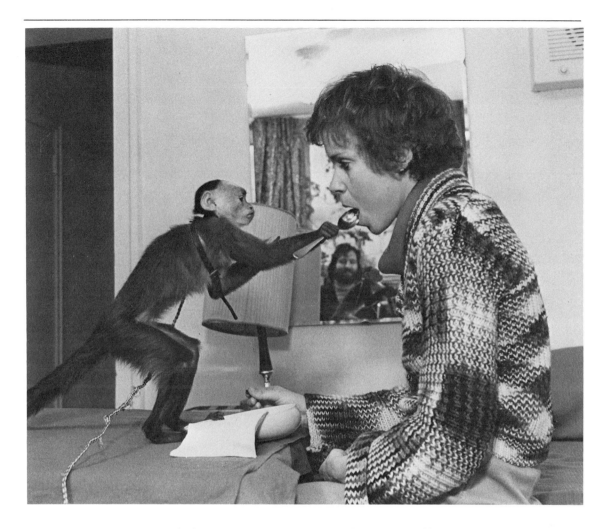

quire extensive training, and of course their actions are not entirely predictable. But these animals may provide invaluable aid in certain rehabilitation cases.

Social adjustment

Spinal cord injury centers have an important role in psychological as well as physical rehabilitation. Patients are taught to feed, bathe, and clothe themselves, using specially designed braces to support their frail limbs.

There are no private rooms.

Interaction is encouraged. Frequent ward meetings stress that patients discuss their problems with each other. Families and friends are invited.

Courses are conducted on sexual adjustment. As a result, divorce rates for center patients do not differ from those of the general public.

Frequent "out-trips" to bowling alleys, discos, restaurants, and sporting and shopping events all aid adjustment. "The individual has to learn how to do familiar things in a

different way. He learns that he can still enjoy them as before," comments one therapist.

Dr. Murray Freed had a special feel for the problems of his patients because he, too, has a disability. He suffered severe burns and the loss of a leg in the Battle of the Bulge during World War II. After eighteen months at Walter Reed Hospital in Washington, D.C., he went on to medical school and specialty training in rehabilitation medicine.

He is one of many handi-

Hospices

capped people who work in the rehabilitation field. Many are in wheelchairs themselves. Paraplegic engineer Ralph Hotchkiss of Washington, D.C., has designed a device that enables a paralyzed person to stand without assistance. Dr. Joseph Panzarella, a quadriplegic as a result of multiple sclerosis, directs a sixty-four-bed rehabilitation hospital at the Brunswick Medical

Social rehabilitation is as important as physical adjustment. These patients have paralyzed legs, but can still enjoy bowling. (Courtesy Boston University Medical Center)

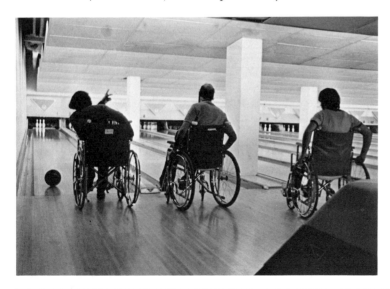

center in Amityville, New York. The American Association for the Advancement of Science lists more than 600 handicapped scientists active in research and patient care within its organization.

As one researcher, herself handicapped, says, "Aerodynamically a bumblebee is not supposed to fly." The presence of handicapped individuals within the rehabilitation field adds an unusual sensitivity and serves as an example that people can, indeed, surmount a disability—and perhaps even fly.

To learn to die is better than to study the ways of dying.

Sir Thomas Browne
Christian Morals, 1642

The past few decades have witnessed the development of extraordinary and innovative ways to diagnose and treat illness. Lifesaving machinery and techniques are becoming ever more sophisticated. Defibrillators, radiation therapies, cardiopulmonary resuscitation programs, and countless other innovations characterize modern medical care. But for all its advances, today's health care system has generally failed patients who face terminal illness. Too often, lifesaving efforts focus on the body as an electrochemical machine, ignoring the emotions and souls of whole persons and their families. Too often, the system persists in prolonging the death process, rather than making more meaningful the life that remains. Too often, says Elisabeth Kübler-Ross, "death becomes lonely and impersonal."

"Death is a necessary end," said Shakespeare in *Twelfth Night*. "It will come when it will come." Today, the hospice movement provides care for travelers on the final phase of life's journey—the dying. The hospice movement, begun in England in 1967, is rapidly spreading across Europe and the United States. In medieval times a hospice was a way station, a place where footsore and weary travelers could receive hospitality and care. A hospice is not necessarily a site where care occurs; it is rather a philosophy of care, where the emphasis shifts from cure to caring, to helping patients maintain a high quality of life in their remaining days. Counseling, symptom control, sound medical attention, and a comforting environment minimize discomfort and allow the terminally ill to maintain control over their lives. They may remain at home much longer, avoid the impersonal hospital or nursing home environment, and, along with their families, approach death with dignity.

The hospice concept

Hospitals and nursing homes, where people with cancer and other terminal illnesses usually die, do not accommodate the needs of dying patients and their families. Staffs are not trained to deal with their physical and emotional demands. The needs of the institution often come before the needs of the patient. This may be translated to "No more than two people in the room at once, please"; or, "It's not time for your next pain shot yet"; or, "You'll have to leave because visiting hours are over." Worst of all, dying patients in hospitals and nursing facilities are separated from the people and surroundings that have given meaning to their lives. And they often die alone.

Even though most patients may wish to die at home, fulfilling that wish has become difficult in America. Most families are not structured to allow for the full-time care of a dying relative; and the American health care system has been gradually shifting toward the hospital as the locus of care.

The hospice movement recognizes that the emotional and physical needs of the dying patient are equally important. Hospices allow patients to die a natural death, emphasizing that they are alive until they die and that each minute of remaining life deserves care, attention, and grace.

Dr. Cicely Saunders began the revolution in care for the dying when she founded St. Christopher's Hospice in London in 1967. A former nurse, she became frustrated by patients who spent their last days lying in unfamiliar, sterile hospital beds, attached to monitors, fed and drained by tubes, and alone, separated from their families and friends. She became a physician to "look into the problems of pain in the dying patient." The results of her work influenced the way her country's health care system responded to fatal illness, an influence that is spreading rapidly all over the world. "If I were dying of a terminal illness, I'd like to die at St. Christopher's," says Harvard psychologist Dr. William Worden, reflecting the ultimate accolades that health care professionals have given to Dr. Saunders's work.

The hospice concept implies a facility to care for patients with an inevitably fatal illness. Sometimes it is an inpatient facility, where people are admitted when they require more involved care. In these cases it is usually free-standing, physically separate from a hospital. Most often, though, a hospice is a facility that supports home care. Facility-based physicians, nurses, and social workers take their expertise into the home to support, assist, and teach family and friends to care for and live with the patient. So it is at St. Christopher's and twenty-six other hospices in Great Britain. In the United States there are only three hospices that provide inpatient and outpatient care from a free-standing facility: the Hillhaven Hospice in Tucson, Arizona; the Kaiser-Permanente Medical Care Program in Los Angeles, California; and Hospice, Inc., in New Haven, Connecticut. All are funded by the National Cancer Institute and similar organizations. While much of the beauty of the hospice concept lies in its separation from the traditional hospital setting, the large number of unoccupied hospital beds has made it difficult to justify the construction of British-type free-standing facilities in the United States. Furthermore, the United States has no national health service to absorb even part of the operating and treatment costs. The United States hospice system, therefore, has focused on home care with tie-ins to local hospitals. Two hundred such units exist today.

How hospices work

Hospices try to arrange for home care by integrating various community agencies with the hospice staff. They draw on the expertise of the Visiting Nurse Association and other support and service groups. Twenty-four-hour-per-day, seven-day-per-week emergency help is also available. Although most emergencies can be dealt with by telephone conversations with a concerned hospice worker, physician, or nurse, house calls are made when necessary. Alarming and frightening symptoms can occur at any time, day or night, and can make the patient and family feel quite helpless. Dr. Sylvia Lack recalls the time a husband reluctantly placed his wife in a nursing home for the last three months of her life after the stress of trying to replace a gastrostomy tube (a stomach tube for feeding) by following the directions of a physician on the telephone. The tube had accidentally fallen out, an event that happens all too frequently. "A physician house visit could have saved three months of institutional therapy," Dr. Lack commented.

Hospices operate on a team philosophy. The patient, family, doctor, nurse, social worker, clergyman, friends, and volunteers are all part of the team. Problem-solving approaches are used and plans of actions developed for each patient or family need. While the physician may be a key member of the hospice team and integral to the patient's care, often the greatest discomforts derive from concerns other than medical ones. The other team members can be instrumental in helping the patient and family cope with interpersonal relationships, fear of pain, isolation, and financial and social worries.

Patients are admitted to hospice programs only after reasonable treatments have been exhausted and death is only a matter of months away.

But hospices are not one-way escalators to death, inattentive to potential or real improvements in patients' conditions. Medical direction is important in a hospice, to remain vigilant for evidence of remission, misdiagnosis, inappropriate referrals, and any treatment advances.

Hospice, Inc., in New Haven, Connecticut, was the first American hospice. It began in 1974 as an outpatient, home care service exclusively. In 1980 forty-four beds are under construction in a free-standing facility, designed to provide a better place for patients to die. The facility offers four-bedded rooms to create "a community of share and support between people with similar problems," says Dr. Sylvia Lack, originally with St. Christopher's and now medical director of Hospice, Inc. Private rooms are available, however, for patients who are disruptive or very ill, or those with large families. The private rooms also serve the sexual needs of the terminal patient, "even if they are used for nothing more than emotional closeness between husband and wife." The rooms are cheery, and large windows and skylights give the patients a reference to the outside world. The rooms can be furnished with plants, furniture, and artifacts from the patients' homes. Whatever form they take, hospice settings stress a homelike environment, to foster security and the participation of families. There are also places to view the body when a patient dies, and the recently dead are not hidden from view.

If the inpatient facility is unique and innovative, the focus of care at the Connecticut hospice remains the home. "Patients want to stay at home," emphasizes Dr. Lack, "and families want to care for their relatives. They do the most amazing things. All they need is advice, encouragement, and support." Knowing that inpatient care is available when needed often enables the patient to stay at home much longer, until symptoms can no longer be controlled or until the family is no longer able to continue the level of care required. Or the patient may go back and forth between home and the facility, staying at the latter to give families an occasional break from the exhausting day-to-day chores of home care.

Symptom control

There has been a good deal of writing in the United States in recent years on death and dying; and much of it has concerned the emotional and psychological needs of the dying patient. Many people feel that this is the major emphasis of hospices. "They are missing the point about hospices," states Dr. Lack. "First and foremost, the patient must be kept comfortable. Any group concerned with service to the dying must be talking about smoothing sheets, rubbing bottoms, relieving constipation, and sitting up at night. Such concerns loom large in the lives of dying patients and must be important to the physician if the physician is to treat the whole person. Counseling a patient in a wet bed is ineffective."

Although they do deal in depth with emotional crises and support, hospices don't zero in on death and hospice workers don't hold hands or tell patients to keep their chin up. Hospices work with the unpleasant, sometimes agonizing symptoms of terminal ill-ness—nausea, weakness, breathing troubles, and, most of all, pain.

Pain is the single greatest threat to the daily existence of patients approaching death; not only the pain of their ill-ness, but the intensified pain brought on by fear of dying, a sense of isolation, and the dis-tress of loved ones. Healthy individuals wake up in the morning with back pain and imagine that they did too much the day before. A cancer patient who wakes up with back pain assumes and fears that the disease has spread to the back. Both the pain and the fear of what it implies must be dealt with.

Hospices pay meticulous at-tention to pain and look for medications that control symptoms but do not sedate the patient. St. Christopher's Hospice has popularized the use of a centuries-old formula called Brompton's mixture. Containing diamorphine (heroin), cocaine, and gin in chloroform water, it relieves pain without sedation or un-comfortable side effects. United States hospices like Hospice, Inc., use "cocktails"

containing morphine and a medication for nausea, usually given by mouth. Morphine can be carefully regulated to keep the patient pain free, yet men-tally alert.

The key to pain relief in a hospice is not the traditional prescription direction *p.r.n.* (*pro re nata*, meaning "as needed"), but rather the use of medication *before* it is needed. Giving medications on a schedule and before pain be-comes intolerable prevents the dependency of having to ask for relief in order to get it, pro-vides more continuous control, and diminishes the fear and expectation of pain.

According to Dr. Lack, 85 percent of patients in Hospice are on oral pain medication until their death. Narcotics are reserved for severe pain but, unlike in traditional hospital settings, are not withheld until the patient has hours or days to live. Hospices are not worried about addiction; nar-cotics are used when needed, when nonnarcotic medications and measures such as nerve blocks no longer control the pain.

Dying patients have many other distressing symptoms:

incontinence, constipation, vomiting, bedsores. Such prob-lems are very important to pa-tients and their families and receive much attention in a hospice. Solving them brings great relief for emotional as well as physical states.

Hospices encourage physical and social activity. Small, appetizing meals are provided; and the emphasis is switched from nutrition to eating as a pleasurable experience. With "little" details taken care of, the dying patient has less to worry about and emotional peace is closer at hand.

Financial aspects of hospices

Experts have differing views about the economics of hos-pice care in comparison to acute hospital care. They gen-erally agree that a hospice costs less, but how much less remains to be determined. Dr. Zimmerman at the Church Hospital Hospice-Care Pro-gram in Baltimore, Maryland, is convinced that hospice care is economically efficient. "In-patient care in the program is admittedly intensive. Although it is a relatively low level of technological care, with far fewer diagnostic and therapeutic measures than traditional hospital programs, it does require a high level of personal attention." In his hospice, the average daily cost for a hospice care inpatient is about 80 percent of that for the average intermediate care hospital patient. Even when lower daily inpatient costs, shorter stays, and higher outpatient treatment costs are added, the total is still economically more appealing than traditional terminal care. "If hospice care is compared with conventional treatment for the terminally ill, including prolonged hospitalization, numerous diagnostic tests, and the liberal use of radiation and chemotherapy, hospice care is almost certainly more economically attractive. On the other hand, if it is compared with virtually no care at all (also very common for the terminally ill), it is clearly more expensive."

Other figures uphold the idea that hospice care is a less expensive alternative. In one study of 500 patients at Hospice, Inc., the average cost for a three-month stay was $750, "less than the cost of one week in a typical hospital,"

Dr. Lack says.

Despite the fact that insurance firms and the government now cover more than two-thirds of all health care spending, such coverage is limited, for the most part, to patients who have suffered acute illness and have been hospitalized. Hospices do not receive payment for home care services, which are the focus of their involvement. Given the nature of the hospice service, and the vital need it fills, reimbursement systems must be changed.

The hospice alternative

The hospice system of care is not for everyone with a terminal illness. There are those who want medical technology to give them every last minute of life, regardless of cost and physical or emotional suffering to themselves or their families. For them, traditional hospitals, intensive care units, and research facilities are more appropriate places for care. Hospices, on the other hand, allow patients to die a "natural" death, a death without struggle. Hospices stress palliation rather than cure, low rather than high technology. In

a world that is often too technical, too efficient, and indeed too frightened to accept dying as a phase of life, the hospice movement is a redefinition of life and death and a return to human concerns.

Resources

■ Information about hospices in your area can usually be obtained from your local health planning agency, health systems agency, doctor, or hospital.

■ The National Hospice Organization (NHO) has developed a set of standards for hospice care. The NHO coordinates the activities of hospices around the country and disseminates information on the concept. The national office is:

National Hospice Organization
Tower Suite 506
301 Maple Avenue West
Vienna, Virginia 22180
703-938-4449

■ Also contact:

National Council on Aging
1828 L Street
Washington, D.C. 20036
202-223-6250

Allergy Allergy Al

Aah-CHOO!

Anonymous allergy sufferer

Scratching, sneezing, weeping, wheezing, coughing, nose blowing—the miseries of allergy are well known to some 35 million Americans, according to the National Institute of Allergy and Infectious Diseases. Allergy is a major health problem, being treated today by 3,000 card-carrying specialists and several times that many pediatricians, internists, and family physicians. The millions of allergy sufferers react to airborne pollens from grasses and trees, spores of molds, insect bites, milk, eggs, and other foods, chemicals, house dust, and countless other agents. They experience asthma, eczema, hives, hay fever, and sometimes fatal anaphylactic shock. They pay over $1 billion for advice, drugs, doctors' visits, hospital care, and desensitizing injections, and lose another $1 billion from days they are unable to work. Although diagnostic methods have progressed little beyond the standard skin test, a new understanding of why a person is allergic has led to the development of more specific and effective drugs. There is now hope that the desensitization techniques (allergy shots) so commonly used today will soon be obsolete.

About allergy

The term *allergy* was coined in 1906 by Clemens von Pirquet, who recognized that it was possible for an individual to develop a reaction—indeed, a state of reactivity—to a foreign substance. It was assumed that this condition was caused by something in the blood or serum of an allergic person that was not in the blood of a nonallergic person. Evidence came in 1919, when a person was reported to have developed an allergy to horses after receiving a blood transfusion from an individual with that allergy. Using for the first time a technique that has come to be the reference for defining an allergy, two German physicians in 1921 proved the existence of that "something in the serum." Dr. Heinz Küstner was allergic to fish. A colleague, Dr. Carl Prausnitz, an early practicing allergist, was himself not allergic to fish and ate it regularly without problems. Prausnitz took a small amount of Küstner's serum and injected it into his own skin. Twenty-four hours later, he injected a small amount of fish extract into the same spot. The skin immediately became red, raised, and inflamed. Clearly something in the serum—Prausnitz called the substance *reagin*—was responsible for temporarily transferring to himself Küstner's fish allergy and, presumably, all the symptoms that people even today commonly associate with their allergies.

In the years that followed, when a person was suspected of having an allergy to a particular grass, mold, food, or other substance, an extract of that substance was injected into his or her skin just as Prausnitz had done to himself. Red, raised skin at the site was proof of allergy and the reagin presumed responsible for it. To moderate the intense reaction that often occurred in highly allergic people, the skin test was modified to the current "prick test." Instead of being injected into the skin, a drop of the extract is applied to the skin, and the skin is scratched or pricked slightly through the drop.

But what is this mysterious reagin that accounts for the misery of allergy? In 1966 Dr. Kimishige Ishizaka and Dr. Teruko Ishizaka, a husband-and-wife team, demonstrated that it was a protein, an immunoglobulin that was not previously known. They called it immunoglobulin E or, as it is now commonly called, IgE. The discovery that IgE is responsible for allergic reactions has opened new vistas in allergy. Allergy-prone people can now be identified by the presence of IgE in their blood, and the chemicals that work against IgE may be the answer to allergic symptoms.

CASE HISTORY

J. C. is a seven-year-old girl with no past history of serious medical problems. She was bottle fed and received good neonatal care. In her early months and years she had frequent upper respiratory infections which responded well to decongestants, antihistamines, and antibiotics. On vacation trips or when staying the night at a friend's house, she would occasionally experience runny nose, cough, and swelling around the eyes. Her parents suspected allergy after a while, as there was a family allergic tendency. Several relatives had similar symptoms and one was treated with allergy shots. At a county fair one day J. C. developed sudden facial swelling and wheezing while riding a horse. Subsequent testing at her pediatrician's office confirmed allergy to horse hair at age five. By avoiding anything related to horses, J. C. has been free of symptoms now for two years.

Why some people are allergic and others are not is unclear. Yet much is known about how an allergic response occurs. For clarity, a brief definition of two words used in allergy is necessary. The foreign substance—pollen, hair, molds, spore, or whatever—that provokes an allergic response is called an *antigen*. The body's defense against that foreign substance is called an *antibody*.

When an individual is exposed to a foreign antigen such as a particular chemical, pollen, or dust, by either inhaling it or eating it, plasma cells lining the gastrointestinal tract, nose, and bronchial tubes produce an antibody—a protein that neutralizes that antigen. It is the protein antibody IgE that was isolated and identified by the Drs. Ishizaka. Although the antibody response is normal and common to all people, in an allergic person the body overdoes its protection and produces much more IgE than is needed. Presumably the overproduction of IgE is genetic in nature, but the exact mechanism involved is not completely understood.

Once IgE has been produced, it attaches itself to mast cells, a specialized type of cell that is found throughout the body along blood vessels in the lining of the nose and respiratory tract and just under the skin. Inside each mast cell are many small granules containing the chemical histamine. When a person is again exposed to the same antigen, the reaction of the IgE, now attached to the mast cells, and that antigen causes the mast cells to release large amounts of histamine into the tissues. Histamine's normal function is to help repair tissues, but when large amounts of it are released during the antigen-antibody reaction, it works on blood vessels to cause redness, swelling, and itching. It works on the nerve endings of smooth muscle to cause spasms and wheezes in the bronchial tubes, and it works on the mucus glands of the nose to produce nasal drainage—the common allergic symptoms.

Mast cells are like bombs waiting to explode and release their histamine. An antigen-IgE antibody response can cause histamine release, but not all excess histamine release is from allergy. Some sensitive people can have reactions that mimic allergy from certain drugs, infection, exposure to cold or heat, or even nervous tension. Whereas histamine probably has the major role in allergic symptoms, other factors have also been identified. SRS-A (slow reacting substance of anaphylaxis) with reactions similar to histamine is one of many substances that is provoking great research interest.

Advances in skin testing and desensitization injections

Some specialists say that allergies are best handled by environmental control and occasional antihistamine or decongestant medication, but if antihistamines are needed every day or if medications do not control the symptoms, skin testing should be done to establish the exact allergies. Other allergists are more aggressive and like to have the hard evidence that a skin test provides before administering medication. Although skin testing is the *sine qua non* of allergic diagnosis today, the development of more sensitive and specific extracts for testing and desensitization have made it more reliable. Dr. Paul Hannaway and Dr. David Hopper, allergists at the Tufts–New England Medical Center in Boston, point out the problem with some of today's allergy extracts. "Some are hardly diagnostic," they report. "Up to 70 percent of people react to a skin test, when far fewer, only 10 percent or so, actually have symptoms."

Work is under way to develop more sensitive skin testing, for the better the test, the better the results, and the more accurate the therapy. Bee venom allergies are a good example of how more sensitive testing is accomplished.

Insect bites inevitably accompany warm weather. Although often a mere aggravation, they can also produce serious allergic reactions. Drs. Hannaway and Hopper point out that up to 1 million people may experience allergic reactions to insect stings; at least forty people in the United States die from them each year. For years people have been skin tested for insect sting allergies by using extracts made from the whole bodies of insects. Failures were and are common with whole-body extracts, probably because of contamination and the relatively small amount of venom in each insect. Now there is a new, purified bee venom extract that gives more accurate diagnosis and subsequently better desensitization therapy.

Charles Mraz operates an apiary in Pleasant Valley, Vermont. He is one of the suppliers of honeybee venom to the U.S. Food and Drug Administration's Bureau of Biologics. Outside his beehives are small electric grids covered with plastic wrap. When a bee lands on the grid, a slight electric shock causes it to sting through the grid, releasing venom. As other bees are attracted to the grid, they too are shocked and release venom. Since the insects are not killed, the process can be repeated again and again and a large volume of venom collected. Replacing the tedious task of dissecting out individual venom sacs, the grid method of venom collection has made it possible to test people more reliably for insect sting allergy.

Similar work to purify extracts is going on for ragweed pollen, for which the actual offending agent is still unknown; poison ivy, oak, and sumac, in which chemicals known as uroshiols are felt to be responsible for the reaction (poison plant dermatitis is actually an allergic reaction), as well as house dust. House dust obviously has many components, including lint, wool, and animal danders, and manufacturers sell more house dust extracts than any other. The actual allergic substance in house dust may be any one or all of its components. In 1964 a mite the size of a pencil point, *Dermatophagoides farinae*, was discovered and, subsequently, has been found in house dust worldwide. But the organism's role in causing allergic symptoms is still unknown.

New medications for asthma

Doctors recognized many years ago that allergic reactions could be aborted by stimulating the sympathetic, or adrenergic, nervous system to counter the effect of histamine. Epinephrine (Adrenalin) is one drug that effectively performs this stimulation and has been the mainstay of treatment in allergic reactions since its development in 1910. But Adrenalin stimulates the sympathetic nervous system throughout the body, so its effects are seen in virtually all body organs. This is not desirable if the allergic reaction is limited to one or two organs. As an example, someone with an acute attack of asthma due to allergy has tight, wheezing respiration. Epinephrine quickly stops the wheezing in many cases by relaxing the muscles in the bronchial wall and opening them for greater air flow, but it also causes increased heart rate, pale skin, shaking, and nervousness. The ideal medication would affect only the asthmatic lungs.

This is now possible, for it has been discovered that the sympathetic nervous system can be selectively stimulated. The sympathetic nerves deliver messages to their target organs by means of chemicals that pass from nerve endings to receptor sites on the organ cells. Within the sympathetic nervous system there are different kinds of receptors for different kinds of activity. So-called alpha receptors mediate blood vessel narrowing and uterus contractions; B1 receptors mediate heart rate and the force of its contractions; B or beta-2 receptors mediate bronchial tube openings. Epinephrine affects all these receptors. Isoproterenol (Isuprel), another drug commonly used for asthma, affects B1 and B2 receptors.

In a recent issue of *Pediatric Annals*, Dr. John Anderson, a Detroit immunologist, discusses the newer drugs for asthma and points out that they affect only the B2 receptors. "With these B2 agonists breathing is improved without unpleasant cardiovascular side effects, a substantial improvement of particular importance to people with asthma who also have coexisting high blood pressure or heart disease."

It is now possible to treat asthma without complicating or worsening heart disease. The currently available B2 drugs include inhalants—Metaproterenol (trade names Alupent and Metaprel) and isoetharine (trade names Bronkosol and Bronkometer); and oral or injectable drugs—terbutaline (trade names Brethine and Bricanyl).

Beta 2 drugs are not completely selective, however. Muscle tremors and anxiety are frequently seen along with their bronchial side effects. "Other B2 drugs," adds Dr. Anderson, "are in use outside the United States and are similar to terbutaline but are not available here yet."

Unlike those drugs which abort an allergic reaction, cromolyn sodium, a white powder that is inhaled four times a day to coat the mast cells, is a preventive drug only. Although the drug's functions not completely understood, it is thought to inhibit the release of histamine by the mast cell. When administered during pollen season or before exercise or exposure to any allergen or trigger mechanism such as smoke or vapor, the drug can prevent an acute attack. When first released in 1965, cromolyn sodium was greeted as a "miracle drug," but subsequent use has tempered this enthusiasm.

"Steroids [cortisone] are the most effective inhibitors of allergic and asthmatic reactions available today," according to Dr. Philip Norman, allergist and immunologist at Johns Hopkins University School of Medicine, in a recent survey article on advances in allergy research in the journal *Drug Therapy*. Cortisone inhibits histamine synthesis or release, directly relaxes smooth muscles in the bronchial and blood vessel walls, and makes the receptor sites more sensitive. Its anti-inflammatory abilities are also well known. Applied topically, cortisone has revolutionized the treatment of allergic skin disorders such as eczema. There are twenty different topical cortisones on the market today, including sprays, gels, lotions, and ointments. Oral and injectable cortisone has also been used for allergic asthma. But long-term systemic cortisone use has debilitating results—fluid retention, intestinal bleeding, weakness, physiological dependence—and it complicates diabetes, high blood pressure, chronic infection, and some psychological disorders.

Dr. Norman comments that it isn't necessary to experience these symptoms anymore: "The single most important advance in the drug treatment of asthma has been the development of inhaled steroids." Beclomethasone with daily use substantially reduces symptoms of asthma with few side effects. Available by prescription only under the trade names Beclovent and Vanceril, beclomethasone occasionally leads to yeast infections, but careful use can prevent this complication. None of the other complications of cortisone seem to be a problem with this drug.

New approaches using IgE

The discovery of IgE as the mediator for allergic reactions is altering current concepts of diagnosis. Although there are exceptions, most allergic people have elevated levels of IgE in their serum. With a highly specific blood examination called RAST (radioallergosorbent test), IgE antibodies against specific allergens can be detected in the serum even if they are present in extremely small amounts. Skin testing is still more sensitive, efficient, and certainly cheaper, but the future may see an increased use of RAST, particularly in patients with skin conditions that prevent scratch testing or who object to it for personal reasons. The RAST test costs $5 to $10 for each allergy test, which adds up quickly if tests are run for multiple allergies.

The future may also bring an end to desensitization injections, the commonly used allergy shots, to control allergic reactions. Desensitization injections work by gradually building up protection against IgE in an allergic person's serum. Animal studies suggest, however, that it may be possible to control or suppress IgE formation rather than deal with it after it has formed, as is the current method. At the Scripps Foundation in La Jolla, California, a single injection of an allergen modified to stimulate the body's immune or suppressive reaction rather than IgE formation has been successful in preventing allergic sensitivity. If the technique can be found to work in humans, it will in effect turn off the allergy before it begins, and the ritual of allergy shots and other medications may become a thing of the past.

In the future

The so-called big five allergic diseases are allergic rhinitis (stuffy, draining nose), asthma, eczema (dermatitis), urticaria (hives), and anaphylaxis (allergic collapse or shock). Studies of these problems have suggested that it may be possible in the near future to predict who will develop allergic disease in early childhood and to prevent the allergy from developing. Currently, allergic symptoms are seen in one of every five children, and the percentage is even higher when one or both parents have an allergic history.

It is here that the significance of the Ishizakas' discovery of IgE is most profound. High serum IgE levels correlate well with the presence or future development of allergic disease. Putting in-

Steering clear of environmental sources of allergy

Around the bedroom

Pillows, blankets, and mattresses: Encase mattress, box spring, and pillows in plastic covers that close with a zipper. Avoid cotton-filled quilts and comforters and use electric or synthetic blankets instead. No chenille bedspreads. No feathers allowed anywhere in the house.

Rugs: Use linoleum or floor tile instead.

Furniture: Avoid stuffed furniture in the bedroom. Use only wooden chairs or those padded with rubber.

Curtains, shades, and drapes: Use only plastic or washable drapes. If fabric drapes are used, wash at least every two weeks.

Stuffed animals: Remove from the entire house. Favorite stuffed animals can be restuffed with old nylon stockings or shredded foam rubber.

Other helpful tips: Do not smoke or keep cosmetics, flowers, or plants in the bedroom. Do not use wax or antiseptic sprays on floors or furniture. Damp mop only. Wash walls and floor frequently. Keep windows closed and use air conditioners. Clean frequently behind pictures. Keep closet doors closed and clothes in plastic bags. Allergex or Dust Seal can be sprayed on floors and drapes to keep dust down.

Around the workplace and garden

Paints and varnishes: Leave the house during painting, moving, or decorating and for two weeks afterward. Do not do painting yourself. Never paint in an enclosed space, such as a closet. Oil-base paints are the worst offenders, but even water-base paints are irritating.

Fumes and odors: Avoid auto exhaust, cleaning supplies, and products with strong odors.

Occupational sources: Those at risk for occupational asthma are farm workers, bakers, furriers, florists, janitors, and barbers.

Outdoor sources: Insect bites can trigger asthma, as can hay, wind, rain, cold air, trees, gardens, and flowering plants. Use an artificial Christmas tree in your house.

---

fants at high risk for allergy as determined by family history and IgE on strict allergy prevention programs just may reduce the incidence of allergic symptoms. The program as defined by many investigators includes (1) exclusive breast feeding for the first six months; (2) strict attention to dust and mold in the house; (3) no house pets; (4) properly balanced diet and moderation for the breast-feeding mother and avoidance of all eggs, milk, and foods known to give her allergic symptoms (see "Perspectives," pages 264–266). Dr. Robert Hamburger of the Department of Pediatrics of the University of California, San Diego, has reported much success with this protocol.

Of course, if further studies determine a method for suppressing the IgE allergic response to begin with, the hope of conquering or at least controlling allergy may at last be realized. Dr. I. Leonard Bernstein, a Cincinnati allergist, commented in an interview in *Medical World News* recently, "If this happens, the Nobel Prize may be given to the Ishizakas for their discovery—and they will have deserved it."

Around the house

Rugs: Use as few as practical. Always use rubber pads beneath them.

Drapes: Use as few as possible. Wash frequently.

Animal danders: Remove all pets from the household, even those kept outdoors. Change clothes before entering the house if you've had contact with animals (i.e., riding horses, farm animals).

Furniture and pillows: Use only synthetic pillows; encase in plastic first. Board up bottoms of furniture with linoleum. Avoid furniture filled with horse hair, cotton, or kapok. Preferred materials are plastic, leather, or nylon. Upholstered furniture should be covered with plastic and then with cotton or nylon.

Clothes and closets: Check the labels on "imitation furs"; these may contain fur of "cheaper" animals, and not be synthetic. Avoid moth balls. Check labels for sweaters of mohair that contain goat hair. Avoid fluffy wool sweaters.

Furnaces: Avoid coal heat. Radiator or radiant heat is ideal. Keep furnace filters clean and changed every two weeks. Each fall, clean registers and air vents thoroughly before turning on heat. With forced air heat, cover registers with dampened cheesecloth or steel wool filters for the first week. Use humidifier in winter.

Cosmetics: Avoid perfumes, face powders, sachets, scented soaps and talcum powders, and toilet waters. Nonallergenic products such as those made by Marcelle, Almay, or Ar-Ex may be substituted.

Fumes and odors: Avoid mustard plasters, medication in vaporizers, aerosol deodorizers, air fresheners, decongestant sprays, floor wax, or furniture polish.

Dampness and moldy areas: Keep basement as dry as possible; avoid flooding. Look for and remove molds from the basement. Continuous lighting keeps mold growth down. Keep basement and attic as clean as rest of the house.

Resources

■ National Institute of Allergy and Infectious Diseases
Office of Research Reporting and Public Response
Room 7A32, Building 31
National Institute of Health
Bethesda, Maryland 20205
301-496-5717

■ Referrals to an allergist can also be obtained from a family doctor or local hospital.

CANCER

THE PERSONAL WAR

Cancer:
the personal war

"Man is man and master of his fate."

Alfred Lord Tennyson
Idylls of the King, 1859–1885

Cancer is the disease that people fear most.

People fear cancer because it often causes a slow and miserable death, eroding and replacing one normal tissue after another, sapping strength until the body literally wastes away.

People also fear cancer because it seems indefensible. The disease may strike thirty years or more *after* exposure to a carcinogenic substance. And researchers seem to identify cancer-causing agents with frightening regularity in our environment today.

Cancer is the second greatest killer, after cardiovascular disease, in the United States. The number of cancer deaths in 1979 was eight times the number of deaths in six years of fighting in Vietnam, six times the number killed in auto accidents each year, and greater than the total number of Americans killed in all four years of World War II.

"Yet there is a paradox here," says Dr. Vincent DeVita, the director of the National Cancer Institute. "Cancer is one of the most curable diseases in the country today." New advances in chemotherapy have produced spectacular cures and brought about remission in acute leukemia in children, Hodgkin's disease, Wilms'

kidney tumor, breast and bone cancer, and others. Combinations of chemotherapy, surgery, and irradiation have successfully managed many other cancers. Modalities of therapy still on the horizon or in their infancy—heat treatments, immunology, and interferon among them—will doubtless contribute to the progressive success in the fight against cancer.

Despite the enormous advances in cancer therapy, one statistic still stands out with frightening clarity: two-thirds of all patients with cancer die of their disease within five years of their diagnosis. The greatest tragedy of cancer is that many of these deaths occur needlessly. The American Cancer Society estimates that 130,000 people each year could be saved through early diagnosis.

But if more lives are to be saved, another approach must clearly be developed. As the medical community slowly begins to understand cancer's causes, research can show us how to prevent the disease. Many doctors are beginning to emphasize prevention as well as cure.

Most Americans disregard the concept of cancer prevention today, a feeling prompted perhaps by cancer's long latency factor. Exposure to certain carcinogens may not take effect for twenty-five years or more. Ingrained habits that promote the disease continue because cancer's onset seems too far in the future to be considered a real possibility.

Yet many cancers *are* preventable. Cigarette smoking alone causes more than 100,000 cancer deaths per year. "If cigarette smoking were eliminated, 80 percent of all cancers of the lung, 50 percent of the bladder, and high percentages of cancers of the larynx, esophagus, pancreas, and mouth would be eliminated," states a recent Surgeon General's report.

The International Agency for Research on Cancer in Lyon, France, under the auspices of the World Health Organization, has determined that environmental factors cause 85 percent of all cancers. Under its director, Dr. John Higginson, the IARC has analyzed data from five continents on more than 550 suspected chemicals, many of which have been found to cause cancer.

The best defense against cancer today is knowledge. By avoiding proven cancer risks and recognizing cancer's warning signs, everyone can participate in the fight against cancer. And our efforts will benefit each of us in return.

About cancer

Cancer is not a single disease. Rather, cancer is a group of highly unique diseases that can strike any organ or any part of the body at any time.

Cancer can begin in any of the body's cells. Perhaps programmed by a genetic error and triggered by a toxic chemical, excess radiation, or virus, the cell undergoes an abnormal change and begins a process of unbridled growth and spread. One abnormal cell divides into two; those redivide into four; then eight, sixteen, and so on in geometric progression. The process can begin slowly but may move quickly, without pattern.

Unlike normal cells that reproduce in an orderly manner to replace worn-out cells or repair small injuries, cancer cells grow uncontrollably into masses that successfully compete with normal cells for nutrition. Cancer cells destroy and replace normal tissue: few tissue boundaries or defenses can stop them. Not all cell growths are cancerous. Some can develop and cause no harm to the patient; these are said to be benign. Malignant growths are always cancerous—and always harmful to patients.

Cancer passes through several stages. Initially the cancer cells remain clumped at the original site, the so-called localized cancer. Later the abnormal cells invade neighboring tissues and organs and eventually enter lymph channels or blood vessels, spreading through them to reach more distant sites—in this stage the disease is known as metastatic cancer. Metastatic cancer can be regional, confined to a particular area of the body, or generalized and thereby spread throughout the body. But cancer spread can never be predicted. Some cancers spread when they are microscopic in size; other cancers never spread at all.

With each advancing stage cancer becomes more difficult to control. A localized cancer is therefore more treatable and curable than a generalized cancer. Indeed, with most generalized cancers, death cannot be too far away.

Risk factors for cancer

"Everything I like is either amoral, illegal, fattening, or causes cancer."

This quote typifies the feeling of the well-read consumer today. Doubtless we've all shared the gnawing suspicion that nothing is safe to eat, drink, smoke, or wear. In recent months, reports have appeared linking cancer to almost everything, it seems, from cosmetics, insecticides, and aerosol sprays to red dye, soft drinks, bacon, and even the air we breathe.

Although some of the risks may be exaggerated, certain factors definitely contribute to cancer development. The factors that increase the risk of cancer are known as "carcinogens." They can appear in almost every phase of our life, both indoors and out, with and without our knowledge. Following are some of the ways these risk factors are transmitted to us.

Smoking: Cigarette smoking is responsible for more cancer deaths than any other known factor. Cigarette smokers have twenty-five times the frequency of lung cancer of nonsmokers, five times the frequency of cancer of the mouth, and three times the frequency of bladder, pancreas, and intestinal cancers.

Cigarette smoke contains dozens of chemical agents that directly affect the lungs and spread through the bloodstream to affect other areas of the body. Scientists still do not know, however, *which* of the chemicals in the smoke cause the damage.

Although the American tobacco industry would deny it, many cancer experts feel that a filter and low-tar cigarette offers little or no reduction in cancer risk. And the smug smoker of filter cigarettes should realize that the smoke from the burning end of the cigarette is not filtered; that secondhand smoke, breathed in by other people in the room, increases the cancer risk of family members and friends.

In particular more women are smoking now, and, even more alarming, the rate is highest among younger women and teenagers in particular. One can't help but make the association that the death rate of women from lung cancer has also grown —quadrupled, in fact, in the past twenty years. Death rates among men from lung cancer have doubled in that same period. Cigar and pipe smokers have generally lower malignancy rates for lung cancer, but equal rates for mouth and lip cancer.

Actions that are believed to reduce cancer risk

bladder: not smoking; reducing intake of saccharine

breast: reducing intake of meat, dairy products, and all other fats; having a child before the age of thirty; self-examining breasts monthly; maintaining moderate body weight

cervix: not having intercourse before the age of eighteen; limiting the number of sexual partners; maintaining good genital hygiene; having pap test as recommended

colon-rectum: eating a well-balanced diet, low in fat, high in fiber; maintaining moderate body weight; having annual proctological exam after the age of forty

esophagus: not smoking; limiting alcohol consumption to less than three ounces daily

gastro-intestinal (including stomach): not smoking; maintaining moderate body weight; limiting intake of highly processed, pickled, cured, or smoked foods; limiting alcohol consumption to less than three ounces daily; limiting the intake of charcoal-cooked foods

larynx: not smoking

liver: limiting alcohol consumption to less than three ounces daily

lung: not smoking

mouth: maintaining good oral hygiene; not smoking; limiting alcohol consumption to less than three ounces daily

pancreas: not smoking

prostate: maintaining a low-fat, low-cholesterol diet; having an annual prostate exam after the age of forty

skin: avoiding excessive sun exposure

thyroid: avoiding unnecessary X-ray exposure

uterus: avoiding unnecessary post-menopausal estrogenic therapy; maintaining moderate body weight; having pap test as recommended

whole body: not smoking; becoming an "aware" consumer; avoiding known carcinogens; eating a well-balanced, low-fat, low-cholesterol diet that includes green, leafy vegetables, fresh fruit and whole grains; limiting alcohol consumption; avoiding unnecessary X-rays; avoiding unnecessary drugs, especially if pregnant; following safety guidelines at work; acknowledging early warning signs; having an annual check-up

Smoking can also multiply the risks associated with other carcinogenic agents. Asbestos exposure coupled with cigarette smoking increases the rate of cancer of the lung by ninety times.

The data speak clearly. Smoking is the greatest cancer risk going. And when one considers smoking's contribution to heart disease and stroke, cigarette smoking may be the single greatest health risk.

Diet: Most of the information about dietary relationship to cancer is based so far on animal studies, but these nevertheless should raise a red flag.

Saccharin is one case in point. In a 1978 report, the National Academy of Sciences voiced concern about the risk of bladder cancer from the use of saccharin, based on its effects on laboratory mice. Subsequent studies, however, have not demonstrated this marked effect in humans. Harvard researchers Dr. Alan S. Morrison and Julie E. Buring studied 1,200 patients and reported their findings in a 1980 issue of the *New England Journal of Medicine.* The researchers found that "users of artificial sweeteners have little or no increased incidence of bladder cancer."

But saccharin worries cancer specialists. Cancer can take decades to develop, and the major users of saccharin in diet soft drinks are the young. Dr. Robert Hoover of the National Cancer Institute, commenting on the Harvard study, concluded that sufficient time for an obvious carcinogenic effect to appear may not have elapsed. He noted that "since artificial sweeteners have little objective benefit, excessive use by anyone is ill advised and should be actively discouraged."

Dietary influences on cancer certainly merit a hard look. Diet-restricting Mormons and Seventh-Day Adventists, for example, have half the cancer incidence of the general United States population. Researchers have found that a diet heavy in fiber (bran, seeds, nuts, fresh fruits, and raw vegetables) and low in beef and fat results in a lower incidence of cancer of the large intestine. Most experts feel that dietary fiber increases bulk in the stool, which passes through the intestine much more quickly and thereby reduces the exposure of the intestinal lining to any products in the food.

Individuals who eat large amounts of pickled and prepared foods that contain nitrates, nitrosamines, and the preservative BHT have higher rates of stomach cancer. Studies show that when these people change their dietary habits, their cancer rates change as well. So the dietary elements themselves must be the factor influencing cancer rates.

The typical American diet includes foods with many additives to enhance taste, add color, preserve, and retard spoilage, or as residues of packaging materials. Since these agents have been used only in the past decade, studies have not conclusively linked preservatives to cancer. But many scientists suspect that future studies will bear out suspicions that food additives trigger cancer. And doctors and researchers alike agree that careful dietary scrutiny certainly benefits general good health.

While conclusive results are not yet available, many cancer specialists recommend that the following dietary guidelines be followed to avoid unnecessary cancer risks:

- Limit consumption of preserved foods.
- Limit consumption of prepared meats —bacon, luncheon meats, hot dogs, and so on.
- Avoid artificial sweeteners.
- Reduce intake of beef, dairy, and other fats.
- Reduce intake of pickled and charcoal-broiled foods.
- Limit foods with artificial flavors and colors.
- Increase dietary fiber or bulk.
- Maintain a reasonably normal weight.

Radiation: Madame Marie Curie discovered the radioactive material radium in the late nineteenth century and later died from cancer caused by radiation. Scientists have recognized a connection between X-ray exposure and cancer ever since malignancies began to appear in scientists and technicians who received large radiation doses in their work with radium and early X-ray tubes.

Today researchers agree that everyone should avoid unnecessary X rays and radiation exposure at all costs. All radiation poses a risk that accumulates with each exposure. For example, X-ray treatments commonly given for tonsil infections and skin problems in the 1940s and 1950s are resulting in increased incidence of thyroid cancer in those patients today. And radiology specialists currently estimate that each mammogram, or X ray of the breast, increases a woman's cancer risk by .02 percent.

Many individuals feel they need an X ray for every cough and to evaluate every lump or bump. But the need for a specific X ray should always be carefully discussed with a physician in order to guard against overexposure to diagnostic X rays.

Sunlight: Doctors once felt that sun exposure promoted good health. But today, even as sun worshiping approaches a national pastime, irrefutable evidence links excessive sun exposure to cancer.

Individuals whose occupations or recreational pursuits expose them to the sun year round commonly have increased rates of skin cancer. The problem is magnified in people with fair skin or freckles who burn rather than tan. "Fair-skinned sun worshipers should beware," says Dr. Michael Greenwald, a prominent Boston dermatologist who practices at the New England Deaconess Hospital. "Excess sun exposure will give [these individuals] rough skin at early ages and skin cancer by age fifty." Dermatologists also share concern that the recently popular suntanning centers where people seek a year-round tan certainly increase their chances of developing skin cancer.

Quite simply, doctors agree that excess sun exposure should be avoided. When the sun cannot be avoided, sunscreen preparations with high protective factors should be used to reduce the skin cancer risk.

Alcohol: Large amounts of alcohol increase the rates of cancer of the larynx (voice box), mouth, liver, and esophagus. Nutritional deficiencies often associated with drinking may contribute to these higher rates, but doctors also feel that contaminants accumulated during the manufacturing of alcoholic beverages promote cancer in heavy or consistent drinkers.

Occupational Carcinogens: In 1775 the English physician Dr. Percivall Pott made the observation that chimney sweeps were more likely to contract scrotal cancer then men in the general population. Subsequent work demonstrated that some cases did not occur until more than twenty years after the chimney sweeps began work. These observations were the first to recognize the latency period of cancer and the first to point out the susceptibility of the body to certain chemicals, in this case charcoal in the soot.

Today the American Cancer Society estimates that 2 million people are exposed to carcinogens in the work place. Not everyone develops cancer after exposure to cancer-causing substances; length and intensity of exposure and the individual's susceptibility all influence cancer rates. The frequency of tumor formation does decline as exposure is reduced, but the risk of cancer doesn't disappear until the exposure reaches zero.

CASE HISTORY

Z. P., a fifty-five-year-old accountant, had a cough that had lasted two weeks. He has never been a smoker.

When his symptoms persisted, he

visited his physician, who found what he presumed to be pneumonia on a chest X ray. Z. P. was started on antibiotics, but returned to the doctor ten days later when there was no improvement. Another chest X ray showed a slightly larger area of pneumonia in the lung. Analysis of Z. P.'s sputum was negative, and the doctor began to suspect malignancy.

Through fiber optic bronchoscopy, the doctor identified a tumor by looking directly into the lung. A small sample was taken and the laboratory found mesothelioma, a relatively rare cancer, but one known to be associated with exposure to asbestos.

Z. P.'s occupational and social history were obtained, and the asbestos exposure was finally traced to one summer's work as a plumber's apprentice thirty-seven years before.

Clearly, then, one cannot safely be exposed to a known carcinogen.

Thousands of new chemicals are added to the American work place each year. Finding those that are carcinogenic is no small task, but the Federal Hazardous Substances Act gives the government authority to study and identify potential carcinogens. Today the federal government regulates seventeen carcinogens, and many other chemicals are being closely monitored.

"To a degree we've zeroed in on certain chemical families," said Donald Kennedy, the former commissioner of the United States Food and Drug Administration. "Many of the occupational bad actors come from those families. There are obviously still compounds that we don't know about, but the more we study, the more we're able to screen out those harmful compounds." Local offices of the National Institute for Occupational Safety and Health and the Occupational Safety and Health Administration offer help to people who suspect they are being exposed to carcinogens in their work.

A list of carcinogenic agents found in the workplace and their known effects follows on page 296.

Early detection

Not all cancers can be prevented. But when cancer is discovered early, treatment is far more likely to succeed. Cancer grows and develops long before the disease causes symptoms. If cancer is detected during these early stages while still localized to a single area, the disease can often be successfully treated.

After an eighteen-month study aided by a committee of prominent specialists, the American Cancer Society recently revised its guidelines for checkups designed to detect early cancer.

To detect cancer of the cervix: Although its incidence has declined since 1950, invasive cancer of the cervix still affects 20,000 women per year and kills 7,500. The risk of cervical cancer is higher in women who have early and frequent sexual activity, multiple sexual partners, or multiple childbirths.

All women over the age of twenty and women below twenty who are sexually active should have two Pap smears a year apart. If both are negative, Pap smears can then safely be done every three years thereafter. This screening frequency should be increased for women taking oral contraceptives or on estrogen therapy.

The Pap smear involves an analysis of cells obtained by scraping the cervix (the visible end of the uterus) during the pelvic examination. The Pap smear can detect cells with cancer potential before they invade the uterus itself. This localized cancer of the cervix is called carcinoma in situ.

Since it may take five to ten years for carcinoma in situ to invade the uterus, and since carcinoma in situ is virtually 100 percent curable, the American Cancer Society feels that Pap smears every three years of-

Occupational cancer hazards

Agent	Organ Affected	Occupation
Wood	Nasal cavity and sinuses	Woodworkers
Leather	Nasal cavity and sinuses; urinary bladder	Leather and shoe workers
Iron oxide	Lung; larynx	Iron ore miners; metal grinders and polishers; silver finishers; iron foundry workers
Nickel	Nasal sinuses; lung	Nickel smelters, mixers, and roasters; electrolysis workers
Arsenic	Skin; lung; liver	Miners; smelters; insecticide makers and sprayers; tanners; chemical workers; oil refiners; vintners
Chromium	Nasal cavity and sinuses; lung; larynx	Chromium producers, processors, and users; acetylene and aniline workers; bleachers; glass, pottery, and linoleum workers; battery makers
Asbestos	Lung (pleural and peritoneal mesothelioma)	Miners; millers; textile, insulation, and shipyard workers
Petroleum, petroleum coke, wax, creosote, shale, and mineral oils	Nasal cavity; larynx; lung; skin; scrotum	Contact with lubricating, cooling, paraffin or wax fuel oils or coke; rubber fillers; retort workers; textile weavers; diesel jet testers
Mustard gas	Larynx; lung; trachea; bronchi	Mustard gas workers
Vinyl chloride	Liver; brain	Plastic workers
Bis-chloromethyl ether, chloromethyl methyl ether	Lung	Chemical workers
Isopropyl oil	Nasal cavity	Isopropyl oil producers
Coal soot, coal tar, other products of coal combustion	Lung; larynx; skin; scrotum; urinary bladder	Gashouse workers, stokers, and producers; asphalt, coal tar, and pitch workers; coke oven workers; miners; still cleaners
Benzene	Bone marrow	Explosives, benzene, or rubber cement workers; distillers; dye users; painters; shoemakers
Auramine, benzidine, alpha-Naphthylamine, magenta, 4-Aminodiphenyl, 4-Nitrodiphenyl	Urinary bladder	Dyestuffs manufacturers and users; rubber workers (pressmen, filtermen, laborers); textile dyers; paint manufacturers

fer sufficient protection for most women. (It should be noted, however, that the American College of Obstetrics and Gynocology continues to recommend an annual examination, concluding in a recent report: "The annual physical examination and pap smear give the opportunity for the earliest possible diagnosis of a potentially lethal condition and at the same time encourage an ongoing dialogue between doctor and patient." Clearly this issue will generate controversy for some time to come.)

To detect cancer of the rectum and large intestine (colo-rectal cancer): Cancer of the colon and rectum accounts for 15 percent of all cancers; it affects 80,000 people each year and causes 40,000 deaths, the second most common cause of death from malignancy. Men and women over the age of fifty should have a digital rectal examination and a stool guaiac test each year, and two sigmoidoscopy exams one year apart. If both examinations are negative, sigmoidoscopy examination can safely be done every three years thereafter. Sigmoidoscopy exams need to be more frequent in patients with a family history of colo-rectal cancer, polyps, or ulcerative colitis. (Many cancer specialists feel a three-year interval between sigmoidoscopies is not enough and recommend it every year. The American Cancer Society formerly agreed with this assessment, but relaxed its recommendation to every three years, feeling that frequent performance of this occasionally painful examination may discourage people from having it at all.)

Sigmoidoscopy is the visual examination of the last ten inches of the bowel with a metal or flexible tube. Another instrument called the colonoscope can visualize the entire large bowel. Polyps can easily be seen and safely removed with either instrument. Since 50 to 75 percent of all bowel cancers begin as polyps, these procedures can be very effective.

The stool guaiac test detects blood which can ooze in very small amounts from intestinal cancer or other bowel disease. The test is performed by adding a guaiac chemical to a stool specimen. Fifty percent of all colo-rectal cancer lies beyond the reach of the sigmoidoscope, so the stool guaiac examination is a valuable screening procedure.

To detect breast cancer: Breast cancer is the most common malignancy affecting American women. Breast cancer will strike one out of thirteen women, resulting in 110,000 new cases and 36,000 deaths each year. Twenty-eight percent of breast cancer occurs in women below the age of fifty. All women over the age of twenty should examine their own breasts each month. Before the age of forty, they should have a breast examination by a physician every three years. Between the ages of forty and fifty that examination should occur every year. After the age of fifty, women should have a mammogram once a year. There are certain exceptions to this:

■ All women with a breast mass should have a mammography to evaluate that mass. All suspicious masses should be biopsied. The real value of mammography lies in detecting other masses in the same or opposite breast, because more than one cancer can occur at the same time.

■ All women who have had previous breast cancer should have annual mammography.

■ Women with blood relatives who have cancer of the breast should have mammography each year after age forty.

Women themselves find most breast cancers through breast self-examination. Because of hormonal changes in breast tissue, menstruating women should examine themselves just after each menstrual period. Most lumps or irregularities found on examination are benign, but they should nevertheless be checked by a physician.

Mammography has been the subject of

some controversy since X-ray exposure alone increases cancer risk. Data from the Cincinnati and Milwaukee Breast Cancer Detection Projects and the New York Health Insurance Plan Survey, each of which examined many thousands of patients, demonstrate that mammography is valuable. It can detect cancer early when cure is a possibility. In the New York study, for example, patients with cancer detected by mammography had an 80 percent ten-year cure rate.

Notably absent in the American Cancer Society recommendations is any statement about chest X ray or lung cancer detection. Both the American Cancer Society and the United States surgeon general's office feel that chest X ray does not promote the early detection of lung cancer. By the time the disease is visible on chest X ray, lung cancer has usually spread.

Lung cancer is the most common lethal malignancy, causing 120,000 new cases and 108,000 deaths each year. Eighty percent of all these deaths, however, could be prevented by eliminating cigarette smoking, and more by eliminating occupational carcinogens.

Warning signs

The American Cancer Society does not intend its guidelines to become the last word in cancer prevention. Consultation with a physician may result in a tightening or relaxing of the recommendations in an individual case. Furthermore, the guidelines are intended for healthy people who have no symptoms.

Despite the most elaborate preventive measures, cancer may still strike, so in addition to preventive efforts, each of us should learn to recognize the early warning signals. If you detect any of these symptoms, see your doctor immediately.

- A change in bowel or bladder habits.
- A sore that doesn't heal.
- Unusual bleeding or discharge.

- A thickening or lump in the breast or anywhere else.
- Indigestion or difficulty swallowing.
- A change in a wart or mole.
- Nagging cough or hoarse voice.

The hopeful side of cancer

Cancer is not a cause for resignation. Much *can* be done.

In all cases, the best defense against cancer is a strong offense. Support of cancer research programs and the investigation of cancer-causing agents will help make the environment safer, and more effective treatments for cancer available. Investigation of symptoms and attention to early diagnostic guidelines can point out many early cancers while they may still be cured. Attention to habits that can increase cancer risk can prevent many cancers.

As the American Cancer Society states in its current annual report, ''Americans have the power to prevent more than one-half the major cancers by simply altering behavior patterns already under their control.'' It's not easy to change lifelong habits, but all of us owe it to ourselves to try.

As Mark Twain said, ''Habit is habit, and not to be flung out the window by any man, but cast down stairs a step at a time.''

Resources

Information on cancer is available from:

■ American Cancer Society
National Headquarters
777 Third Avenue
New York, New York 10017
212-371-2900

(Also contact the state and regional chapter offices in most major cities, listed in the telephone directory.)

■ National Cancer Institute
National Institutes of Health
Office of Cancer Communication
Building 31, Room 10A18, Bethesda, Maryland 20205
301-496-4000
Tollfree Hotline 800-638-6694

(The National Cancer Institute also sponsors 27 regional information centers, listed in the telephone directory under cancer Information Service.)

Information on occupational hazards is available from:
■ Occupational Safety and Health Administration (OSHA)
New Department of Labor Building
Publications Office
3rd Street and Constitution Avenue
Washington, D.C. 20210
202-523-8148 (Office of Informational Services)
523-8151 (Office of Public and Consumer Affairs)

(OSHA also has several state and regional offices listed in the telephone directory under the United States Government, Department of Labor section.)

■ Clearinghouse for Occupational Safety and Health
National Institute for Occupational Safety and Health (NIOSH)

Center for Disease Control
Robert A. Taft Laboratory
4676 Columbia Parkway
Cincinnati, Ohio 45226
513-684-8326

Cancer and smoking information is available from:

■ Office of Smoking and Health
Department of Health and Human Services
Room 1–16, Park Building
5600 Fishers Lane
Rockville, Maryland 20857
301-443-1690

American Lung Association
1740 Broadway
New York, New York 10019
212-245-8000

(The American Lung Association also has state chapters and regional chapters listed in the telephone directory.)

Bibliography

Articles and information from the following professional journals provided much of the information for this book:

American Family Physician
American Heart Journal
American Journal of Cardiology
American Journal of Diseases of
Children
American Journal of Medicine
American Journal of Nursing
American Journal of Obstetrics and
Gynecology
American Journal of Public Health
American Journal of
Roentgenology
Annals of Otology, Rhinology, and
Laryngology
Annals of Plastic Surgery
Annals of Surgery
Archives of Internal Medicine
Archives of Ophthalmology
Archives of Otolaryngology
Archives of Surgery
Behavioral Medicine
British Medical Journal
CA—A Cancer Journal
Cardiovascular Medicine
Circulation
Clinical Orthopedics and Related
Research
Clinical Symposia—CIBA
Clinics in Plastic Surgery
Connecticut Hospice Seminars
Connecticut Medicine
Consultant
Contemporary Orthopedics
Continuing Education for the
Family Physician
Critical Care Medicine
Current Concepts in
Gastroenterology
Current Prescribing
Current Therapeutic Research
Cutis
Dermatology
Diabetes Forecast
Diagnosis
Drug Therapy
Emergency Medicine
Gastroenterology
Hospital Practice
Hospital Topics

Journal of the American Medical
Association
Journal of Bone and Joint Surgery
Journal of Cardiovascular Medicine
Journal of Continuing Education in
Family Medicine
Journal of the Louisiana State
Medical Society
Journal of Molecular Medicine
Journal of Pediatrics
Journal of Reproductive Medicine
Lahey Clinic Proceedings
Lancet
Mayo Clinic Proceedings
MD—Medical News Magazine
Medical Clinics of North America
Medical Digest
Medical Dimensions
Medical Times
Medical Tribune
Medical World News
Medico-Legal News
M.I.T. Reports and Research
Modern Medicine
National Association of Social
Workers News
New England Journal of Medicine
Nursing Research
Orthopedic Clinics of North
America
Orthopedics Digest
Patient Care
Pediatric Annals
Pediatrics
Perinatal Care
Perspectives on Aging
Pharmacy Times
Postgraduate Medicine
Primary Cardiology
Primary Cardiology Clinics
Psychiatric Annals
Radiology/Nuclear Medicine
Science
Scientific American
Seminars in Roentgenology
Surgery, Gynecology and
Obstetrics
Surgical Clinics of North America
The Female Patient
The Physician and Sports
Medicine
Today's Health
Transactions of the Academy

of Ophthalmology and
Otolaryngology
Urban Health
Virginia Medical
Western Journal of Medicine

Information was also obtained
from these additional
periodicals and pamphlets:
American Academy of Orthopedic
Surgeons Instructional Material
Atlanta Constitution
Boston Globe
Boston Magazine
Business Week
Cancer Facts and Figures—1980
Cancer News
Children's World
Consumer Reports
Dimensions of the Massachusetts
Rehabilitation Hospital
Family Circle
Focus—The Harvard Medical Area
Fortune Magazine
Good Housekeeping Magazine
Introduction to Computerized
Tomography (The General
Electric Co.)
Kurzweil Reading Machine Update
LaLeche League information sheets
Lynn (Lynn Hospital)
McCalls Magazine
Newsweek Magazine
New York Magazine
New York Times Magazine
Parade Magazine
Parents Magazine
Rush-Presbyterian St. Luke's
Hospital Magazine
Time Magazine
Union Hospital Monitor
United States Department of
Health and Human Services
physician newsletter
University of Michigan Medical
Center Report
Yale alumni magazine
Wellbeing (Beth Israel Hospital)
Public relations and informational
newsletters from countless
medical foundations

Index